Organic Acidurias

Organic Acidurias

Proceedings of the 21st Annual Symposium of the SSIEM, Lyon, September 1983

The combined supplements 1 and 2 of *Journal of Inherited Metabolic Disease* Volume 7 (1984)

edited by
G. M. Addison, R. A. Chalmers,
P. Divry, R. A. Harkness
and R. J. Pollitt

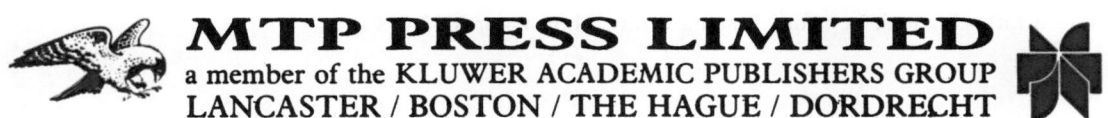

MTP PRESS LIMITED
a member of the KLUWER ACADEMIC PUBLISHERS GROUP
LANCASTER / BOSTON / THE HAGUE / DORDRECHT

Published in the UK and Europe by
MTP Press Limited
Falcon House
Lancaster, England

British Library Cataloguing in Publication Data

Society for the Study of Inborn Errors of
    Metabolism. *Annual Symposium (21st: 1983: Lyon)*
    Organic acidurias.
    1. Acids, Organic—Metabolism—Disorders
    2. Urine
    I. Title   II. Addison, G. M.
    616.6'3   RB147

ISBN-13:978-94-010-8975-3   e-ISBN-13:978-94-009-5612-4
DOI: 10.1007/978-94-009-5612-4

Published in the USA by
MTP Press
A division of Kluwer Boston Inc
190 Old Derby Street
Hingham, MA 02043, USA

Typeset by Speedlith Photo Litho Limited, Longford Trading Estate, Manchester M32 0JT.

Contents

Index of Authors

Subject Index

J. Inher. Metab. Dis. 7 Suppl. 1 (1984) 1

Preface

The first symposium of the Society for the Study of Inborn Errors of Metabolism (SSIEM) on the organic acidurias was held in Leeds in 1971 and published by the Society in 1972 (the 9th Annual SSIEM Symposium). Although relatively few of these disorders were recognized at that time, the symposium was prompted by the then recent identification between 1966 and 1970 of isovaleric acidaemia, methylmalonic aciduria, propionic acidaemia, pyroglutamic aciduria and 3-methylcrotonylglycinuria. Identification and diagnosis of diseases of this kind had greatly improved primarily through the application of gas chromatography and mass spectrometry to medicine, although the complexity of the underlying biochemistry and the genetic heterogeneity of the organic acidurias was not then realised. Since 1971 there has been a dramatic increase in the number of recognized organic acidurias caused by defects in the metabolic pathways of amino acids, lipids and carbohydrates with some 50 disorders of this kind now being recorded. Rapid advances have been made, particularly during the last few years, in our understanding of these diseases, their clinical course and management and of their underlying molecular and biochemical aetiology. Much remains unclear however and new avenues open each year for further research and discovery. The rapid evolution of this field and the impact of these diseases upon paediatric medicine and biochemistry made the subject a primary choice for a second symposium (the Society's 21st Annual Symposium) which was held in Lyon in September 1983.

The scope of the field is now too great and the subject matter too complex to cover all the known organic acidurias in a single symposium. The decision was taken therefore to concentrate upon those complex areas of greatest current interest and development not covered in previous symposia of the Society: the dicarboxylic acidurias and the congenital lactic acidurias. In addition, the clinical aspects and management of these diseases are of primary importance and are again areas in which there is much current interest with an urgent need for recording and discussing collectively experience from different centres. These subjects were thus also chosen to be a major part of the symposium. It was therefore most appropriate that Professor J. M. Saudubray gave the Society's Hudson Lecture on neonatal management of the organic acidurias, collating his extensive experience and putting into perspective the difficulties and practicalities of treating the acutely ill newborn with these diseases. The difficulties of longer term management were indicated by the following lectures by Dr Guibaud and Dr Leonard. Prenatal diagnosis thus remains very important in these diseases and Dr Sweetman has provided a valuable overview of advances in the application of chemical analysis of amniotic fluid to their early prenatal diagnosis. The continuing complexity of diagnosis, biochemistry and aetiology of the dicarboxylic acidurias has been admirably reduced by the papers from Dr Gregersen and Dr Goodman, with Dr Goodman clearly identifying the primary defect in the polycystic variant of multiple acyl CoA dehydrogenase deficiency ("glutaric aciduria type II") as a deficiency of electron transfer flavoprotein (ETF) dehydrogenase. Dr Engel's paper also provides a useful overview from currently available data of the place of L-carnitine in the organic acidurias, an area in which rapid developments are occurring. The emerging understanding of the aetiologies of the congenital lactic acidoses was evident at the 1971 symposium: the outstanding advances made since that time are clearly shown in the papers from Drs Robinson, Clark, Bartlett and Chalmers. In a symposium concerned with some of the developing areas in the organic acidurias it seems appropriate that three complementary papers on a newly identified disorder, 4-hydroxybutyric aciduria, should be included in the main program. Other areas of current interest and development are indicated by the scope of the relevant free communications presented at the Symposium.

The 21st Symposium of the Society provided a stimulating and valuable forum for a large number of participants. The efficiency of the organisation and the overwhelming success of the meeting were due to our President for 1983, Professor Cotte, Dr Priscille Divry and their colleagues in Lyon and to Mrs Anne Green, Meetings Secretary. We are particularly grateful to our friends and colleagues in Lyon for their warm and generous hospitality given in superb and traditional style. Our thanks and those of the Society are due to many organisations who provides support for the meeting, especially to the Institut Merieux for most generous support. Our thanks are also due to the Université Claude Bernard, the Institut de Physique Nucléare, U.E.R. de Chimie Biochimie, Hôspices Civils de Lyon, the Conseil Général du Rhône, the Chambre de Commerce de Lyon, the Association pour le développement économique de la Region Lyonnaise and the Association française pour le déspitage et la prévention de maladies métaboliques et des handicaps de l'enfant. Our especial thanks go to Mr J. G. Jones and Scientific and Hospital Supplies Ltd of Liverpool who have provided such generous support to the SSIEM over many years, including sponsorship of the Hudson Lecture.

G. M. Addison   *R. A. Chalmers*   *R. J. Pollitt*
P. Divry   *R. A. Harkness*

J. Inher. Metab. Dis. 7 Suppl. 1 (1984) 2–9

Hudson Memorial Lecture

Neonatal Management of Organic Acidurias. Clinical Update

J. M. SAUDUBRAY, H. OGIER, C. CHARPENTIER*, E. DEPONDT, F. X. COUDÉ, A. MUNNICH, G. MITCHELL, F. REY, J. REY and J. FRÉZAL

Clinique et Unité de Recherche de Génétique Médicale Inserm U 12, Département de Pédiatrie, Hôpital Necker Enfants Malades, 149 Rue de Sèvres, 75730 Paris Cédex 15, France
* *Laboratoire de Biochimie CHU, 94720 Kremlin Bicêtre, France*

Therapeutic guidelines have been obtained from a restrospective review of 41 patients affected with organic acidaemias, 16 patients with neonatal maple syrup urine disease (MSUD), 11 methylmalonic acidaemia, (MMA) seven propionic acidaemias (PA) and seven isovaleric acidaemias (IVA), and by comparing this personal series with similar reported cases. The emergency treatment of these organic acidurias in the neonate has to main goals: toxin removal and anabolism. Anabolism is always promoted by early diet therapy. The best method of toxin removal depends on the nature of the defect; peritoneal dialysis with exchange transfusions or multiple or prolonged exchange transfusions in MSUD and in PA, diuresis and exchange transfusions in MMA and glycine supplementation in IVA. Vitamin supplementation (thiamine 20 mg, biotin 10 mg, B_{12} 2 mg and riboflavin 100 mg) should be tried in all cases although the neonatal forms of these defects are very rarely vitamin responsive. Additional treatments such as carnitine or insulin may prove to be useful.

INTRODUCTION

The description by Menkes *et al.* (1954) of maple syrup urine disease (MSUD) represented the first report of an organic aciduria due to an inborn error of branched chain amino acid (BCAA) metabolism: branched chain ketoaciduria (BCKA) (Menkes, 1959; Dancis *et al.*, 1960). In 1961, Childs *et al.* described the ketotic hyperglycinaemia syndrome, which was later broken down into several precise aetiological entities involving BCAA metabolism: isovaleric acidaemia (IVA) (Tanaka *et al.*, 1966), methylmalonic acidaemia (MMA) (Oberholzer *et al.*, 1967; Stokke *et al.*, 1967) and propionic acidaemia (PA) (Hommes *et al.*, 1968). Over the past three decades, several hundred of these patients have been described and major progress has been made in understanding the biochemical and genetic mechanisms underlying these conditions. Many modes of therapy have been suggested in the acute phase of these diseases. Evidence is accumulating that the severe central nervous system dysfunction often associated with such organic acidurias can be prevented by dietary restriction of precursor amino acids. Despite the abundance of case reports, however, few studies have adequately compared these different treatment modalities on large numbers of patients (Snyderman, 1967; Committee, 1976; Farriaux, 1980; Wolf *et al.*, 1981; Naughten *et al.*, 1982; Saudubray *et al.*, 1980, 1982a,b; Bremer *et al.*, 1981; Chalmers and Lawson, 1982; Tanaka and Rosenberg, 1983; Matsui *et al.*, 1983).

Over the last 15 years, we have treated more than 60 patients with inborn errors of BCAA catabolism. Forty-one of these had severe neonatal disease. None of this latter group were vitamin-responsive. The clinical course and treatment of these children was retrospectively reviewed and compared with similar reported cases. On this basis, we have attempted to draw certain therapeutic guidelines.

METHODS

The patients in our series and those reported in the literature underwent initial toxin removal by one or more of the following methods.

(1) Exchange transfusion: 1.5–3 volume exchanges repeated four to six times (Frézal *et al.*, 1965; Schuchman *et al.*, 1972; Hammersen *et al.*, 1978) or performed one or two times immediately before and after peritoneal dialysis (Snyderman, 1974; Saudubray *et al.*, 1979), or alternatively continuous exchange over 15–20 hours involving 8–12 blood volumes (Wendel *et al.*, 1982b).

(2) Peritoneal dialysis with 2.5–3 litres per day of isotonic solution over 1–3 days (Rey *et al.*, 1969; Sallan and Cottom, 1969; Gaull, 1969; Saudubray *et al.*, 1971).

(3) Forced diuresis with intravenous volume loads of $150–200 \, ml \, kg^{-1} \, d^{-1}$ of 10% glucose solution with or without associated diuretic administration (Saudubray *et al.*, 1979).

(4) In some cases of isovaleric acidaemia, glycine therapy, $250 \, mg \, kg^{-1} \, d^{-1}$ orally (Krieger and Tanaka, 1976). In all of our cases, specific diet therapy given by nasogastric tube was started as soon as possible in order to promote anabolism.

Journal of Inherited Metabolic Disease. ISSN 0141-8955. Copyright © SSIEM and MTP Press Limited, Queen Square, Lancaster, UK.

PATIENTS

All of our patients were diagnosed on the basis of their clinical presentation and routine laboratory tests (Saudubray *et al.*, 1978, 1983). Organic acidurias were considered in all full-term neonates who, after a symptom free interval, developed rapidly progressive and unexplained feeding refusal, lethargy, hypertonia, abnormal movements or ketosis. The clinical diagnosis was confirmed by amino acid ion exchange chromatography and by organic acid gas–liquid chromatography–mass spectrometry of serum and urine samples. The average age at diagnosis varied from a maximum of 10 days for MSUD (range 6–21 days) to a minimum of 4.6 days for MMA (range 1–8 days). The average duration of the symptom-free period was 5 days for MSUD and 2.8 days for MMA, yielding a mean delay of diagnosis of 5 days and 2 days respectively. This discrepancy reflects the striking difference in the clinical severity of these two conditions. In addition to the features shared with MSUD (Table 1), the presentation of MMA, PA and to a lesser extent IVA includes severe dehydration, metabolic acidosis, hyperammonaemia and hypocalcaemia.

RESULTS AND DISCUSSION

Overall

Thirty of 41 patients were alive at 1 month. Of the 11 who died, most had been diagnosed late or developed sepsis. The 30 survivors were intubated for an average of 3–4 days and remained in the intensive care unit for 5–6 days. Coma disappeared and primitive reflexes were obtainable within 6 days of the institution of specific treatment. In MSUD the abnormal movements and hypertonia persisted for 12 and 23 days respectively but disappeared more rapidly in the other diseases (Table 2).

Weight gain was observed within 8 days in MSUD, MMA and PA and within 3 days in IVA. Plasma metabolites decreased to the near normal range by the seventh day of treatment of MSUD and MMA and by the third day of treatment of PA and IVA. Precursor amino acid-free feedings were started by the end of the first day and adequate caloric intake was obtained between the second and fifth days of treatment. Precursor amino acids were introduced by the ninth day of treatment in MSUD (leucine) and by the third day in MMA, PA and IVA (Table 3).

The efficacy of the various methods of toxin removal differs greatly among these diseases.

Maple syrup urine disease

In MSUD forced diuresis was consistently found to be inefficient. The total amount of toxic metabolites removed by diuresis was negligible, as would be expected from the low renal clearances reported for leucine (0.01–0.12 ml/min per 1.73 m^2) (Ghisolfi *et al.*, 1973) and for ketoleucine (0.0355 ml/min per 1.73 m^2) (Langenbeck *et al.*, 1979). Although this urinary excretion is quantitatively ineffective it is related to serum leucine concentrations. Determination of urine keto-acids with 2,4 dinitrophenylhydrazine (Scriver and Rosenberg, 1973) can be used for rapid bedside monitoring of the progress of other methods of toxin removal (Wendel *et al.*, 1982b).

In most of our dialysed MSUD patients dialysis was found to be effective as judged by the decrease of blood BCAAs and by the amount of leucine removed by the dialysate. In two cases, however, we found no leucine in the dialysate while the same order of decrease was observed in blood leucine, suggesting that the improvement was due to another endogenous process, such as anabolism. Dialysis failed in two cases, in which blood leucine levels remained elevated and dialysate leucine and ketoleucine

Table 1 Clinical presentation before treatment

	MSUD n = 16	*MMA* n = 11	*PA* n = 7	*IVA* n = 7
Symptom-free period (days)	5 (3–8)	2.8 (1.5–5)	2 (0.25–4)	3.5 (1–9)
Age at diagnosis (days)	10 (6–21)	4.6 (1–8)	7.6 (5–13)	7.2 (1–20)
Feeding refusal	100	55	100	100
Coma	100	100	100	100
Hypertonia abnormal movements	100	100	86	86
Ketosis	100	82	83	100
Dehydration	12	100	100	14
(% loss of BW)	(8 ± 5%)	(14 ± 4%)	(13 ± 2%)	(10%)
Acidosis pH ⩽ 7.30	0	100	86	80
Hyperammonaemia	18	100	100	100
⩾ 100 μmol/l	120 (90–130)	360 (165–670)	340 (165–705)	353 (145–780)
Hypocalcaemia	0	67	71	67
⩽ 1.7 mmol/l		1.59 ± 0.17	1.56 ± 0.2	1.56 ± 0.2

Data in upper part of table expressed as mean and range

Data in lower part of table expressed as the percentage of the total number of patients. (Mean ± SD where appropriate)

Table 2   Clinical course

	MSUD	MMA	PA	IVA
Intensive care unit	5.5	6.2	6	8
	(2.5–8)	(4–9)	(4–9)	(3–13)
Intubation	2.8	4.5	4.2	3.3
	(1.5–5)	(0–7)	(2–8)	(3–4)
Coma	5.5	6	6.2	4.8
	(3–8)	(3–8)	(5–9)	(3–6)
Absent primitive reflexes	5.3	5.8	6.2	5
	(4–8)	(4–8)	(5–8)	(3–6)
Abnormal movements	12	7	9	5
	(5–21)	(3–10)	(5–14)	(3–6)
Hypertonia	23	7	6.5	4
	(7–30)	(5–10)	(4–12)	(3–6)
One month survival*	15	8	3	4
Presently alive*	14	0	1	4
	(16–0.5 y)		(5 y)	(12–0.5 y)

Data expressed as days (mean and range) from the beginning of the specific treatment

* Number of patients

were low. Both patients had sepsis and the failure of dialysis may have been related to tissue catabolism or to an inadequate splanchnic blood flow (Fine, 1982). As demonstrated by Wendel *et al.* (1980) the removal by dialysis of each BCAA approximatively equalled that of the corresponding BCKA. Similarly, blood levels of corresponding BCAAs and BCKAs were closely related. Approximately 2 mmol of both leucine and ketoleucine were dialysed over a 14 h period. As previously described (Rey *et al.*, 1969; Clow *et al.*, 1981) blood leucine levels during dialysis tended to plateau around 1–1.5 mmol/l (13–20 mg/100 ml). In some cases a small postdialysis rebound was observed. Typically, these concentrations were attained by 24 hours, suggesting that it is not useful to prolong the dialysis beyond this time (Rey *et al.*, 1969; Saudubray *et al.*, 1971, 1979).

In the seven of our MSUD patients in whom exchange transfusions were performed, significant decreases in blood leucine were observed. These were, however, transient unless peritoneal dialysis was performed as well. In four patients, very good results were obtained by 'sandwiching' peritoneal dialysis between two exchange transfusions, as performed by Snyderman (1974).

Sustained decrease in blood leucine levels, sometimes more rapid than those obtained by peritoneal dialysis, have been described with the use of multiple (Frezal *et al.*, 1965; Schuchman *et al.*, 1972; Snyderman, 1974; Hammersen *et al.*, 1978) and prolonged (Wendel *et al.*, 1982b) exchange transfusions. In these cases as well, a tendency to stabilization between 1.0 and 1.5 mmol/l concentrations of leucine and ketoleucine was observed, suggesting that further transfusions may not be useful.

Table 3   Nutrition

	MSUD	MMA	PA	IVA
Caloric intake	1.5	4	0.5	3.5
i.v. + PO ⩾ 100 kcal/kg	(0–4)	(1–10)		(2–7)
Introduction of oral feeding	1.2	1	1.2	0.9
	(0–3)	(0.25–3)	(0.5–2)	(0.25–1.5)
Oral intake	3	5.5	2	4.2
> 100 kcal/kg	(1.5–6)	(2–10)	(1–4)	(1–5)
Introduction of precursor	8.9			
amino acids	(6–15)			
	(leucine)			
	2	3.5	2.8	3.5
	(val + ileu)	(0.5–6)	(0.5–4)	(1–5)
Weight gain	8.6	8	9.3	3.3
	(2–18)	(2–15)	(7–11)	(2–5)
Normal plasma	7.3	7.2	3.25	3.3
metabolite levels	(1–13)	(2–17)	(1.5–5)	(2–5)
	(leu ⩽ 6.5 mg/	(⩽ 1.5 mg/	(⩽ 1.5 mg/	(trace)
	100 ml)	100 ml)	100 ml)	

Data expressed as mean and range in days from the beginning of specific treatment

leu ⩽ 6.5 mg/100 ml ≃ 0.5 mmol/l

MMA ⩽ 1.5 mg/100 ml ≃ 0.01 mmol/l

PA ⩽ 1.5 mg/100 ml ≃ 0.02 mmol/l

Although Wendel *et al.* (1982b) obtained excellent results with a continuous blood exchange of 130–140 ml/h via a superior vena cava catheter over a 15–20 h period, the technical expertise necessary for safe performance of this procedure is not widely available. A comparison of the percentage reduction of blood leucine obtained in five patients treated with multiple exchange transfusions, 14 with peritoneal dialysis and eight with a combination of both methods, showed a small but statistically significant superiority of multiple exchange transfusions and of the combined therapy over peritoneal dialysis alone (Table 4). Exogenous methods such as exchange transfusions and peritoneal dialysis are thus effective in rapid initial removal of toxic metabolites but do not totally normalize serum concentrations.

The preponderant role of anabolism in the treatment of metabolic disease was recognized very early (Westall, 1963; Snyderman *et al.*, 1964; Costil *et al.*, 1971). Urea nitrogen excretion is one index of protein catabolism. In critically ill children without nitrogen intake urinary urea nitrogen is linearly related to the body surface area (Mickell, 1982) and can be estimated to be 1–1.5 g per day in the neonate. Assuming that urea accounts for 85% of urine nitrogen and nitrogen 16% of animal proteins, net daily protein catabolism of neonates in the acute phase of organic acidurias can be estimated to be 7–10 g. Since leucine forms 10% by weight of mammalian proteins this represents an endogenous liberation of 5.4–7.7 mmol (700–1000 mg) leucine per day. In a 3.2 kg neonate with an estimated 2.5 litres of body water, this could result in an increase of 2–3 mmol/l (28–40 mg/100 ml) in serum leucine. Conversely, the same amount could be removed by a protein anabolism of 7–10 g, corresponding to a muscle weight gain of 35–50 g.

In agreement with these theoretical speculations we found a close correlation between delay before weight gain and the time required for normalization of serum leucine in our 15 MSUD patients (Figure 1). Normalization of serum leucine levels preceded the onset of weight gain in most cases and may thus be the more sensitive indicator of tissue anabolism (Figure 2). The essential role of anabolism in the metabolite equilibration in organic acidurias has been emphasized by several authors. Initially calories are supplied by high concentrations intravenous glucose (Snyderman *et al.*,

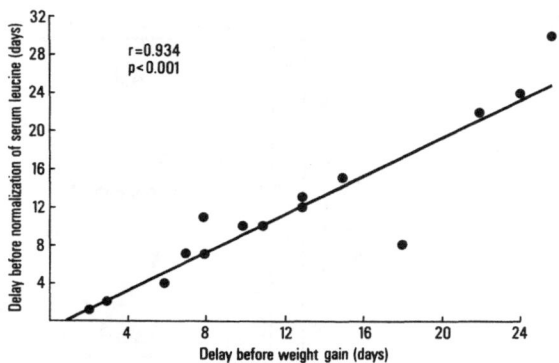

Figure 1 Normalization of serum leucine versus weight gain

1964; Costil *et al.*, 1971; Hammersen *et al.*, 1978; Saudubray *et al.*, 1982b), sometimes with lipid emulsions as well (Clow *et al.*, 1981). Enteral feedings are introduced as soon as possible. The adjunction of insulin to further stimulate anabolism has been suggested and initial results are encouraging (Wendel *et al.*, 1982a). As stated by Clow *et al.* (1981) the superiority of current methods of toxin removal over a regimen of complete protein withdrawal with adequate hydration and caloric intake has not been proven in the acute phases of MSUD. Very few case reports of the treatment of neonatal MSUD by diet alone are available. Normalization of leucine levels within 3–6 days has been reported (Westall, 1963; Snyderman *et al.*, 1964 (case CLB); Gaull, 1969). However, in other reports (patients 2 and 7 of the Canadian Committee, 1976, case No. 1 of Hammersen *et al.*, 1978), and in our experience with two patients, 7–30 days were required for normalization. Furthermore, leucine concentrations after 2 days of treatment remained quite elevated.

In conclusion, it seems reasonable at present to recommend that a method of exogenous toxin removal be used in addition to diet therapy in the initial treatment of neonatal MSUD. However, the precise treatment protocol must be individualized according to local expertise in the various procedures.

METHYLMALONIC ACIDAEMIA

The most prominent feature of the initial course of our MMA patients was the striking efficiency of urinary

Table 4 Effects of treatment on serum leucine levels (mg/100 ml) (130 mg = 1 mmole)

	Before	*After*	*% Decrease*	*Significance*
Multiple or prolonged ET* (*n* = 5)	40 ± 8	13.8 ± 3	65 ± 6%	0.05 ⩾ *p* ⩾ 0.02
Peritoneal dialysis† (*n* = 14)	43 ± 12	21.6 ± 7	49 ± 15%	
Peritoneal dialysis + ET‡ (*n* = 8)	34.6 ± 9	11.6 ± 5	64 ± 21%	0.10 ⩾ *p* ⩾ 0.05

ET = exchange transfusion

* Schuchmann *et al.*, 1972; Hammersen *et al.*, 1978; Wendel *et al.*, 1982b

† Personal series; Sallan and Cottom, 1969; Costil *et al.*, 1971; Astruc *et al.*, 1977; Clow *et al.*, 1981; Harris, 1971

‡ Personal series; Snyderman, 1974

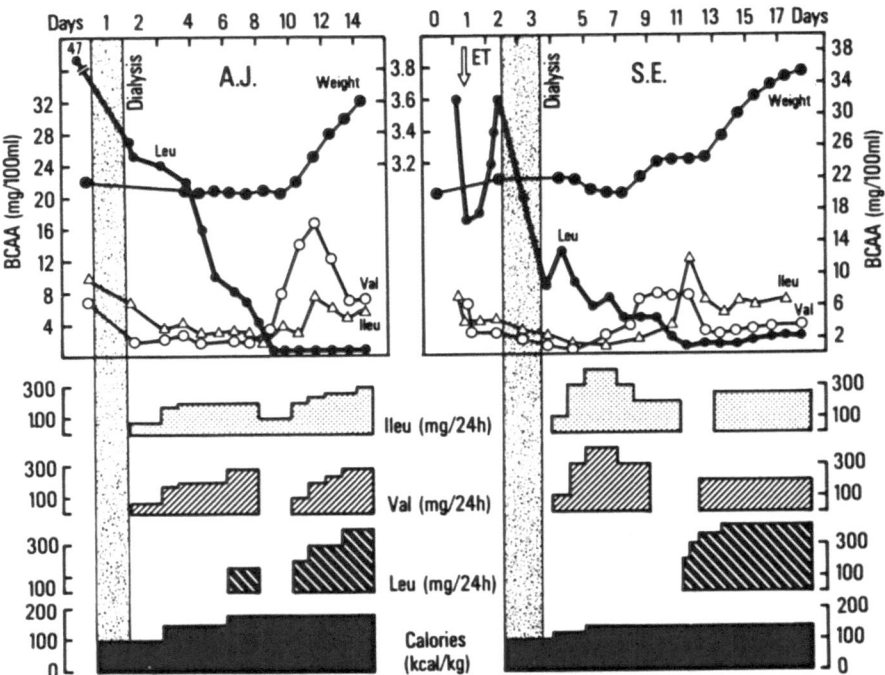

Figure 2 Role of anabolism. Observe the decrease of blood leucine whereas weight curve remains flat. Leucine: 1 mmol ≈ 130 mg

MMA excretion which was much greater than the quantities removed by peritoneal dialysis. The renal clearance of MMA was 22 ± 9 ml/min and the average MMA excretion before and during therapy was 6 and 4.3 mmol/24 h respectively, compared with 2.22 mmol extracted by dialysis (Table 5).

Interestingly, 24 h urinary MMA bore no relation to urine volume, as shown in Figure 3. For example, patient 6 (dialysed) excreted 5.5 mmol of MMA in a 24 h urine volume of 100 ml, whereas patient 7, treated by forced diuresis, excreted 5.4 mmol in 420 ml. In contrast, we found a linear relationship between pretreatment excretion and birth weight (Figure 4), which suggests that daily MMA excretion, like urea nitrogen (Mickell, 1982), may be correlated linearly with body surface area.

This large MMA excretion was often associated with a

persistent diuresis which was undoubtedly instrumental in the development of the marked dehydration seen in all our cases (Table 1) and noted by others (Matsui *et al.*, 1983). It probably results from a functional tubular nephropathy (see review in Broyer *et al.*, 1974; Whelan *et al.*, 1979; Saudubray *et al.* in Farriaux, 1980). Because of these findings, we have recently abandoned the use of peritoneal dialysis in management of MMA for a less aggressive protocol involving hydration, partial initial correction of metabolic acidosis with isotonic bicarbonate solution and one or two exchange transfusions. Our most recent patient, number 7 in Figure 3, was

Table 5 Effects of treatment on blood and urinary metabolites in MMA and PA

	MMA	*PA*
Urinary excretion (mmol/24 h)		
Before	6 ± 1.6	<0.15
During	4.32 ± 1.12	<0.10
Dialysis extraction (mmol)	2.22 ± 0.4	2.86 ± 2.7
Renal clearance (ml/min per		
$1.73 \,\mathrm{m}^2$)	22 ± 9	<0.03
Organic acid blood level		
(mmol/l)		
Before	2.08 ± 1.07	3.9 ± 1.5
After	0.88 ± 0.78	0.26 ± 0.04
Blood NH_3 (μmol/l)		
Before	360 ± 156	340 ± 190
After	135 ± 100	76 ± 37

Data as mean $\pm$ SD

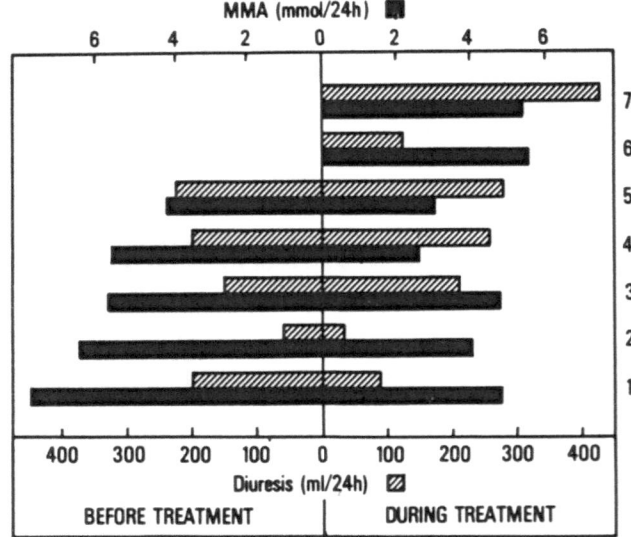

Figure 3 Urinary MMA excretion before and during treatment. Patients 1 to 6 were dialysed and received one or two exchange transfusions. Patient 7 was treated by exchange transfusion and hydration

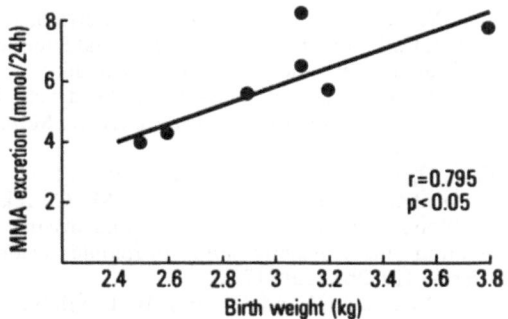

Figure 4 MMA excretion before treatment versus birthweight

treated by this method. Within 28 hours blood methylmalonate and ammonia levels were reduced from 2.4 mmol/l and 620 µmol/l to 0 mmol/l and 20 µmol/l respectively (Figure 5).

PROPIONIC ACIDAEMIA

In contrast to methylmalonic acid, the urinary excretion of propionic acid is negligible (Table 5). In PA methylcitrate and 3-hydroxypropionate excretion (Ando *et al.*, 1972a,b) may represent a quantitatively important method of detoxification but few data are available (Wadlington *et al.*, 1975; Sweetman *et al.*, 1978; Cartigny in Farriaux, 1980; Delvalle *et al.*, 1982; Wadman and Duran, personal communication). Our seven PA patients presented with very severe disease, four were diagnosed at more than 1 week of age and died before or despite the institution of specific therapy. As in MSUD, we performed exchange transfusion immediately before and after a 24 h peritoneal dialysis. In accordance with the results of other investigators (Robert *et al.*, 1972; Russell *et al.*, 1974; Costil *et al.*, 1979), we obtained an improvement over 36 hours in blood propionate and ammonia levels, which fell from mean values of 4 mmol/l and 340 µmol/l to 0.26 mmol/l and 76 µmol/l respectively. In three of the five dialyses between 3 and 6 mmol of propionic acid were removed in 24 hours but in the other two cases, less than 1 mmol was

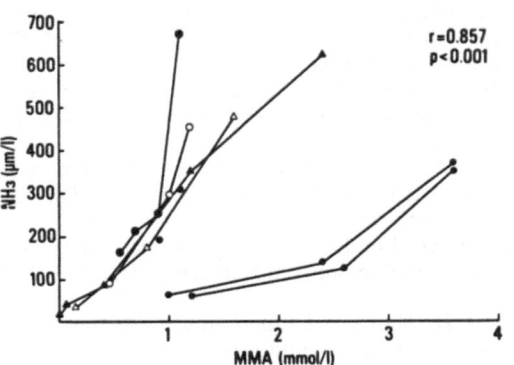

Figure 5 Blood MMA versus blood NH_3 during the acute treatment stage in seven different patients. (Each patient is represented by a different symbol.) Patient No. 7 described in the text is represented by black triangles

present in the dialysate. As for methylmalonic acid in MMA, the normalization of blood ammonia paralleled the descent of blood propionate (Wolf *et al.*, 1978; Cathelineau *et al.*, 1981; Coudé *et al.*, 1982b). This suggests that sodium benzoate administration and other specific treatments for hyperammonaemia (Wolf *et al.*, 1981) are, in addition to possibly being dangerous, not useful in these organic acidurias. In addition, because of the urea cycle inhibition known to be caused by organic acids (Coudé *et al.*, 1979; Walser and Stewart, 1981), we feel that precursor-free amino acid mixtures should be avoided while blood organic acid concentrations remain elevated.

Because of the low serum carnitine levels described in organic acidurias (Coudé *et al.*, 1982a) and in some unaffected neonates (Schmidt-Sommerfeld *et al.*, 1983) carnitine therapy may be of interest. No data of its use in the neonatal period are available, but there is suggestive evidence of a long-term beneficial effect (Roe and Bohan, 1982).

ISOVALERIC ACIDAEMIA

In neonatal-onset isovaleric acidaemia, therapy by diet alone (Levy *et al.*, 1973) and by peritoneal dialysis alone (Saudubray *et al.*, 1976) or with exchange transfusions (Winokur *et al.*, 1978) have proven successful. However, the safest and most effective method seems to be glycine therapy (Krieger and Tanaka, 1976; Yudkoff *et al.*, 1978; Cohn *et al.*, 1978). This treatment enhances the conjugation pathway whereby isovalerylglycine is formed from isovaleryl-CoA and glycine (Tanaka and Isselbacher, 1967; Bartlett and Gompertz, 1974). Using doses of 250 mg/kg per day by nasogastric tube, Cohn *et al.* (1978) obtained a dramatic normalization of serum isovalerate within 3 days. A concomitant increase in urinary isovalerylglycine excretion was observed. Clinically, neurological examination became normal after 2 weeks of therapy and an initial severe pancytopenia was corrected after 3 weeks.

CONCLUSION

In conclusion, the emergency treatment of organic acidurias in the neonate has two main goals, toxin removal and anabolism. Anabolism is always promoted by early diet therapy. The best method of toxin removal depends on the nature of the defect; peritoneal dialysis with exchange transfusions or multiple or prolonged exchange transfusions in MSUD and in PA, diuresis and exchange transfusions in MMA and glycine supplementation in IVA. Vitamin supplementation (thiamine 20 mg, biotin 10 mg; B_{12} 2 mg and riboflavin 100 mg) should be tried in all cases although the neonatal forms of these defects are very rarely vitamin responsive (Saudubray in Farriaux, 1980; Wolf *et al.*, 1981; Tanaka and Rosenberg, 1983; Matsui *et al.*, 1983). In our experience (Table 2) and in that of others (Wolf *et al.*, 1981; Matsui *et al.*, 1983), the long-term prognosis of MMA and PA is very guarded, emphasizing the importance of prenatal diagnosis in pregnancies at risk for such conditions.

The patients were managed in the intensive care units of: Dr J. Canet, Hôpital Intercommunal, Creteil; Dr Checouri, Hôpital Saint Vincent de Paul, Paris; Professor M. Cloup, Hôpital des Enfants Malades, Paris; Dr J. P. Fournet, Hôpital Intercommunal, Montreuil; Professor A. Huault, Hôpital d'Enfants, Bicêtre; Professor J. Laugier, Hôpital Clocheville, Tours.

We thank Drs Asensi, Brissaud, Coffin, Delaitre, Demenibus, Denavit, Despres, Feron, Gerbeaux, Greninger, Hayat, Herouin, Hoppeler, Lauzecker, Leroux, Menget, Mouzard, Peters, Piussan, Raffi, Saint Martin and Tupin, for referring the reported patients to us, and Francis Rocchiciolli for the mass spectrometric identification of metabolites in some of the patients.

References

Ando, T., Rasmussen, K., Wright, J. M. and Nyhan, W. L. Isolation and identification of metabolic product of propionate in patients with propionic acidemia. *J. Biol. Chem.* 247 (1972a) 2200–2204

Ando, T., Rasmussen, K., Nyhan, W. L. and Hull, D. Hydroxypropionate: significance of β oxidation of propionate in patients with propionic acidemia and methylmalonic acidemia. *Proc. Natl. Acad. Sci. USA* 69 (1972b) 2807–2811

Astruc, J., Froye, E., Luciani, J. M., Bellet, H., Magnan de Bornier, P. and Brunel, D. Leucinose néo-natale d'évolution favorable: problemes évolutifs et thérapeutiques. *Ann. Pediatr.* 24 (1977) 605–610

Bartlett, K. and Gompertz, K. The specificity of glycine-N-acylase and acylglycine excretion in the organic acidaemias. *Biochem. Med.* 10 (1974) 15–23

Bremer, H. J., Duran, M., Kamerling, J. P., Przyrembel, H. and Wadman, S. *Disturbances of Amino Acid Metabolism: Clinical Chemistry and Diagnosis.* Urban and Schwarzenberg, Baltimore, Munich, 1981

Broyer, M., Guesry, P., Burgess, E. A., Charpentier, C. and Lemonnier, A. Acidemie methylmalonique avec nephropathie hyperuricémique. *Arch. Fr. Pédiatr.* 31 (1974) 543–555

Cathelineau, L., Briand, P., Ogier, H., Charpentier, C., Coudé, F. X. and Saudubray, J. M. Occurrence of hyperammonemia in the course of 17 cases of methylmalonic acidemia. *J. Pediatr.* 99 (1981) 279–280

Chalmers, R. A. and Lawson, A. M. L. *Organic Acids in Man.* Chapman & Hall, London, New York, 1982

Childs, B., Nyhan, W. L., Borden, M., Bard, L. and Coore, R. Idiopathic hyperglycinemia and hyperglycinuria: a new disorder of amino-acid metabolism. 1. *Pediatrics* 27 (1961) 522–537

Clow, C., Reade, T. and Scriver, C. Outcome of early and long-term management of classical maple syrup urine disease. *Pediatrics* 68 (1981) 856–862

Cohn, R., Yudkoff, M., Rothman, R. and Segal, S. Isovaleric acidemia: use of glycine therapy in neonates. *N. Engl. J. Med.* 299 (1978) 996–999

Committee for Improvement of Hereditary Disease Management. Management of maple syrup urine disease in Canada. *CMA Journal* 115 (1976) 1005–1111

Costil, J., Debard, A., Guilhaume, A., Charpentier, C., Pousset, J. L. and Brissaud, H. E. Acidémie propionique: à propos de deux observations. *Ann. Pédiatr.* 26 (1979) 283–288

Costil, J., Aymard, P., Repesse, G., Richardet, J. M. and Brissaud, H. E. Leucinose aiguë, développement psychomoteur normal à un an. *Ann. Méd. Interne.* 122 (1971) 1273–1278

Coudé, F. X., Ogier, H., Carrier, H., Berthillier, G., Charpentier, C., Pham Dinh, D., Aicardi, J. and Saudubray, J. M. Myopathy in methylmalonic acidemia: a new secondary carnitine deficiency syndrome (abstract). *Fifth international congress on neuromuscular diseases.* Marseille, 12–13 September 1982a

Coudé, F. X., Ogier, H., Grimber, G., Parvy, Ph., Pham Dinh, D., Charpentier, C. and Saudubray, J. M. Correlation between blood ammonia concentration and organic acid accumulation in isovaleric and propionic acidemia. *Pediatrics* 69 (1982b) 115–117

Coudé, F. X., Sweetman, L. and Nyhan, W. L. Inhibition by propionyl coenzyme A of N-acetylglutamate synthetase in rat liver mitochondria: a possible explanation for hyperammonemia in propionic and methylmalonic acidemia. *J. Clin. Invest.* 64 (1979) 1544–1548

Dancis, J., Levitz, M. and Westall, R. Maple syrup urine disease: branched-chain ketoaciduria. *Pediatrics* 25 (1960) 72–79

Delvalle, J. A., Merinero, B., Jimenez, A., Garcia, M. J. and Ugarte, M. Dietary treatment and biochemical studies on a neonatal case of propionyl-CoA carboxylase deficiency. *J. Inher. Metab. Dis.* 5 (1982) 121–124

Farriaux, J. P. *Les Anomalies Héréditaires du Métabolisme des Acides Aminés à Chaine Ramifiée.* Doin, Paris, 1980

Fine, R. Peritoneal dialysis update. *J. Pediatr.* 100 (1982) 1–7

Frézal, J., Gabilan, J. C., Rey, J., Vis, H., Roy, C., Olivennes, M. and Lamy, M. Deux observations de leucinoses. *Arch. Fr. Pédiatr.* 22 (1965) 1226–1227

Gaull, G. Pathogenesis of maple-syrup urine disease: observations during dietary management and treatment of coma by peritoneal dialysis. *Biochem. Med.* 3 (1969) 130–149

Ghisolfi, J., Augier, D., Dalous, A. and Regnier, C. Les clearances rénales endogènes des acides aminés. *Arch. Fr. Pédiatr.* 30 (1973) 131–143

Hammersen, G., Wille, L., Schmidt, H., Lutz, P. and Bickel, H. Maple syrup urine disease: treatment of the acutely ill newborn. *Eur. J. Pediatr.* 129 (1978) 157–165

Harris, R. J. Infection in maple syrup urine disease. *Lancet* 2 (1971) 813–814

Hommes, F. A., Kuipers, J. R. G., Elema, J. D., Jansen, J. F. and Jonxis, J. H. Propionicacidemia, a new inborn error of metabolism. *Pediatr. Res.* 2 (1968) 519–524

Krieger, I. and Tanaka, K. Therapeutic effects of glycine in isovaleric acidemia. *Pediatr. Res.* 10 (1976) 25–29

Langenbeck, U., Wendel, U. and Luthe, H. Renal clearance of branched-chain 2-oxo-acids in maple syrup urine disease. *J. Clin. Chem. Clin. Biochem.* 17 (1979) 176–177

Leonard, J., Umpleby, A. M., Naughten, E. M., Boroujerdi, M. A. and Sonksen, P. H. Leucine turnover in maple syrup urine disease (abstract). *20th annual symposium of SSIEM*, Manchester, 8–10 September 1982

Levy, H., Erickson, A., Lott, I. and Kurtz, D. Isovaleric acidemia: results of family study and dietary treatment. *Pediatrics* 52 (1973) 83–94

Matsui, S., Mahoney, J. and Rosenberg, L. The natural history of the inherited methylmalonic acidemias. *N. Engl. J. Med.* 308 (1983) 857–861

Menkes, J. H. Maple syrup urine disease: isolation and identification of organic acids in urine. *Pediatrics* 23 (1959) 348–353

Menkes, J. H., Hurst, P. L. and Craig, J. M. New syndrome: progressive familial infantile cerebral dysfunction associated with unusual urinary substance. *Pediatrics* 14 (1954) 462–470

Mickell, J. Urea nitrogen excretion in critically ill children. *Pediatrics* 70 (1982) 949–955

Naughten, E. R., Jenkins, J., Francis, D. and Leonard, J.

Outcome of maple syrup urine disease. *Arch. Dis. Child.* 57 (1982) 918–921

Oberholzer, V. G., Levin, B., Burgess, E. and Young, W. Methylmalonic aciduria: an inborn error of metabolism leading to chronic metabolic acidosis. *Arch. Dis. Child.* 42 (1967) 492–504

Rey, F., Rey, J., Cloup, M., Feron, J. F., Dore, F., Labrune, B. and Frézal, J. Traitement d'urgence d'une forme aigüe de leucinose par dialyse péritonéale. *Arch. Fr. Pédiatr.* 26 (1969) 133–137

Robert, M. F., Schultz, D. J., Wolf, B., Cochran, W. D. and Schwartz, A. L. Treatment of a neonate with propionic acidaemia and severe hyperammonemia by peritoneal dialysis. *Arch. Dis. Child.* 54 (1972) 962–965

Roe, C. R. and Bohan, T. P. Carnitine therapy in propionic acidaemia. *Lancet* 1 (1982) 1411–1412

Russell, G., Thom, H., Tarlow, M. J. and Gompertz, D. Reduction of plasma propionate by peritoneal dialysis. *Pediatrics* 53 (1974) 281–283

Sallan, S. E. and Cottom, D. Peritoneal dialysis in maple syrup urine disease. *Lancet* 2 (1969) 1423–1424

Saudubray, J. M., Fournet, J. P. and Cloup, M. Intérêt de la dialyse péritonéale dans le traitement d'urgence des maladies métaboliques d'origine constitutionnelle révélées dans la période néo-natale. *Ann. Med. Intern.* 122 (1971) 1279–1283

Saudubray, J. M., Sorin, M., Depondt, E., Herouin, C., Charpentier, C. and Pousset, J. L. Acidémie isovalérique: étude et traitement chez trois frères. *Arch. Fr. Pédiatr.* 33 (1976) 795–808

Saudubray, J. M., Charpentier, C. and Coudé, F. X. Urgences néonatales en rapport avec une maladie héréditaire du métabolisme des acides aminés et des hydrates de carbone. *Rev. Pédiatr.* 14 (1978) 611–621

Saudubray, J. M., Amédée Manesme, O., Lavaud, J., Mselati, J. C., Besson Leaud, M., Ogier, H., Checouri, A., Leraillez, J., Ferre, P., Coudé, F. X. and Charpentier, C. Traitement d'urgence des amino-acidopathies à révélation néonatale. *Arch. Fr. Pédiatr.* 36 (1979) 969–980

Saudubray, J. M., Charpentier, C., Coudé, F. X., Ogier, H., Pham Dinh, D., Bartlett, K. and Gompertz, D. Pronostic des aciduries méthylmaloniques héréditaires. Corrélation entre la tolérance protéique, la sensibilité à la vitamine B12 et le déficit enzymatique. *Arch. Fr. Pédiatr.* 37 (1980) IX–XIV

Saudubray, J. M., Ogier, H., Charpentier, C., Amédée Manesme, O., Coudé, F. X. and Frézal, J. Acute and long-term management of infants with amino-acidopathies and organic acidurias. In Bonne-Tamir, B. (ed.) *Human Genetics. Part B: Medical Aspects,* Liss, New York (1982a), pp. 589–596

Saudubray, J. M., Amédée Manesme, O., Munnich, A., Ogier, H., Depondt, E., Charpentier, C., Coudé, F. X., Rey, F. and Frézal, J. Hétérogénéité de la leucinose. Corrélations entre l'aspect clinique, la tolérance protéique et le déficit enzymatique. *Arch. Fr. Pédiatr.* 39 (1982b) 735–740

Saudubray, J. M., Ogier, H., Charpentier, C., Coudé, F. X., Munnich, A., Cathelineau, L. and Frézal, J. A programmed screening for hyperammonemias: strategy and results. In Naruse, H. and Irie, M. (eds.) *Neonatal Screening,* Excerpta Medica, Amsterdam, Oxford, Princeton, 1983, pp. 382–387

Schmidt-Sommerfeld, E., Penn, D. and Wolf, H. Carnitine deficiency in premature infants receiving total parenteral nutrition: effect of L-carnitine supplementation. *J. Pediatr.* 102 (1983) 931–935

Schuchmann, L., Witt, I., Schulz, P., Schumacher, H. and Rudiger, H. Multiple exchange transfusions as treatment during the acute period in maple syrup urine disease. *Helv. Paediatr. Acta* 27 (1972) 449–456

Scriver, C. R. and Rosenberg, L. E. Methods of amino-acid analysis and diagnosis of amino-acidopathies. In *Amino-acid Metabolism and its Disorders,* Saunders, Philadelphia, 1973

Snyderman, S. E. The therapy of maple syrup urine disease. *Pediatrics* 113 (1967) 68–73

Snyderman, S. E. Maple syrup urine disease. In Nyhan, W. L. (ed.) *Heritable Disorders of Amino-acid Metabolism,* Wiley, New York, 1974, pp. 17–31

Snyderman, S. E., Norton, P. M., Roitman, E. and Holt, L. E. Jr. Maple syrup urine disease, with particular reference to dietotherapy. *Pediatrics* 34 (1964) 454–472

Stokke, O., Eldjarn, L., Norum, K. R., Steen Johnsen, J. and Halvorsen, S. Methylmalonic acidemia: a new inborn error of metabolism which may cause fatal acidosis in the neonatal period. *Scand. J. Clin. Lab. Invest.* 20 (1967) 313–328

Sweetman, L., Weyler, W. and Nyhan, W. L. Abnormal metabolites of isoleucine in a patient with propionyl-CoA carboxylase deficiency. *Biomed. Mass Spectrom.* 5 (1978) 198–207

Tanaka, K., Budd, M. A., Efron, M. L. and Isselbacher, K. J. Isovaleric acidemia: a new genetic defect of leucine metabolism. *Proc. Natl. Acad. Sci. USA* 56 (1966) 236–242

Tanaka, K. and Isselbacher, K. J. The isolation and identification of N-isovaleryl glycine from urines of patients with isovaleric acidemia. *J. Biol. Chem.* 353 (1967) 2966–2972

Tanaka, K. and Rosenberg, L. E. Disorder of branched-chain amino-acid and organic-acid metabolism. In Stanbury, J. B., Wyngaarden, J. B., Frederickson, D. S., Goldstein, J. L. and Brown, M. S. (eds.) *The Metabolic Basis of Inherited Diseases,* McGraw Hill, New York, 1983, pp. 440–473

Wadlington, W. B., Kilroy, A., Ando, T., Sweetman, L. and Nyhan, W. L. Hyperglycinemia and propionyl CoA carboxylase deficiency and episodic severe illness without consistent ketosis. *J. Pediatr.* 86 (1975) 707–712

Walser, M. and Stewart, P. M. Organic acidaemia and hyperammonaemia: review. *J. Inher. Metab. Dis.* 4 (1981) 177–182

Wendel, U., Becker, K., Przyrembel, H., Bulla, M., Manegold, C., Mench-Hoinowxki, A. and Langenbeck, U. Peritoneal dialysis in maple syrup urine disease: studies on branched-chain amino and keto-acids. *Eur. J. Pediatr.* 134 (1980) 57–63

Wendel, U., Langenbeck, U., Lombeck, I. and Bremer, H. J. Maple syrup urine disease. Thereapeutic use of insulin in catabolic states. *Eur. J. Pediatr.* 139 (1982a) 172–175

Wendel, U., Langenbeck, U., Lombeck, I. and Bremer, H. J. Exchange transfusion in acute episodes of maple syrup urine disease. *Eur. J. Pediatr.* 138 (1982b) 293–296

Westall, R. G. Dietary treatment of a child with maple syrup urine disease (branched-chain keto-aciduria). *Arch. Dis. Child.* 38 (1963) 485–491

Whelan, D. T., Ryan, E., Spate, M., Morris, M., Hurley, R. M. and Hill, R. Methylmalonic acidemia: 6 years' clinical experience with two variants unresponsive to vitamin B12 therapy. *CMA Journal* 19 (1979) 1230–1234

Winokur, P. A., Vashista, K. and Seshamawi, R. Isovaleric acidemia: a case report. *Pediatrics* 61 (1978) 902–907

Wolf, B., Hsia, D. Y., Tanaka, K. and Rosenberg, L. E. Correlation between serum propionate and blood ammonia concentrations in propionic acidemia. *J. Pediatr.* 93 (1978) 471–473

Wolf, B., Hsia, E., Sweetman, L., Gravel, R., Harris, D. J. and Nyhan, W. L. Propionic acidemia: a clinical update. *J. Pediatr.* 99 (1981) 835–846

Yudkoff, M., Cohn, R. M., Puschak, R., Rothman, R. and Segal, S. Glycine therapy in isovaleric acidemia. *J. Pediatr.* 92 (1978) 813–817

J. Inher. Metab. Dis. 7 Suppl. 1 (1984) 10–12

Long Term Outcome of Organic Acidurias: Survey of 105 French Cases (1967–1983)

R. ROUSSON and P. GUIBAUD
Unité de Génétique et d'Etude des maladies métaboliques de l'Enfant – Hôpital Debrousse, 29 rue Soeur Bouvier, 69322 Lyon Cédex 05, France

The French experience in the long term follow-up of 105 cases of organic aciduria (45 maple syrup urine disease, 12 isovaleric acidaemia, 19 propionic acidaemia, 24 methylmalonic aciduria and some rare allied disorders) is reported. Main conclusions drawn from this survey are the poor overall prognosis and the slow improvement in the outcome of such disorders over the last 15 years. In MSUD, while early diagnosis and early management remain a basic requirement, intellectual development did not improve as much as expected. In propionic and methylmalonic acidaemia modern treatment does not prevent a fatal outcome in the classical neonatal forms. It should be also emphasized that in the rare cases where a coenzyme deficiency has been demonstrated, vitamin therapy is very often ineffective *in vivo*.

In this work we summarize the long term follow-up of 105 cases of organic acidurias we have been able to collect in France since 1967. This survey has been conducted as a retrospective study through a detailed questionnaire sent to paediatricians concerned with metabolic diseases. Maple syrup urine disease (MSUD) has been included in addition to isovaleric, propionic and methylmalonic acidurias. We also collected a few cases of rare variants. Numbers of each type are given in Table 1.

As Table 1 shows, the first finding of this review is the high overall mortality of over 50%. Half of these are children who had survived the neonatal period. For the isovaleric, propionic, methylmalonic group the mortality rises to 65% and again, half of the deaths occurred after the neonatal period. Detailed analysis gives the following results.

MAPLE SYRUP URINE DISEASE

Out of the seven patients who died during infancy and childhood, two patients who had late diagnoses (made in 1967 and 1969) were already severely retarded and for

this reason were not treated. In two others, despite an early diagnosis, therapeutic attempts never corrected the amino acid profile sufficiently and they died at 5 and 6 months. The last three died during a ketoacidotic episode at the ages of 5 years 6 months, 6 years and 7 years although their development and their biochemical control were satisfactory.

Among the 29 living patients, 25 have survived more than 2 years and the eldest is 16. Twenty cases showed a classical type starting soon after birth but five are different. Two may be classified as having an intermittent form and one had a late presentation (2 months) but then evolved like the classical form. The remaining two belong to a peculiar family in which the first case presented as a classical form (decarboxylase activity 1.9% of control) but the next two siblings have residual decarboxylase levels of 8% and were able to stop their synthetic diet at 30 and 17 months respectively.

Tolerance to dietary leucine in the classical form (Figure 1) hardly changes. At 6 months, dietary intake only exceptionally reaches 500 mg per day and in the great majority of the cases there is only a slight increase in tolerance by 2 and even 10 years. Even after 10 years

Table 1 Outcome of French patients with organic aciduria 1967–1983

	Total	Died in neonatal period	Died in infancy– childhood	Alive
Maple syrup urine disease	45	9	7	29
Isovaleric acidaemia	12	4	1	7
Propionic acidaemia	19	10	4	5
Methylmalonic aciduria	24	4	13	7
Dicarboxylic aciduria	2	—	—	2
Glutaric type II aciduria	1	—	1	—
4-Hydroxybutyric aciduria	1	—	—	1
3-Methylglutaconic aciduria	1	—	—	1

Journal of Inherited Metabolic Disease. ISSN 0141–8955. Copyright © SSIEM and MTP Press Limited, Queen Square, Lancaster, UK.

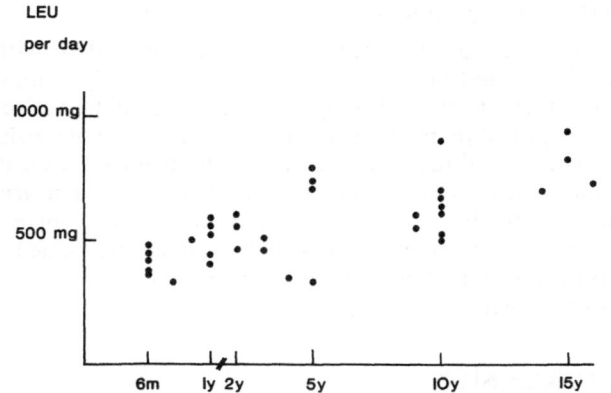

Figure 1 Tolerance to dietary leucine in the classical forms of MSUD

these patients cannot tolerate more than 1 g leucine. In contrast, normal or low protein diets (i.e. 2 g/kg per day) are soon tolerated in the intermittent and the atypical forms. None of the patients shows a clearly thiamine responsive type.

Long term results on psychomotor development (Table 2) are not as good as expected. In the classical form only three patients have completely normal development, while most of the others have levels ranging from mildly retarded to low average. On the other hand, only five children are severely retarded and only one case could not be explained by late diagnosis or dietary problems. All the patients with the intermittent and atypical forms have a normal mental level.

When considering the ketoacidotic episodes the study has been limited to those which required at least intravenous infusion. In the classical forms crises occurred in all cases with a mean frequency of one to two per year. However, their incidence is influenced by parental education. They are more frequent during the first year of life and after 3 years of age, classically precipitated by infections and dietary errors. We did not find any correlation between serum level of branched chain amino acids and clinical manifestations. No clear mental deterioration can be related to a single episode but, out of the 12 patients with abnormal electro-encephalograms, five have had more than six crises. In contrast, no severe ketoacidotic crisis has been observed in the intermittent and the atypical cases since they have been diagnosed.

ISOVALERIC ACIDAEMIA

Out of the 11 reported cases, eight were alive after the neonatal period. Two show severe encephalopathy because of late diagnosis. Two with neonatal presentation are presently less than 1 year old; they have normal development and tolerate 600 mg/day of dietary leucine with 125 mg/kg of additional glycine since the third month of life.

The last four are between 2 and 9 years of age. Two have benefited from immediate management since birth because of a positive family history, while two others had presented later, at 4 months of age. Tolerance to dietary leucine was more than 800 mg/day at 1 year and a low protein diet has sufficed since their second year of life. In all cases development is normal. Three of these children have ketotic attacks (about two per year) even if two of them receive additional glycine. Crises are very difficult to anticipate because of the absence of detectable ketonuria at their outset but they are usually easy to treat, with complete recovery.

PROPIONIC ACIDAEMIA

Eleven patients out of the 19 cases were metabolically uncontrollable and died during the neonatal period (eight) or the first few months of life (three). Severe infections have frequently complicated the course of the disease. Three who had a later presentation (between 3 and 4 months) survived several years (between 2 years 6 months and 4 years 6 months): two showed recurrent crises and progresssive deterioration in spite of all therapeutic attempts. The third had an apparently milder form with only two ketoacidotic attacks during the first 3 years; however, he died during a third crisis without any response to therapy.

Table 2   Mental evaluation of patients with organic acidurias

	Retarded	Mildly retarded to low average	Normal
Maple syrup urine disease			
classical type	5	12	3
other	—	—	4
Isovaleric acidaemia	2	—	6
Propionic acidaemia			
classical form	—	1	1
late form	1	1	1
Methylmalonic acidaemia			
mutase O form	—	1	—
other	—	—	4

The five surviving patients form a heterogeneous group. One is the brother of the last case mentioned. He has shown only one crisis and his development is perfectly normal. However, he is still only 2 years old. The second surviving patient had a neonatal presentation and she is now 4 years old. She is mildly retarded, has neurological symptoms, is under average in weight and height and might be partially deficient in carnitine.

The last three patients belong to the late form. One was perfectly normal till 2 years 10 months when the first acidotic attack happened, leaving a very severe encephalopathy. During the family study another case was recognized before any clinical manifestation. Unfortunately this child was already mildly retarded because of neonatal anoxia. The third patient is normal at 21 years of age. He has presented only three crises at 3 months of age and during his fourth year when the diagnosis was made. He is presently on a normal diet but shows a classical aversion to meat.

METHYLMALONIC ACIDURIA

The outcome of this group is not much better than the propionic acidaemias, since only seven patients out of 24 are alive. Most of the cases (15) have had a neonatal presentation but deaths occurred usually during infancy and childhood (Table 1). Direct causes of death are acidotic crises but they are often complicated by severe infections and poor nutritional status. Twelve patients have had enzymatic studies: mutase activity was zero in 11 cases, while in the twelfth case cbl B (Rosenberg, 1981) was involved.

Among the seven living patients a late presentation, between 4 and 14 months, has been observed in six cases: at least two of these, and probably two others, are cbl B and cbl A mutants. In the fifth and the sixth cases, mutase activities are respectively 20% of normal and zero. The last patient had a neonatal presentation; his enzymatic study is still incomplete but apoenzyme activity is normal. B_{12} sensitivity is positive *in vitro* in the cases where the cofactors are involved and in the mut – patient. However, *in vivo*, only the cbl A mutant is responsive. Mental development is abnormal in three cases, namely the mut 0, the mut – and cbl B mutants.

Finally it should be mentioned that the mut – patient showed a decrease of serum carnitine (approximately 50% of normal). Therapy with oral DL-carnitine corrected the serum level but did not produce any obvious clinical improvement.

MISCELLANEOUS

Two cases of dicarboxylic aciduria presented with clinical symptoms of recurrent ketotic hypoglycaemia; they have a normal development and have not had crises during the 2 years following the reorganization of meals.

The last three patients with 4-hydroxybutyricuria glutaricuria type II and 3-methylglutaconic aciduria were already severely retarded when the correct diagnosis was made. No conclusions could be made on the evolution of the diseases or the effects of a low protein diet.

CONCLUSION

The main features drawn from this survey are the poor overall prognosis and the slow improvement in the outcome of such disorders over the last 15 years. In MSUD, modern management does not prevent ketoacidotic episodes and intellectual development remains in most of the cases below average. Moreover, some cases still escape from treatment and in other cases diagnosed early, on the basis of a family history, prognosis is not strikingly different. However, early recognition and early management remain a basic requirement for future progress. In propionic and methylmalonic acidaemias modern treatment does not prevent a fatal outcome in the classical form and even treatment itself could be questionable after the correct diagnosis is made. The more recently recognized mutants, where a coenzyme is involved, are uncommon and it should be emphasized that vitamin therapy is very rarely effective *in vivo*, even if it has to be systematically tried. Finally, amongst all these disorders isovaleric acidaemia seems to be the mildest, at least with regard to the patients who survive the neonatal period.

This study of French cases was possible thanks to the collaboration of Professor Saudubray and Dr Ogier (Paris), and Professors Piussan (Amiens), Farriaux (Lille), Bimar (Marseille), Bonnet (Montpellier) and Vidailhet (Nancy). We also thank Drs Bourgeois, Collet, Dutruge, Floret, Hermouet and Plauchu, who provided us with information on some cases followed in Lyon.

Reference

Rosenberg, L. E. The inherited methylmalonic acidaemias: A model system for the study of vitamin metabolism and apoenzyme–coenzyme interactions. In Bolton, N. R. and Toothill, C. (eds.) *Transport and Inherited Disease*, MTP Press, Lancaster, 1981, pp. 3–32

J. Inher. Metab. Dis. 7 Suppl. 1 (1984) 13–17

The Management and Long Term Outcome of Organic Acidaemias

J. V. Leonard, P. Daish, E. R. Naughten and K. Bartlett*
*The Institute of Child Health, 30 Guilford Street, London WC1N 1EH, The Hospital for Sick Children, Great Ormond Street and *Department of Clinical Biochemistry, The Royal Victoria Infirmary, Newcastle upon Tyne NE1 4LP, UK*

We review the outcome of patients with maple syrup urine disease (14 classical patients and three variants), biotinidase deficiency (two patients) and non-cofactor-responsive variants of methylmalonic acidaemia (eight patients), propionic acidaemia (eight patients) and isolated 3-methylcrotonyl CoA carboxylase deficiency (three patients). Their survival, growth, intellectual development and other clinical problems are analysed. With the exception of isolated 3-methylcrotonyl CoA carboxylase deficiency the outcome of patients with disorders that are not cofactor responsive is disappointing. Twelve patients have died (five maple syrup urine disease, two methylmalonic acidaemia, five propionic acidaemia) and many of the survivors are developmentally retarded. The outlook is worst for patients with propionic acidaemia presenting in the neonatal period but a good outcome is possible for patients with maple syrup urine disease if the diagnosis is made early.

INTRODUCTION

The presenting features and initial biochemical findings in the more common organic acidaemias are now well documented. However, there is still considerable uncertainty surrounding the long term management and eventual outcome of patients with these disorders.

In this paper we report our experience at the Hospital for Sick Children of patients with maple syrup urine disease (MSUD), non-cofactor-responsive variants of methylmalonic acidaemia (MMA), propionic acidaemia (PA) and isolated 3-methylcrotonyl CoA carboxylase deficiency, and biotinidase deficiency.

PATIENTS

The review of patients with MSUD includes all those diagnosed since 1969. Patients with the other disorders are included only if they have attended the Hospital for Sick Children since 1978. Patients diagnosed here but not admitted have been excluded.

RESULTS

Maple syrup urine disease

In MSUD plasma concentrations of the branched chain amino acids parallel those of the corresponding 2-oxo-acids (Langenbeck *et al.*, 1978) and metabolic control may be assessed by measurement of the plasma branched chain amino acid concentrations. The management of MSUD is therefore quite distinct from that of the other organic acidaemias in which at present only indirect indices of control are available.

The intake of branched chain amino acids from natural protein is adjusted to maintain the plasma leucine concentration between 100 and 700 µmol/l and plasma isoleucine and valine concentrations between 100 and 400 µmol/l. Since this results in a natural protein intake much lower than the minimum recommended for normal growth (Figure 1) it is necessary to supplement the diet with an amino acid mixture free of the branched chain amino acids. The supplemented diet provides a total amino acid intake equivalent to more than 2 g protein/kg per day (Figure 1).

The control of the plasma branched chain amino acid concentrations in our 17 patients with MSUD (14 classical, three variants) has been generally satisfactory. Since 1978 patients have required few hospital admissions; the major exception is a child with β-thalassaemia major whose control has been erratic partly owing to the need for regular blood transfusions.

Five patients with classical and one with variant MSUD have died. The ages of death varied between 2 and 13 years. Two died after short and overwhelming illnesses and the other four during the recovery phase of apparently minor infections.

Overall the children with MSUD have grown normally despite short periods of poor growth associated with feeding difficulties at the time of introduction of solids (see Figure 3, patient A). Prolonged nasogastric tube feeding has never been required. Poor growth may also be associated with psychosocial problems: this is well illustrated by patient B (Figure 2) who failed to thrive and was taken into care at the age of 2 because her mother was unable to cope; subsequently the child grew rapidly.

We have recently reported the outcome of our patients with MSUD (Naughten *et al.*, 1982). Of those children with classical MSUD still alive only one is unequivocally normal (Figure 3). This child was diagnosed in the neonatal period within 24 hours of the onset of symptoms. He had a developmental quotient of 115 at the age of 4.25 years and now attends normal school. The others are all handicapped but none has deteriorated intellectually since the start of treatment; indeed all the late-treated patients have tended to show some improvement.

Journal of Inherited Metabolic Disease. ISSN 0141–8955. Copyright © SSIEM and MTP Press Limited, Queen Square, Lancaster, UK.

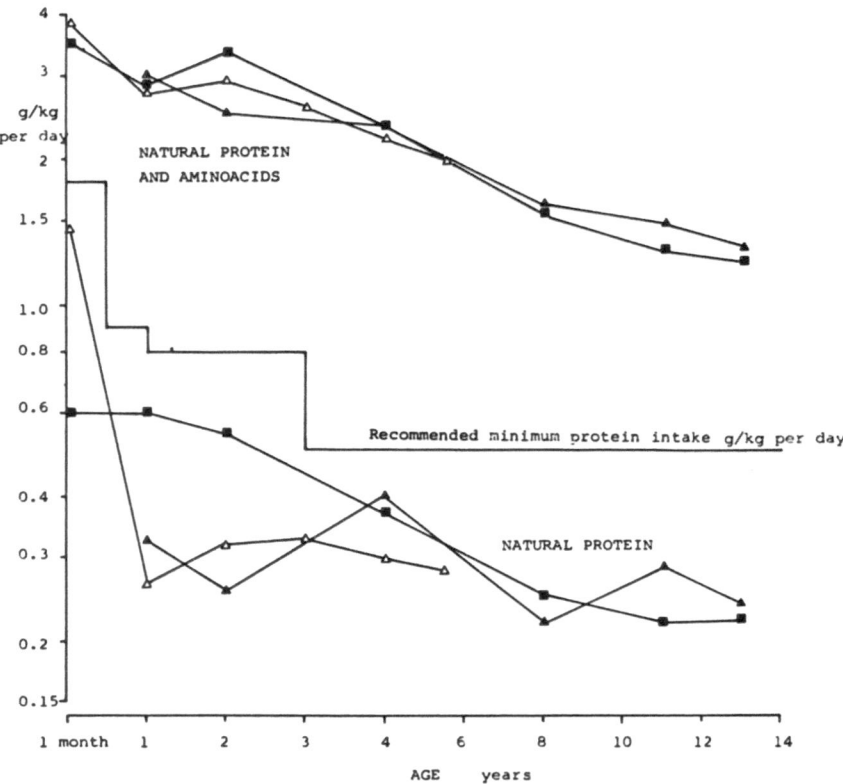

Figure 1 Intake of natural protein and supplementary amino acids for three patients with maple syrup urine disease. Minimum protein intakes adapted from WHO and DHSS recommendations. All intakes are expressed in g/kg body weight per day. Patient A ▲; Patient B ■; Patient C △

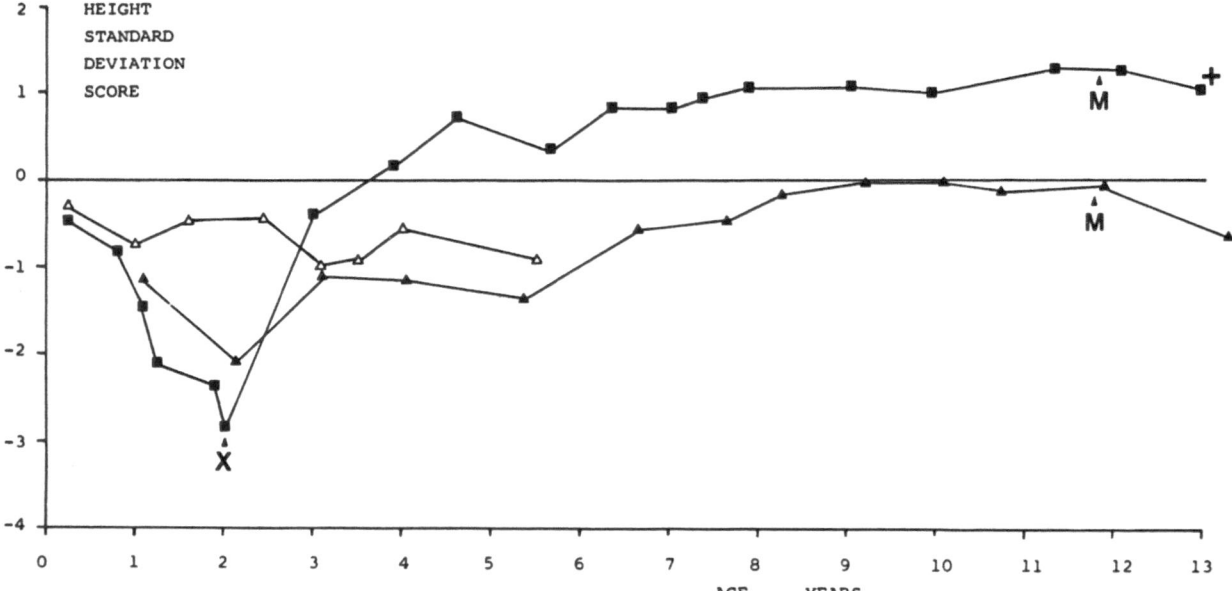

Figure 2 Longitudinal height data expressed as height standard deviation score of three patients with maple syrup urine disease. Patient A ▲; Patient B ■; Patient C △. X = taken into care; M = menarche; + = death

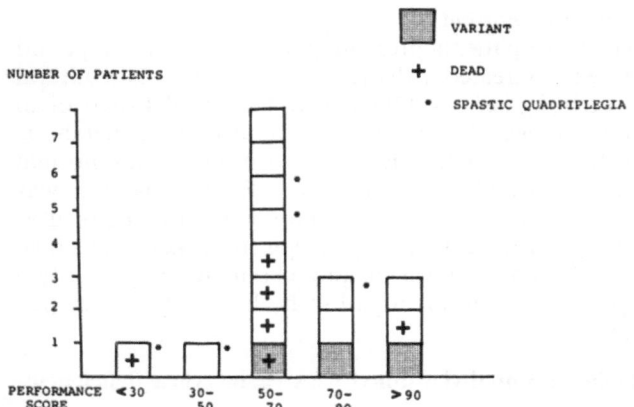

NUMBER OF PATIENTS

☐ VARIANT

✛ DEAD

• SPASTIC QUADRIPLEGIA

Figure 3 Performance scores and outcome of patients with maple syrup urine disease

Two patients with classical MSUD have marked hypotonia which has persisted since the neonatal period. By contrast the extent of neurological handicap in the five patients with spastic quadriplegia gradually became apparent during the first year of life in a manner similar to the evolution of signs in patients with cerebral palsy.

Analysis of our data yields the important conclusion that very early diagnosis and vigorous treatment are essential if the outcome for patients with MSUD is to improve.

Methylmalonic acidaemia

We have cared for eight patients with non-B_{12}-responsive MMA since 1978.

Two of the three patients who developed symptoms in the neonatal period have since died, one at the age of 4 years after a life punctuated by frequent episodes of acidaemia and ketosis, and another who developed symptoms at age 3 days but remained undiagnosed until his terminal illness 3 months later. By contrast all the five patients with late onset of symptoms are still alive.

The mainstay of management for all patients bar one

is restriction of dietary protein; the exception is patient 8 (Table 1) who tolerates a normal diet. To the most severely affected children we give between 1.0 and 1.2 g natural protein/kg per day often in combination with supplementary amino acids (omitting valine, isoleucine, threonine and methionine). For those less severely affected we increase the dietary protein to around 1.5 g/kg per day. During periods of catch-up growth, higher protein intakes are often tolerated.

We have found feeding problems such as food refusal and self-induced vomiting to be common. Indeed three patients with 'severe' disease have each required nasogastric feeding for well over a year.

Patients with MMA tend to be of short stature. Attempts to promote growth in severely affected patients by increasing energy intake have merely resulted in obesity without increase in growth velocity. Patients diagnosed after the neonatal period who are short at presentation may show catch-up growth following the start of treatment, but this is rarely complete.

Most of the severely affected children show mild or moderate developmental retardation but all those with milder disease are intellectually normal. The majority of patients are hypotonic but none has any other neurological signs.

Even amongst the patients who have no residual methylmalonyl CoA mutase activity (mut^0) there is considerable variation in the severity of disease (Table 1). In preliminary studies we have shown that the plasma propionate concentrations correlate well with the severity of disease; the relationships between plasma methylmalonate and propionate concentrations in three patients (1, 2 and 5 – with severe, moderate and mild disease respectively) are shown in Figure 4.

Propionic acidaemia

Neonatal presentation

Our experience of patients with PA presenting in the neonatal period suggests a gloomy outlook with the

Table 1 Details of patients with methylmalonic acidaemia

Patient	Age at presentation	Enzyme activity	Outcome	Level of development	Height standard deviation score	Feeding problems
1	3 days	mut^0	died 4.1 y	2.5 y at 3.5 y	−2.8	prolonged nasogastric feeding
2	3 days	mut^0	alive	22 months at 33 months	−1.63	prolonged nasogastric feeding
3	3 days	mut^0	died at 3 months (delayed diagnosis)	—	—	—
4	4 months	*	alive	3 y at 3.25 y	−3.8	prolonged nasogastric feeding
5	5 months	mut^0	alive	normal at 2 y except for marked speech delay†	−2.01	mild feeding difficulties†
6	5 months	mut^0	alive	mild delay	−2.65	none
7	3 months	*	alive	normal at 5 y	−1.5	none
8	9 months	*	alive	normal at 2.5 y	−0.42	none

The diagnosis of MMA was based on the presence of characteristic metabolites in blood and urine
* No enzyme data available
† Severe psychosocial problems at home

typical course characterized by intractable feeding problems, frequent episodes of ketoacidaemia, severe retardation of growth and development, and early death. Of our five patients with PA who presented shortly after birth three have died (two of these having survived long enough to be assessed as delayed); the two survivors are retarded.

We have attempted to manage these patients with a diet similar to that employed for patients with MMA but have found if anything that feeding problems are even worse; all children surviving longer than 6 months have required prolonged nasogastric tube feeding. Patients have tended to be hypotonic and one (patient 1, Table 2) had choreoathetosis. Early diagnosis and appropriate management may not necessarily improve the outlook significantly (in contrast to MSUD): patient 4 (Table 2) was diagnosed rapidly but has not done well despite appropriate therapy initiated early in the neonatal period.

Late presentation

The three patients presenting after the neonatal period have been treated with diets containing 1.5–2.0 g natural protein/kg per day. One died at the age of 4 years of an unusual encephalitic illness without marked metabolic disturbance; at the time he had been making normal developmental progress. The second patient was severely retarded and had choreoathetosis; he died at the age of 18 years during an episode of ketoacidaemia. The third patient was diagnosed only recently after two episodes of encephalopathy; he has so far developed normally.

Isolated 3-methylcrotonyl CoA carboxylase deficiency

Our three patients with isolated 3-methylcrotonyl CoA carboxylase deficiency have done well. One patient presented in the neonatal period and has been managed with a dietary protein intake restricted to 2 g/kg per day. She has had only mild episodes of ketoacidosis. The

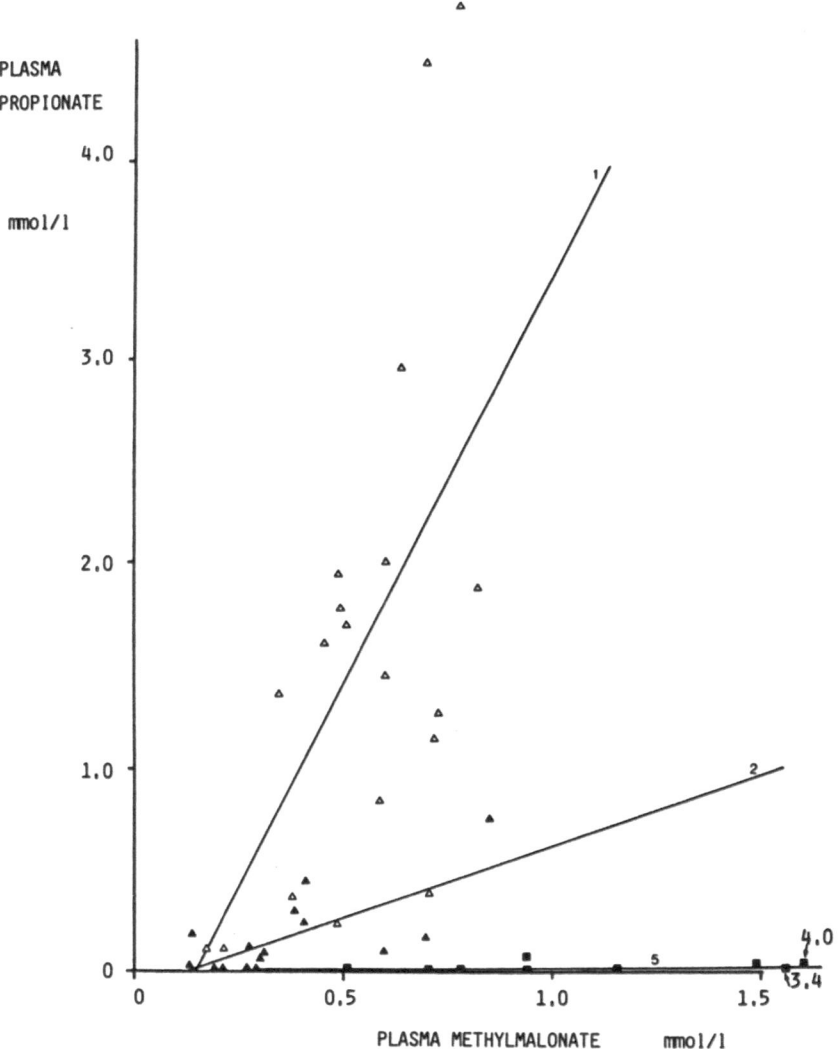

Figure 4 Concentrations of plasma propionate and methylmalonate in three patients with methylmalonic acidaemia (mut⁰). (△ patient 1, ▲ patient 2, and ■ patient 5 in Table 1)

Table 2 Details of patients with propionic acidaemia

Patient	Age at presentation	Outcome	Level of development
1	3 days	died 1.9 y	5–8 months at 1.5 y
2	6 days	died 6 weeks	—
3	3 days	died 1.5 y	<6 months at 1.5 y
4	2 days	alive (3.75 y)	<2 years at 3.75 y
5	4 days	alive (1.5 y)	6–7 months at 1.4 y
6	8 months	died 4 y	normal
7	11 months	died 18 y	retarded and severe choreoathetosis
8	16 months	alive (20 months)	normal

The diagnosis of PA was based upon the presence of characteristic metabolites in plasma and urine

other two patients are siblings, the younger of whom presented at the age of 2.75 years with severe metabolic acidaemia during an episode of gastroenteritis. The asymptomatic sibling, aged 5, was detected on subsequent screening. The family are vegetarians and have a natural protein intake of only 1.8–2.3 g/kg per day.

All three patients are making normal neurodevelopmental progress.

Biotinidase deficiency: late complications

We have recently shown that two of our patients with multiple carboxylase deficiency (Leonard *et al.*, 1981) have absent biotinidase activity (unpublished observations). The children presented with developmental regression, hair loss and skin rashes. Both responded rapidly to oral biotin supplements but one has a severe partial hearing loss (70–80 dB for speech frequencies) and the other optic atrophy with poor visual acuity.

CONCLUSIONS

We have found that the outcome for patients with the more common organic acidaemias is disappointing. The established long term management of patients with MSUD is probably near optimal but it is clear that events in the neonatal period are crucial and that appropriate treatment must be given early if the overall prognosis is to improve.

Although the ideal long term treatment for PA and MMA has yet to be determined it is apparent that additional factors including biochemical function and psychosocial background will profoundly influence the final outcome.

References

Langenbeck, U., Wendel, U., Mench-Hoinowski, A., Kuschel, D., Becker, K., Przyrembel, H. and Bremer, H. J. Correlations between branched-chain amino acids and branched-chain α-keto acids in blood in maple syrup urine disease. *Clin. Chim. Acta* 88 (1978) 283–291

Léonard, J. V., Seakins, J. W. T., Bartlett, K., Hyde, J., Wilson, J. and Clayton, B. Inherited disorders of 3-methylcrotonyl CoA carboxylation. *Arch. Dis. Child.* 56 (1981) 53–59

Naughten, E. R., Jenkins, J., Francis, D. E. M. and Leonard, J. V. Outcome of maple syrup urine disease. *Arch. Dis. Child.* 57 (1982) 918–921

J. Inher. Metab. Dis. 7 Suppl. 1 (1984) 18–22

Prenatal Diagnosis of the Organic Acidurias

L. SWEETMAN

Department of Pediatrics M-009, University of California, San Diego, La Jolla, CA 92093, USA

Prenatal diagnosis for the genetic counselling of families at risk for having children with the life-threatening organic acidurias is advancing rapidly. The two major approaches to prenatal diagnosis are the assay for deficient activity of the enzymes in cultured amniocytes and the measurement of increased concentrations of the organic acids in the amniotic fluid. The latter, when done by stable isotope dilution analysis, is rapid, relatively inexpensive and very reliable.

The availability of reliable methods of prenatal diagnosis is an important component of genetic counselling for families who have had a child with an organic aciduria. Many of these inherited disorders are life-threatening and the treatment and prognosis are less than ideal. Although the incidence of the individual disorders is low, their aggregate incidence is significant. Prenatal diagnosis is generally indicated when the parents are known to be heterozygotes and this is usually established by the birth and diagnosis of an affected child. It is essential for prenatal diagnosis that the disorder of the previously affected children in the family be adequately documented. This is particularly true for the assay of partial deficiencies of enzymes where it is essential to distinguish homozygous affected from heterozygous individuals.

The number of disorders that can be diagnosed prenatally has increased rapidly in the last decade. The inherited organic acidurias are particularly amenable to prenatal diagnosis because the enzymes involved are usually expressed in all tissues and large concentrations of organic acids accumulate in body fluids. It is likely that prenatal diagnosis will become available for all of the organic acidurias.

Two main approaches are being utilized. One is the assay of deficient enzymatic activity in cultured amniocytes (Galjaard, 1980). In general, if an enzyme is normally expressed in cultured fibroblasts and an enzyme deficiency can be demonstrated in fibroblasts of affected patients, the same will be true of cultured amniocytes. The most direct method is a specific assay of the enzyme in cell lysates. The activity can also be determined by incubation of intact amniocytes with ^{14}C-labelled substrates and measurement of the oxidation to [14]CO_2 or incorporation into macromolecules.

Amniotic fluid is derived in part from the mother and in part from the fetus, including fetal urine (Natelson *et al.*, 1974). The organic acidurias characteristically have large elevations of normal or abnormal metabolites in urine. These metabolites are produced in excessive amounts by an affected fetus and generally accumulate in amniotic fluid. Prenatal diagnosis by measurement of elevated levels of organic acids in amniotic fluid requires sensitive, specific and reliable methods. The most suitable method is stable isotope dilution analysis in which an excess of the stable isotopically labelled acid, usually containing 2–6 atoms of deuterium, is added to the amniotic fluid sample as a carrier and internal standard. The acid is extracted, derivatized and the relative amounts of unlabelled compound from the amniotic fluid and the internal standard determined by gas chromatography–mass spectrometry (GC–MS). This method corrects for all losses in the procedure and the detection of the internal standard ensures that the determination was done properly.

A third method for prenatal diagnosis that may be of value is the measurement of increased concentrations of organic acids in maternal urine. This is a less direct method of measuring the production of acids by the fetus than the analysis of amniotic fluid, but has the advantages of being non-invasive and repeated sampling is convenient. However, the urinary excretion of acids in maternal urine appears less reliable as the concentrations may not increase until late in pregnancy and may be more influenced by maternal metabolism than those of the amniotic fluid.

Table 1 summarizes the status of the prenatal diagnosis of a number of organic acidurias. Most of the techniques were developed in the last 10 years, and it is anticipated that successful prenatal diagnosis will be accomplished shortly for the remaining disorders.

Maple syrup urine disease with defective oxidation of isoleucine, valine and leucine, was first diagnosed prenatally by the measurement of decreased oxidation of branched chain amino acids (Dancis, 1972) and 2-oxoacids (Wendel *et al.*, 1973) in intact amniocytes. The most suitable procedure is the microassay with the cells attached to the culture plate (Wendel *et al.*, 1981). These authors have shown that the enzymatic activity is similar in different types of normal cells derived from amniotic fluid and that the assay can be performed within 2 weeks of the amniocentesis. Determination of the concentrations of metabolites in amniotic fluid is not useful for prenatal diagnosis. The branched chain amino acids and 2-oxoacids are normal in the amniotic fluid with an affected fetus (Wendel *et al.*, 1980). The corresponding branched chain 2-hydroxy acids are also normal (Jakobs, Sweetman and Nyhan, unpublished observations).

3-Oxothiolase deficiency or 2-methyl-3-hydroxybutyric 2-methylacetoacetic aciduria, a defect of the

Journal of Inherited Metabolic Disease. ISSN 0141–8955. Copyright © SSIEM and MTP Press Limited, Queen Square, Lancaster, UK.

Table 1 **Prenatal diagnosis of the organic acidurias**

Disorder	McCusick number	Enzyme activity in cultured amniocytes		Metabolite levels in amniotic fluid	
		Potential	Accomplished	Potential	Accomplished
Maple syrup urine disease	24860		+ + +		—
3-Oxothiolase deficiency	20375	+ + +		+ + +	
Propionic acidaemia	23200, 23205		+ + +		+ + +
Methymalonic acidaemia	25100, 25110, 25111		+ + +		+ + +
Isovaleric acidaemia	24350	+ + +		+ + +	
3-Methylcrotonyl-CoA carboxylase isolated deficiency	21020	+ + +		+ + +	
Multiple carboxylase deficiency–biotin responsive	21021, 25327		+ + +		+ + +
3-Methylglutaconic aciduria	25095	???		+ + +	
3-Hydroxy-3-methylglutaryl-CoA lyase deficiency	24645	+ + +		+ + +	
Glutaric aciduria type I	23167		+ + +		+ + +
Glutaric aciduria type II	23168, 30595		+ + +		+ + +
Pyruvate carboxylase deficiency	26615		+ + +		—
4-Hydroxybutyric aciduria	—		—	+ + +	

metabolism of isoleucine, has not been diagnosed prenatally. Recently a specific assay for 2-methylacetoacetyl CoA thiolase has been employed to demonstrate a deficiency of this enzyme in cultured fibroblasts (Middleton and Bartlett, 1983) and it is likely that this will be suitable for prenatal diagnosis with cultured amniocytes. 2-Methyl-3-hydroxybutyric acid has been quantified in normal amniotic fluid (Jakobs, Sweetman and Nyhan, unpublished observations) and is likely to be elevated in the amniotic fluid with an affected fetus. Propionic acidaemia, a defect in the catabolism of isoleucine, valine and other compounds, was first diagnosed prenatally by the demonstration of deficient activity of propionyl CoA carboxylase (EC 6.4.1.3) in cultured amniocytes (Gompertz *et al.*, 1975). Elevated concentrations of the two diastereoisomers of methylcitric acid, metabolites characteristically elevated in the urine of patients with propionic acidaemia, were found in amniotic fluid with an affected fetus (Sweetman *et al.*, 1979). In the first application of stable isotope dilution analysis for prenatal diagnosis of an organic aciduria, methylcitric acid labelled with three deuterium atoms was used as an internal standard (Naylor *et al.*, 1980). The methylcitric acid was isolated from 1–4 ml of amniotic fluid by liquid partition chromatography, methylated and the ratio of methylcitric acid to $[^2H_3]$-methylcitric acid determined by ammonia chemical ionization, selected ion monitoring GC–MS. With this technique, methylcitric acid could be quantified in normal amniotic fluid, demonstrating that this 'abnormal' metabolite is normal and that quantitative rather than qualitative differences need to be determined for reliable prenatal diagnoses of the organic acidurias. Table 2 summarizes our experience with the

measurement of the concentration of methylcitric acid in amniotic fluid by stable isotope dilution for prenatal diagnosis of 34 pregnancies at risk for propionic acidaemia. The mean concentration in affected pregnancies was about 18 times the normal mean or the mean for unaffected pregnancies. The least elevated concentration of methylcitric acid with an affected fetus was 18 standard deviations above the concentration of the unaffected pregnancies. The concentration of methylcitric acid in amniotic fluid has given the correct diagnosis in all cases. In one case in which the elevation of methylcitric acid indicated an affected fetus, propionyl CoA carboxylase in cultured amniocytes was normal. An affected child was born and it was established that the amniocytes had been overgrown with maternal fibroblasts (Buchanan *et al.*, 1980). Thus the measurement of methylcitric acid in amniotic fluid appears more reliable for prenatal diagnosis than the measurement of enzyme activity in cultured amniocytes.

Prenatal diagnosis of the various types of methylmalonic acidaemia has been established. In the first prenatal diagnosis, elevated concentrations of methylmalonic acid were found in amniotic fluid and maternal urine at 25 weeks of pregnancy (Morrow *et al.*, 1970). Subsequently, elevated concentrations of methylmalonic acid in amniotic fluid and decreased activity of methylmalonyl CoA mutase (EC 5.4.99.2) in cultured amniocytes (Gompertz *et al.*, 1974) and decreased oxidation of propionic and methylmalonic acid in intact amniocytes (Mahoney *et al.*, 1975) have been used for prenatal diagnosis. A vitamin B_{12}-responsive fetus was diagnosed prenatally and the mother treated with vitamin B_{12} (Ampola *et al.*, 1975). The elevated concentration of methylmalonic acid in the maternal

Table 2 Stable isotope dilution analysis of organic acids in amniotic fluid

	Methylcitric acid (µmol/l) Mean ± SD	Range
Normal (n = 8)	0.38 ± 0.10	0.24–0.58
At risk for propionic acidaemia		
Not affected (n = 23)	0.42 ± 0.22	0.17–1.13
Affected (n = 11)	7.34 ± 1.94	4.48–10.16
At risk for methylmalonic acidaemia		
Not affected (n = 10)	0.39 ± 0.19	0.23–0.89
Affected (n = 4)	2.72 ± 0.05	2.68–2.78

	Methylmalonic acid (µmol/l) Mean ± SD	Range
Normal (n = 9)	0.29 ± 0.08	0.17–0.44
At risk for methylmalonic acidaemia		
Not affected (n = 7)	0.39 ± 0.20	0.16–0.78
Affected (n = 3)	37.0 ± 32.0	17.6–74.0

urine was significantly decreased with vitamin B_{12} therapy, indicating effective prenatal therapy. Methylmalonic acid may not be elevated in maternal urine with an affected fetus until after 22 weeks of pregnancy (Bakker *et al.*, 1978). This indicates that the other methods of prenatal diagnosis are preferable. Methylmalonyl CoA mutase has been assayed in uncultured amniotic fluid cells which would eliminate the long time needed for culture of amniocytes (Morrow *et al.*, 1977). However, considering the large number of non-viable cells in amniotic fluid and the wide range of activities found, this may not be a reliable diagnostic test. A method which reduces the time required to culture sufficient amniocytes for prenatal diagnosis to two to four passages is the incorporation of 1-^{14}C-propionic acid into macromolecules (Willard *et al.*, 1976). Decreased incorporation occurs in amniocytes of all types of methylmalonic acidaemia and with propionic acidaemia as well.

The most rapid method for reliable prenatal diagnosis of methylmalonic acidaemia is the measurement of methylmalonic acid in amniotic fluid by stable isotope dilution analysis. Three different procedures have been described using [$^2H_3$]-methylmalonic acid as internal standard and the following concentrations of methylmalonic acid (µmoles/litre ± 1 SD) found for normal amniotic fluid: 0.31 ± 0.10 (Trefz *et al.*, 1981), 0.32 ± 0.13 (Zinn *et al.*, 1982) and 0.29 ± 0.08 (Sweetman *et al.*, 1982). This illustrates the very high accuracy of stable isotope dilution analyses, compared to an earlier gas chromatographic method which gave normal levels 20 times higher (Nakamura *et al.*, 1976). The experience in our own laboratory with prenatal diagnosis of methylmalonic acidaemia by stable isotope dilution analysis of methylmalonic acid in amniotic fluid is summarized in Table 2. The elevations with affected fetuses have ranged from 60 to 255 times normal. Methylcitric acid is also elevated about seven times in amniotic fluid with a fetus affected with methylmalonic

acidaemia (Table 2). We routinely measure both methylmalonic acid and methylcitric acid in amniotic fluid of pregnancies at risk for methylmalonic acidaemia to increase the confidence in the prenatal diagnosis.

Isovaleric acidaemia due to a deficiency of isovaleryl CoA dehydrogenase (EC 1.3.99.10) in the catabolism of leucine, has not been diagnosed prenatally. A pregnancy at risk was monitored by the oxidation of 2-^{14}C-leucine to $^{14}CO_2$ in intact amniocytes which suggested a heterozygous fetus which was confirmed in cultured fibroblasts after birth (Blaskovics *et al.*, 1978). Another potentially useful technique is the measurement of decreased incorporation of 1-^{14}C-isovaleric acid into macromolecules (Chalmers and Spellacy, 1979). Isovalerylglycine, the major abnormal urinary metabolite of isovaleric acidaemia, is likely to be elevated in the amniotic fluid of an affected fetus. An increased concentration of isovalerylglycine has been detected in the amniotic fluid at 37 weeks of pregnancy in a case of multiple acyl CoA dehydrogenase deficiency including isovaleryl CoA dehydrogenase (Niederwieser *et al.*, 1983). Another metabolite of isovaleric acidaemia that may be elevated in amniotic fluid from cases with a fetus affected by isovaleric acidaemia is 3-hydroxyisovaleric acid. A stable isotope dilution assay for this acid has been developed (Jakobs *et al.*, 1984a).

An isolated, biotin-resistant deficiency of 3-methylcrotonyl CoA carboxylase (EC 6.4.1.4) has been documented (Beemer *et al.*, 1982). It should be possible to diagnose this prenatally by assay of the enzyme in cultured amniocytes and measurement of 3-hydroxyisovaleric acid in amniotic fluid as has been done for the deficiency of this enzyme in biotin-responsive multiple carboxylase deficiency.

Two enzyme deficiencies are now known to cause biotin-responsive multiple carboxylase deficiency: an abnormal holocarboxylase synthetase (EC 6.3.4.10) in type I of neonatal form (Burri *et al.*, 1981) and biotinidase (EC 3.5.1.12) deficiency in type II or late onset form (Wolf *et al.*, 1983). A fetus with an abnormal holocarboxylase synthetase was diagnosed prenatally by the demonstration of biotin-responsive deficiencies of the carboxylases for propionyl CoA, 3-methylcrotonyl CoA and pyruvate in cultured amniocytes and elevated concentrations of methylcitric acid in amniotic fluid (Packman *et al.*, 1982). Subsequently, highly elevated concentrations of 3-hydroxyisovaleric acid were shown in the amniotic fluid by stable isotope dilution analysis (Jakobs *et al.*, 1984a). Prenatal treatment was done by oral administration of 10 mg of biotin per day to the mother. A clinically well baby was born and has remained asymptomatic with treatment with biotin. In the amniotic fluid of the affected pregnancy, methylcitric acid was about three times normal, while 3-hydroxyiso-valeric acid was eight times normal. Therefore the latter would appear more reliable for prenatal diagnosis. Both acids were normal in the amniotic fluid with an unaffected fetus (Jakobs *et al.*, 1984a).

A fetus with 3-methylglutaconic aciduria would probably have increased concentrations of 3-methyl-glutaconic and 3-hydroxyisovaleric acids in amniotic fluid since these are highly elevated in urine of the patients (Duran *et al.*, 1982). No specific enzyme assay is available and the incorporation of 1-^{14}C-isovaleric acid into macromolecules is not diagnostic in cultured fibroblasts (Sovik, Sweetman, Gibson and Nyhan, unpublished observations) and presumably not in amniocytes.

3-Hydroxy-3-methylglutaryl CoA lyase (EC 4.1.3.4) deficiency has been diagnosed at 23 weeks of pregnancy by demonstration of increased concentrations of 3-hydroxy-3-methylglutaric, 3-methylglutaconic, 3-hy-droxyisovaleric and 3-methylglutaric acids in the maternal urine (Duran *et al.*, 1979). A deficiency of the enzyme can be demonstrated in cultured fibroblasts (Wysocki and Hähnel, 1976) and presumably also in cultured amniocytes. The organic acids that are elevated in the maternal urine of a pregnancy with an affected fetus would be expected to be elevated in the amniotic fluid. 3-Hydroxyisovaleric acid can be determined by a stable isotope dilution assay (Jakobs *et al.*, 1984a).

Glutaric aciduria type I due to a deficiency of glutaryl CoA dehydrogenase (EC 1.3.99.7) has been diagnosed prenatally by a deficiency of this enzyme in cultured amniocytes and increased concentrations of glutaric acid in the amniotic fluid (Goodman *et al.*, 1980). Glutaric aciduria type II or multiple acyl CoA dehydrogenase deficiency has been diagnosed prenatally by deficiencies of oxidation of medium and long chain fatty acids in cultured amniocytes and by increased concentrations of glutaric acid in amniotic fluid (Niederwieser *et al.*, 1983; Mitchell *et al.*, 1983). Increased concentrations of adipic, suberic and sebacic acid in addition to glutaric acid have been found in the amniotic fluid with an affected fetus (Jakobs *et al.*, 1984b).

Pyruvate carboxylase (EC 6.4.1.1) deficiency has been diagnosed prenatally by the demonstration of a deficiency of this enzyme in cultured amniotic cells (Marsac *et al.*, 1982). Pyruvic acid was not elevated in the amniotic fluid with an affected fetus, indicating that prenatal diagnosis of this disorder by analysis of organic acids in amniotic fluids is not possible (Rocchiccioli *et al.*, 1981).

4-Hydroxybutyric aciduria is characterized by increased excretion of 4-hydroxybutyric acid (Jakobs *et al.*, 1981; Divry *et al.*, 1983). Elevated concentrations of this acid would be expected in amniotic fluid with an affected fetus. The enzymatic defect has been shown in lymphocytes to be a deficiency of succinic semialdehyde dehydrogenase (EC 1.2.1.24) (Gibson *et al.*, 1983). However this enzyme is not expressed in normal fibroblasts and therefore it is unlikely that assay of this enzyme in cultured amniocytes will be useful for prenatal diagnosis.

The prenatal diagnosis of the organic acidurias is a rapidly expanding field and it is anticipated that most, if not all, of these disorders will be diagnosable by measurement of enzyme deficiencies in cultured amniocytes or by the more rapid stable isotope dilution analysis of increased concentrations of organic acids in amniotic fluid. The new techniques of molecular biology for demonstrating abnormalities at the level of the gene (Woo *et al.*, 1983) are potentially useful for prenatal diagnosis of the organic acidurias. Their greatest value will be for prenatal diagnosis of disorders for which the enzyme activity cannot be determined in amniocytes and for which there are no diagnostic elevations of metabolites in amniotic fluid.

I thank Jan Holm for her expert assistance in the stable isotope dilution analyses, Dr Cornelis Jakobs, on leave from the Department of Pediatrics, Free University of Amsterdam, for his dedicated development of additional methods, and the many physicians who provided amniotic fluids from patients at risk. Supported by US Public Health Service Grants No. HD04608 from the National Institute of Child Health and Human Development, GM17702 from the National Institute of General Medical Sciences, National Institutes of Health, Bethesda, MD, USA and Grant No. MCJ004007 from the Health Resources and Services Administration, Department of Health and Human Services, Rockville, MD, USA.

References

Ampola, M. G., Mahoney, M. J., Nakamura, E. and Tanaka, K. Prenatal therapy of a patient with vitamin-B$_{12}$-responsive methylmalonic acidemia. *N. Engl. J. Med.* 293 (1975) 313–317

Bakker, H. D., Van Gennip, A. H., Duran, M. and Wadman, S. K. Methylmalonate excretion in a pregnancy at risk for methylmalonic acidemia. *Clin. Chim. Acta* 86 (1978) 349–352

Beemer, F. A., Bartlett, K., Duran, M., Ghneim, H. K., Wadman, S. K., Bruinvis, L. and Ketting, D. Isolated biotin-resistant 3-methylcrotonyl-CoA carboxylase deficiency in two sibs. *Eur. J. Pediatr.* 138 (1982) 351–354

Blaskovics, M. E., Ng, W. G. and Donnell, G. N. Prenatal diagnosis and a case report of isovaleric acidemic. *J. Inher. Metab. Dis.* 1 (1978) 9–11

Buchanan, P. D., Kahler, S. G., Sweetman, L. and Nyhan, W. L. Pitfalls in the prenatal diagnosis of propionic acidemia. *Clin. Genet.* 18 (1980) 177–183

Burri, B. J., Sweetman, L. and Nyhan, W. L. Mutant holocarboxylase synthetase – evidence for the enzyme defect in early infantile biotin-responsive multiple carboxylase deficiency. *J. Clin. Invest.* 68 (1981) 1491–1495

Chalmers, R. A. and Spellacy, E. A method for the pre- and post-natal detection of defects of isovalerate metabolism. *Clin. Sci.* 57 (1979) 25

Dancis, J. Maple syrup urine disease. In Dorfman, A. (ed.) *Antenatal Diagnosis*, University of Chicago Press, Chicago, 1972, pp. 123–125

Divry, P., Baltassat, P., Rolland, M. O., Cotte, J., Hermier, M., Duran, M. and Wadman, S. K. A new patient with 4-hydroxybutyric aciduria, a possible defect of 4-amino butyrate metabolism. *Clin. Chim. Acta* 129 (1983) 303–309

Duran, M., Schutgens, R. B. H., Ketel, A., Heymans, H., Berntssen, M. W. J., Ketting, D. and Wadman, S. K. 3-Hydroxy-3-methylglutaryl coenzyme A lyase deficiency: postnatal management following prenatal diagnosis by analysis of maternal urine. *J. Pediatr.* 95 (1979) 1004–1007

Duran, M., Beemer, F. A., Tibosch, A. S., Bruinvis, L., Ketting, D. and Wadman, S. K. Inherited 3-methylglutaconic aciduria in two brothers – Another defect of leucine metabolism. *J. Pediatr.* 101 (1982) 551–554

Galjaard, H. *Genetic Metabolic Diseases*, Elsevier/North Holland, Amsterdam, 1980

Gibson, K. M., Sweetman, L., Nyhan, W. L., Jakobs, C., Rating, D., Siemes, H. and Hanefeld, F. Succinic semialdehyde dehydrogenase deficiency: an inborn error of gamma-aminobutyric acid metabolism. *Clin. Chim. Acta* 133 (1983) 33–42

Gompertz, D., Goodey, P. A., Saudubray, J. M., Charpentier, C., Chignolle, A. and Girard, S. Prenatal diagnosis of methylmalonic aciduria. *Pediatrics* 54 (1974) 511–513

Gompertz, D., Goodey, P. A., Thom, H., Russell, G., Johnston, A. W., Mellor, D. H., MacLean, M. W., Ferguson-Smith, M. E. and Ferguson-Smith, M. A. Prenatal diagnosis and family studies in a case of propionic acidemia. *Clin. Genet.* 8 (1975) 244–250

Goodman, S. I., Gallegos, D. A., Pullin, C. J., Halpern, B., Truscott, R. J. W., Wise, G., Wilcken, B., Ryan, E. D. and Whelan, D. T. Antenatal diagnosis of glutaric aciduria. *Am. J. Hum. Genet.* 32 (1980) 695–699

Jakobs, C., Bojasch, M., Mönch, E., Rating, D., Siemes, H. and Hanefeld, F. Urinary excretions of gamma-hydroxy-butyric acid in a patient with neurological abnormalities. The probability of a new inborn error of metabolism. *Clin. Chim. Acta* 111 (1981) 169–178

Jakobs, C., Sweetman, L., Packman, S. and Nyhan, W. L. Stable isotope dilution analysis of 3-hydroxyisovaleric acid in amniotic fluid: Contribution to the prenatal diagnosis of inherited disorders of leucine metabolism. *J. Inher. Metab. Dis.* 7 (1984a) 15–20

Jakobs, C., Sweetman, L., Wadman, S. K., Duran, M., Saudubray, J. M. and Nyhan, W. L. Prenatal diagnosis of Glutaric aciduria type II by direct chemical analysis of dicarboxylic acids in amniotic fluid. *Eur. J. Pediatr.* 141 (1984b) 153–157

Mahoney, M. J., Rosenberg, L. E., Lindblad, B., Waldenström, J. and Zetterström, R. Prenatal diagnosis of methylmalonic aciduria. *Acta Paediatr. Scand.* 64 (1975) 44–48

Marsac, C., Augereau, Ch., Feldman, G., Wolf, B., Hansen, T. L. and Berger, R. Prenatal diagnosis of pyruvate carboxylase deficiency. *Clin. Chim. Acta* 119 (1982) 121–127

Middleton, B. and Bartlett, K. The synthesis and characterization of 2-methylacetoacetyl coenzyme A and its use in the identification of the site of the defect in 2-methylacetoacetic and 2-methyl-3-hydroxybutyric aciduria. *Clin. Chim. Acta* 128 (1983) 291–305

Mitchell, G., Saudubray, J. M., Benoit, Y., Rocchiccioli, F., Charpentier, C., Ogier, H. and Boue, J. Antenatal diagnosis of glutaric aciduria Type II. *Lancet* 1 (1983) 1099

Morrow, G. III, Schwarz, R. H., Hallock, J. A. and Barness, L. A. Prenatal detection of methylmalonic acidemia. *J. Pediatr.* 77 (1970) 120–123

Morrow, G. III, Revsin, B., Lebowitz, J., Britt, W. and Giles, H. Detection of errors in methylmalonyl-CoA metabolism by using amniotic fluid. *Clin. Chem.* 23 (1977) 791–795

Nakamura, E., Rosenberg, L. E. and Tanaka, K. Micro determination of methylmalonic acid and other short chain dicarboxylic acids by gas chromatography: use in prenatal diagnosis of methylmalonic acidemia and in studies of isovaleric acidemia. *Clin. Chim. Acta* 68 (1976) 127–140

Natelson, S., Scommegna, A. and Epstein, M. B. (eds.) *Amniotic Fluid*, Wiley, New York, 1974

Naylor, G., Sweetman, L., Nyhan, W. L., Hornbeck, C., Griffiths, J., Mörch, L. and Brandänge, S. Isotope dilution analysis of methylcitric acid in amniotic fluid for the prenatal diagnosis of propionic and methylmalonic acidemia. *Clin. Chim. Acta* 107 (1980) 175–183

Niederwieser, A., Steinmann, B., Exner, U., Neuheiser, F., Redweik, U., Wang, M., Rampini, S. and Wendel, U. Multiple acyl-CoA dehydrogenation deficiency (MADD) in a boy with nonketotic hypoglycemia, hepatomegaly, muscle, hypotonia, and cardiomyopathy. *Helv. Paediatr. Acta* 38 (1983) 9–26

Packman, S., Golbus, M. S., Cowan, M. J., Caswell, N. M., Sweetman, L., Burri, B. J., Nyhan, W. L. and Baker, H. Prenatal treatment of biotin-responsive multiple carboxylase deficiency. *Lancet* 1 (1982) 1435–1439

Rocchiccioli, F., Leroux, J. P. and Cartier, P. Quantitation of 2-ketoacids in biological fluids by gas chromatography chemical ionization mass spectrometry of O-trimethylsilyl-quinoxalinol derivatives. *Biomed. Mass Spectrom.* 8 (1981) 160–164

Sweetman, L., Weyler, W., Shafai, T., Young, P. E. and Nyhan, W. L. Prenatal diagnosis of propionic acidemia. *J. Am. Med. Assoc.* 242 (1979) 1048–1052

Sweetman, L., Naylor, G., Ladner, T., Holm, J., Nyhan, W. L., Hornbeck, C., Griffiths, J., Mörch, L., Brandänge, S., Gruenke, L. and Craig, J. C. Prenatal diagnosis of propionic and methylmalonic acidemia by stable isotope dilution analysis of methylcitric and methylmalonic acids in amniotic fluid. In Schmidt, H.-L., Förstel, H. and Heinzinger, K. (eds.) *Stable Isotopes*, Elsevier Sci. Publ. Co., Amsterdam, 1982, pp. 287–293

Trefz, F. K., Schmidt, H., Tauscher, B., Depène, E., Baumgartner, R., Hammersen, G. and Kochen, W. Improved prenatal diagnosis of methylmalonic acidemia: Mass fragmentography of methylmalonic acid in amniotic fluid and maternal urine. *Eur. J. Pediatr.* 137 (1981) 261–266

Wendel, U., Rüdiger, H. W., Passarge, E. and Mikkelsen, M. Maple syrup urine disease: Rapid prenatal diagnosis by enzyme assay. *Human Genetik* 19 (197) 127–128

Wendel, U., Claussen, U. and Langenbeck, U. Pattern of branched-chain alpha-keto acids in amniotic fluid. *Clin. Chim. Acta* 120 (1980) 267–269

Wendel, U., Gamm, G. and Claussen, U. Maple syrup urine disease: alpha-keto-isocaproate decarboxylation activity in different types of cultured amniotic cells. *Prenat. Diagn.* 1 (1981) 235–240

Willard, H. F., Ambani, L. M., Hart, A. C., Mahoney, M. J. and Rosenberg, L. E. Rapid prenatal and postnatal detection of inborn errors of propionate, methylmalonate, and cobalamin metabolism. *Hum. Genet.* 34 (1976) 277–283

Wolf, B., Grier, R. E., Parker, W. D. Jr., Goodman, S. I. and Allen, R. J. Deficient biotinidase activity in late-onset multiple carboxylase deficiency. *N. Engl. J. Med.* 308 (1983) 161

Woo, S. L. C., Lidsky, A. S., Güttler, F. and Robson, K. J. H. Cloned human phenylalanine hydroxylase gene allows prenatal diagnosis and carrier detection of classical phenylketonuria. *Nature (London)* 306 (1983) 151–155

Wysocki, S. J. and Hähnel, R. 3-Hydroxy-3-methylglutaric aciduria: Deficiency of 3-hydroxy-3-methylglutaryl coenzyme A lyase. *Clin. Chim. Acta* 71 (1976) 349–351

Zinn, A. B., Hine, D. G., Mahoney, M. J. and Tanaka, K. The stable isotope dilution method for measurement of methylmalonic acid: A highly accurate approach to the prenatal diagnosis of methylmalonic acidemia. *Pediatr. Res.* 16 (1982) 740–745

J. Inher. Metab. Dis. 7 Suppl. 1 (1984) 23–27

Symptoms and Signs in Organic Acidurias

N. J. BRANDT

Section of Clinical Genetics, University Department of Pediatrics, Rigshospitalet, Copenhagen, Denmark

Organic acidaemias can present with a wide variety of signs and symptoms. A survey of the clinical presentation of the organic acidurias shows that single symptoms are not characteristic or diagnostic. Clinical awareness coupled with appropriate laboratory investigation is required for the correct diagnosis to be reached.

The aim of this paper is to try to delineate a pattern of clinical symptoms and signs charateristic of organic acidaemias.

Students of inborn errors of metabolism are well aware of the fact that there are few symptoms these diseases cannot cause and there are few signs for which they may not be responsible. In the history of medicine organic acidaemias are certainly a recent addition, and the usual definition is any disease in which there is accumulation of an acid which does not contain an amino group. With such a broad definition the presentation of these disorders might cover the whole medical spectrum. Even enzyme deficiencies in closely connected pathways can result in completely different syndromes, i.e. accumulation of D-glyceric acid results in symptoms completely different from accumulation of L-glyceric acid (Brandt *et al.*, 1976; Wadman *et al.*, 1976; Williams and Smith, 1968).

It is important, however, to obtain as much information as possible from clinical signs and symptoms, not only because very sophisticated bio-medical techniques are less interesting if they are not related to patients, but also for everyday diagnostic purposes. To try to identify a primary organic acidaemia in a patient treated with valproic acid by studying the gas chromatogram of the urine is cumbersome. But are the symptoms suspicious of organic acidaemia? If they are, one must try to convince the paediatrician that valproic acid should be withdrawn for a period eventually to diagnose the primary defect. Another example is a gas chromatogram with large late peaks, e.g. citric acid, 4-hydroxyphenyl-lactic acid and 4-hydroxyphenylpyruvic acid, together with small amounts of lactic acid, pyruvic acid and 3-hydroxy-butyric acid. Perhaps not too alarming, but when we know that the patient suffers from severe liver disease one would specifically look for succinyl acetone which usually is a very small peak and easy to overlook.

Many other examples could be given, but in our decision making it is very important to determine how much time we should spend on identifying unknown peaks. Of course there should be no delay in diagnosis but, on the other hand, GC/MS work is still costly and time consuming. We must also decide on further clinical investigations such as loading tests, 24 hour fasting etc., procedures which are unpleasant to the patient and even potentially dangerous.

MATERIAL

This survey is based on the numerous cases published in the last decade. With few exceptions only cases dealing with a well defined organic acidaemia, where the enzyme defect has been identified or where so many data have been accumulated that we can be quite sure that we are dealing with a specific disease, are included. Such a review is biased for several reasons. First of all by the author but also because the most interesting cases are reported and the first published and second published cases are supposed to be very typical. Later as more cases accumulate the earlier reported cases may turn out to be rather atypical. Also case reports are of varying quality because papers are often centred around the biochemical findings which are easier to describe than clinical signs and symptoms.

In Table 1 a survey of the disorders included in the study is given. Methylmalonic aciduria has been included among the disorders of branched chain amino acids. Also 3-hydroxyisobutyryl CoA deacylase deficiency has been added although only one report to my knowledge has been published so far (Brown *et al.*, 1982).

Dicarboxylic acidurias include the multiple acyl-CoA dehydrogenase deficiencies whether they are riboflavin responsive or not (so-called gluaric aciduria type II), medium chain acyl-CoA dehydrogenase deficiency and finally systemic carnitine deficiency.

Defects in carbohydrate metabolism include pyruvate carboxylase deficiency and pyruvate dehydrogenase deficiency; however, much of the early work is excluded because of the well known difficulties in measuring these enzymes. I have also excluded cases where the deficency of pyruvated dehydrogenase or pyruvate carboxylase has been associated with the clinical symptoms in signs of Leigh's syndrome (subacute necrotizing encephalomyelopathy).

Among the disorders of lysine metabolism glutaric aciduria type I and 2-oxoglutaric aciduria have been studied. Tyrosinaemia due to fumarylacetoacetase deficiency is the only disorder included of phenylalanine metabolism.

Finally a few miscellaneous organic acidurias are included.

Journal of Inherited Metabolic Disease. ISSN 0141–8955. Copyright © SSIEM and MTP Press Limited, Queen Square, Lancaster, UK.

Table 1   Disorders included in survey

Disorders of branched chain amino acids
MSUD (1)
Isovaleric acidaemia (1–3)
3-Methylcrotonyl CoA carboxylase deficiency (4–6)
Multiple carboxylase deficiency (7–10)
Propionyl CoA carboxylase deficiency (11)
3-Hydroxy-3-methylglutaryl CoA lyase deficiency (12, 13)
3-Methylglutaconyl CoA hydratase deficiency (14)
3-Hydroxyisobuturyl CoA deacylase deficiency (15)
2-Methylacetoacetyl CoA thiolase deficiency (16)
Methylmalonic aciduria (11)
Dicarboxylic acidurias
Multiple acyl-CoA DH deficiency (12, 17, 18, 47)
  Riboflavin responsive (19)
  Non-riboflavin responsive glutaric aciduria type II (20–23)
Medium-chain acyl-CoA DH deficiency (24, 25)
Systemic carnitine deficiency (26)
Carbohydrate metabolism.
Pyruvate carboxylase deficiency (27)
Pyruvate dehydrogenase deficiency (28–30)
D-Glyceric acidaemia with hyperglycinaemia (31)
D-Glyceric acidaemia (32)
Hyperoxaluria type II (L-glyceric aciduria) (33)
Glycerol kinase deficiency (34)
Lysine metabolism
Glutaric aciduria type I (Glut-CoA DH deficiency) (35, 36–38)
2-Oxoglutaric aciduria (DH deficiency) (39)
Phenylalanine metabolism
Tyrosinaemia (fumarylacetoacetase deficiency) (40, 41)
Miscellaneous organic acidurias
Succinyl CoA; 3-keto acid CoA transferase deficiency (42, 43)
Acetoacetyl CoA thiolase deficiency (44)
4-Hydroxybutyric aciduria (45, 46)

(1) Tanaka and Rosenberg, 1983; (2) Duran *et al.*, 1979; (3) Truscott *et al.*, 1981; (4) Beemer *et al.*, 1982; (5) Finnie *et al.*, 1976; (6) Leonard *et al.*, 1981; (7) Munnich *et al.*, 1981; (8) Packman *et al.*, 1981; (9) Sander *et al.*, 1980; (10) Sherwood *et al.*, 1982; (11) Rosenberg, 1983; (12) Robinson *et al.*, 1980; (13) Shilkin *et al.*, 1982; (14) Duran *et al.*, 1982; (15) Brown *et al.*, 1982; (16) Daum *et al.*, 1973; (17) Kamerling *et al.*, 1982; (18) Kølvraa *et al.*, 1982; (19) Gregersen *et al.*, 1982; (20) Gregersen *et al.*, 1980; (21) Goodman *et al.*, 1980; (22) Przyrembel *et al.*, 1976; (23) Sweetman *et al.*, 1980; (24) Divry *et al.*, 1983b; (25) Gregersen *et al.*, 1983; (26) Engel, 1980; (27) Atkin *et al.*, 1979; (28) Farrell, 1977; (29) Kohns *et al.*, 1980; (30) Robinson *et al.*, 1977; (31) Brandt *et al.*, 1976; (32) Wadman *et al.*, 1976; (33) Williams and Smith, 1968; (34) Guggenheim *et al.*, 1980; (35) Brandt *et al.*, 1978; (36) Gregersen *et al.*, 1977; (37) Goodman *et al.*, 1975; (38) Leibel *et al.*, 1980; (39) Kohlschütter *et al.*, 1982; (40) Christensen *et al.*, 1981; (41) Lindblad *et al.*, 1977; (42) Spence *et al.*, 1973; (43) Tildon and Cornblath, 1972; (44) Robinson *et al.*, 1979; (45) Divry *et al.*, 1983a; (46) Jakobs *et al.*, 1981; (47) Niederweiser *et al.*, 1983

SYMPTOMS AND SIGNS

Most organic acidaemias have some clinical manifestations in common. Obviously these patients have decreased resistance to infections. Perhaps not in the usual sense that they tend to have repeated infections, but rather that infections, especially viral, tend to have a serious course. In many case reports, early death is characteristic due to unclassified coma or Reye's syndrome or even sudden and unexpected death. In cases where the proband survived there is very often a history of a sibling dying of a similar clinical syndrome. Unexpected death or coma are also seen in patients responding to treatment and who are apparently in good health for long periods. All of these disorders are certainly potentially very dangerous.

Table 2   General clinical manifestations

Decreased resistance to infections
Early death
  Coma – Reye's
  Sudden unexpected
Failure to thrive
Vomiting
Hypotonia
Hypoglycaemia

Failure to thrive also seems to be associated with organic aciduria in most cases. Even more characteristic is unexplained frequent and persistent vomiting. General hypotonia is much more frequent than hypertonia. Hypoglycaemia is very often severe and difficult to treat. Disorders in which this symptom has been described as particularly severe are listed in Table 3.

Looking specifically for neurological symptoms, cerebral palsy has been described most often in branched chain amino acid disorders but also in D-glyceric acidaemia and glycerol kinase deficiency (Table 3). Convulsions have been described in many disorders, most pronounced in branched chain amino acid metabolism disorders and glutaric aciduria type II. Athetosis and ataxia are symptoms described very often not only in disorders of branched chain amino acid metabolism but also in disorders of carbohydrate metabolism and, as mentioned above, in glutaric aciduria type I and 2-oxoglutaric aciduria.

Mental retardation is described in most organic acidurias, seemingly again most pronounced in disorders of branched chain amino acid metabolism and also in glycerol kinase deficiency, 2-oxo-adipic aciduria, glutaric aciduria type I and pyruvate carboxylase deficiency. In several reports it has been pointed out, however, that intelligence is normal; this is probably most characteristic of isovaleric acidaemia, 2-methylacetoacetyl CoA thiolase deficiency, methylmalonic aciduria, glutaric aciduria type I and ethylmalonic–adipic aciduria, so mental retardation is altogether not very characteristic of organic acidaemias.

Tachypnoea and RDS has been described very often in the case reports. The description is usually not very detailed and it is probable that these symptoms in most cases are due to the well known Kussmaul respiration of acidotic patients. In a very few disorders neutropenia and thrombocytopenia have been described and seem to be characteristic of isovaleric acidaemia, methylacetoacetyl CoA thiolase deficiency, methylmalonic aciduria and propionic acidaemia.

Myopathy has been described in glycerol kinase deficiency and carnitine deficiency and in glutaric aciduria type II. Perhaps, when looked for, myopathy might be more frequent and might explain the general hypotonia so often reported in these patients.

Liver disease is part of Reye's syndrome and as such described in many defects. A more specific liver impairment is described in Refsum's disease and tyrosinaemia due to a fumarylacetoacetase deficiency.

Peculiar smell is a characteristic symptom of MSUD, isovaleric acidaemia and glutaric aciduria type II.

Congenital malformations have been described together with several organic acidurias: glutaric aciduria type II, pyruvate dehydrogenase deficiency, Refsum's disease and 3-hydroxyisobutyryl deacylase deficiency.

Table 3   Correlation between symptoms and specific defect

Hypoglycaemia
MSUD, 3-hydroxy-3-methylglutaconyl CoA lyase deficiency, methylmalonic aciduria, glutaric aciduria type I, glutaric aciduria type II, carnitine deficiency, ethylmalonic–adipic aciduria, pyruvate carboxylase deficiency, pyruvate dehydrogenase deficiency

Cerebral palsy
MSUD, 3-methylcrotonyl CoA carboxylase deficiency, 3-methylglutaconyl CoA hydratase deficiency, D-glyceric acidaemia with hyperglycinaemia, glycerol kinase deficiency, glutaric aciduria type I, 2-oxoglutaric aciduria, pyruvate carboxylase deficiency

Convulsions
MSUD, 3-methylcrotonyl CoA carboxylase deficiency (Salaam), multiple carboxylase deficiency, D-glyceric acidaemia with hyperglycinaemia, glutaric aciduria type II, pyruvate carboxylase deficiency

Athetosis and ataxia
MSUD, isovaleric acidaemia, 3-methylcrotonyl CoA carboxylase deficiency, multiple carboxylase deficiency, 3-methylglutaconyl CoA hydratase deficiency, 3-hydroxy-3-methylglutaryl CoA lyase deficiency, pyruvate carboxylase deficiency, pyruvate dehydrogenase deficiency, 4-hydroxybutyric acidaemia, acetoacetyl CoA thiolase deficiency, glutaric aciduria type I, 2-oxoglutaric aciduria

Mental retardation
MSUD, isovaleric acidaemia, 3-methylcrotonyl CoA carboxylase deficiency, 3-methylglutaconyl CoA hydratase deficiency, 3-methylglutaconyl CoA hydratase deficiency, D-glyceric acidaemia with hyperglycinaemia, glycerol kinase deficiency, 2-ketoadipic aciduria, glutaric aciduria type I (?), pyruvate carboxylase deficiency

Normal intelligence
Isovaleric acidaemia, 2-methylacetoacetyl CoA thiolase deficiency, methylmalonic aciduria, glutaric aciduria type I, ethylmalonic–adipic aciduria

Tachypnoea–RDS
3-Methylcrotonyl CoA carboxylase deficiency, multiple carboxylase deficiency, methylmalonic aciduria, propionic aciduria, pyruvate carboxylase deficiency, pyruvate dehydrogenase deficiency, glutaric aciduria type II

Neutropenia and thrombocytopenia
Isovaleric acidaemia, 2-methylacetoacetyl CoA thiolase deficiency, methylmalonic aciduria, propionic aciduria

Myopathy
Glycerol kinase deficiency, carnitine deficiency, glutaric aciduria type II

Liver disease
Reye's syndrome, Refsum's disease, tyrosinosis (fumarylacetoacetase deficiency)

Peculiar smell
MSUD, isovaleric acidaemia, 3-methylglutaconyl CoA deficiency, glutaric aciduria type II

Congenital malformations
3-Hydroxyisobuturyl CoA deacylase deficiency, glutaric aciduria type II, pyruvate dehydrogenase deficiency

Therefore these physiological compounds might be teratogenic in high concentration.

SUMMARY OF CLINICAL SYMPTOMS

In Table 4 a summary of symptoms and signs in organic acidaemias is given. The first seven symptoms either alone or in combination of two or more are very suspicious of organic acidaemia. Symptoms such as cerebral palsy and convulsions will be found in many other disorders but when coinciding with one or more of these first seven symptoms should lead to investigation for organic acidaemia.

Myopathy is included in the list because muscle should be studied more often, including at autopsy.

Another conclusion which can be drawn from the survey is that a single symptom such as mental retardation is not a characteristic of organic acidaemia and screening for organic acidaemias among the mentally retarded will probably not be very profitable.

A review like this does not and cannot for obvious reasons be expected to represent the whole truth; it is merely an approximation. Thorough clinical description of the patients is important for daily clinical practise and more emphasis should be put into this aspect of published papers. A careful clinical examination is still a prerequisite for case finding.

General references

Chalmers, R. A. and Lawson, A. M. *Organic Acids in Man*, Chapman and Hall, London & New York, 1982

Goodman, S. I. and Markey, S. P. *Diagnosis of Organic Acidemias by Gas Chromatrography–Mass Spectrometry*, Liss, New York, 1981

Stanbury, J. B., Wyngaarden, J. B., Fredrickson, D. S., Goldstein, J. L. and Brown, M. S. *The Metabolic Basis of Inherited Disease*, 5th Edn., McGraw-Hill, New York, 1983

Special references

Atkin, B. M., Buist, N. R. M., Utter, M. F., Leiter, A. B. and Barker, B. Q. Pyruvate carboxylase deficiency and lactic acidosis in a retarded child without Leigh's disease. *Pediatr. Res.* 13 (1979) 109

Beemer, F. A., Bartlett, K. Duran, M., Ghneim, H. K., Wadman, S. K. and Bruinvis, L. Isolated biotin-resistant 3-

Table 4   Summary of symptoms suspicious of organic acidaemias

Severe infections
Intermittent coma
Reye's syndrome
Vomiting – failure to thrive
Hypotonia – lethargy
Hypoglycaemia
Athetosis–ataxia
Peculiar smell
Cerebral palsy
Convulsions
Liver disease
Myopathy?
Congenital malformations?
Mental retardation/normal intelligence

methylcrotonyl-CoA carboxylase deficiency in two sibs. *Eur. J. Pediatr.* 138 (1982) 354–357

Brandt, N. J., Rasmussen, K., Brandt, S., Kølvraa, S. and Schønheyder, F. D-Glyceric-acidemia and non-ketotic hyperglycinaemia. *Acta Paediatr. Scand.* 65 (1976) 17–22

Brandt, N. J., Brandt, S., Christensen, E., Gregersen, N. and Rasmussen, K. Glutaric aciduria in progressive chorea-athetosis. *Clin. Genet.* 13 (1978) 77–80

Brown, G. K., Hunt, S. M., Scholem, R., Fowler, K., Grimes, A., Mercer, J. F. B., Truscott, R. M., Cotton, R. G. H., Rogers, J. G. and Danks, D. M. β-Hydroxyisobutyryl-CoA deacylase deficiency – defect in valine metabolism associated with physical malformations. *Pediatrics* 70 (1982) 532

Christensen, E., Jacobsen, B. B., Gregersen, N., Hjeds, H., Pedersen, J. B., Brandt, N. J. and Beakmark, U. B. Urinary excretion of succinylacetone and δ-amino levulinic acid in patient with hereditary tyrosinemia. *Clin. Chim. Acta* 116 (1981) 331–341

Daum, R. S., Scriver, C. R., Mamer, O. A., Delvin, F., Lamm, P. and Goldman, H. An inherited disorder of isoleucine catabolism causing accumulation of α-methylacetoacetase and α-methyl-β-hydroxybutyrate, and intermittent metabolic acidosis. *Pediatr. Res.* 7 (1973) 149–160

Divry, P., Baltassat, P., Rolland, M. O., Cotte, J., Hermier, M., Duran, M. and Wadman, S. K. A new patient with 4-hydroxybutyric aciduria a possible defect of 4-aminobutyrate metabolism. *Clin. Chim. Acta* 129 (1983a) 303–309

Divry, P., David, M., Gregersen, N., Kølvraa, S., Christensen, E., Collet, J. P., Dellamonica, C. and Cotte, J. Dicarboxylic aciduria due to medium chain acyl CoA dehydrogenase defect. *Acta Paediatr. Scand.* 72 (1983b) 943–949

Duran, M., van Sprang, F. J., Drewes, J. G., Bruinvis, L., Ketting, D. and Wadman, S. K. Two sisters with isovaleric acidemia, multiple attacks of ketoaccidsosis and normal development. *Eur. J. Pediatr.* 131 (1979) 205–211

Duran, M., Beemer, F. A., Tibosch, A., Bruinvis, L., Ketting, D. and Wadman, S. K. Inherited 3-methylglutatonic aciduria in two brothers–another defect of leucine metabolism. *J. Pediatr.* 101 (1982) 551–554

Engel, A. G. Possible causes and effects of carnitine deficiency in man. In Frenkel, R. A. and McGarry, J. D. *Carnitine Biosynthesis, Metabolism, and Functions*, Academic Press, New York, 1980

Farrell, D. F. Pyruvate dehydrogenase (E₁) deficiency associated with congenital acidosis. In Mittler, P. *Research to Practice in Mental Retardation, Biomedical Aspects*, Vol. III, I.A.S.S.M.D., New York, 1977

Finnie, M. D. A., Cottrall, K., Seakins, J. W. T. and Snedden, W. Massive excretion of 2-oxoglutaric acid and 3-hydroxyisovaleric acid in a patient with a deficiency of 3-methylcrotonyl-CoA carboxylase. *Clin. Chim. Acta* 73 (1976) 513–519

Goodman, S. I., Markey, S. P., Moe, P. G., Miles, B. S. and Teng, C. C. Glutaric aciduria: and 'new' disorder of amino acid metabolism. *Biochem. Med.* 12 (1975) 12–21

Goodman, S. I., McCabe, Edvard, R. B., Fennessey, Paul W. and Mace, John W. Multible acyl-CoA dehydrogenase deficiency (glutaric aciduria type II) with transient hypersarcinemia and sarcosinuria; possible inherited deficiency of an electron transfer flavoprotein. *Pediatr. Res.* 14 (1980) 12–17

Gregersen, N., Brandt, N. J., Christensen, E., Grøn, I., Rasmussen, K. and Brandt, S. Glutaric aciduria: clinical and laboratory findings in two brothers. *J. Pediatr.* 90 (1977) 740–745

Gregersen, N., Kølvraa, S., Rasmussen, K., Christensen, E., Brandt, N. J., Ebbesen, F. and Hansen, F. H. Biochemical studies in a patient with defect in the metabolism of acyl-

CoA and sarcosine: another possible case of glutaric aciduria type II. *J. Inher. Metab. Dis.* 3 (1980) 67–72

Gregersen, N., Wintzensen, H., Kølvraa, S., Christensen, E., Christensen, M. F., Brandt, N. J. and Rasmussen, K. C₆–C₁₀-dicarboxylic aciduria: investigations of a patient with riboflavin responsive multiple acyl-CoA dehydrogenation defects. *Pediatr. Res.* 16 (1982) 861–868

Gregersen, N., Kølvraa, S., Rasmussen, K., Mortensen, P. B., Divry, P., David, M. and Hobolth, N. General (medium-chain) acyl-CoA dehydrogenase deficiency (non-ketotic dicarboxylic aciduria): Quantitative urinary excretion pattern of 23 biologically significant organic acids in three cases. *Clin. Chim. Acta* 132 (1983) 181–191

Guggenheim, M. A., McCabe, E. R. B., Roig, M., Goodman, S. I., Lum, G. M., Bullen, W. W. and Ringel, S. P. Glycerol kinase deficiency with neuromuscular, skeletal, and adrenal abnormalities. *Ann. Neurol.* 7 (1980) 441–49

Jakobs, C., Bojasch, M., Mönch, E., Rating, D., Siemes, H. and Hanefeld, F. Urinary excretion of gamma-hydroxybutyric acid in a patient with neurological abnormalities. The probability of a new inborn error of metabolism. *Clin. Chim. Acta* 111 (1981) 169–178

Kamerling, J. P., Duran, M., Bruinvis, L., Ketting, D., Wadman, S. K. and Vliegenthart, J. F. The absolute configuration of urinary 5-hydroxyhexanoic acid – a product of fatty acid (Ω-1)-oxidation – in patients with non-ketotic dicarboxylic aciduria. *Clin. Chim. Acta* 125 (1982) 247–254

Kohlschütter, A., Behbehani, A., Langenbeck, U., Albani, M., Heidemann, P., Hoffmann, G., Kleineke, J., Lehnert, W. and Wendel, U. A familial progressive neurodegenerative disease with 2-oxoglutaric aciduria. *Eur. J. Pediatr.* 138 (1982) 32–37

Kohns, U., Havers, W., Andler, W., Fischer, E. and Berger, R. Familiärer partieller Pyruvat dehydrogenase-Mangel. *Klin. Padiatr.* 192 (1980) 565–572

Kølvraa, S., Gregersen, N., Christensen, E. and Hobolth, N. In vitro fibroblast studies in a patient with C₆–C₁₀-dicarboxylic aciduria: evidence for a defect in general acyl-CoA dehydrogenase. *Clin. Chim. Acta* 126 (1982) 53–67

Leibel, R. L., Shih, V. E., Goodman, S. I., Bauman, M. L., McCabe, E. R. B., Zwerdling, R. G., Bergman, I. and Costello, C. Glutaric acidemia: a metabolic disorder causing progressive choreoathetosis. *Neurology* 30 (1980) 1163–1168

Leonard, J. V., Seakins, J. W. T., Bartlett, K., Hyde, J., Wilson, J. and Clayton, B. Inherited disorders of 3-methylcrotonyl CoA carboxylation. *Arch. Dis. Child.* 56 (1981) 53–59

Lindblad, B., Lindstedt, S. and Steen, G. On the enzymatic defect in hereditary tyrosinemia. *Proc. Natl. Acad. Sci. USA* 74 (1977) 4641–4645

Munnich, A., Saudubray, J. M., Cotisson, A., Coudé, F. X., Ogier, H., Charpentier, C., Marsac, C., Carré, G., Bourgeay-Causse, M. and Frézal, J. Biotin dependent multiple carboxylase deficiency presenting as a congenital lactic acidosis. *Eur. J. Pediatr.* 137 (1981) 203–206

Niederwieser, A., Steinmann, B., Exner, U., Neuheiser, F., Redweik, U., Wang, M., Rampini, S. and Wendel, U. Multiple acyl-CoA dehydrogenation deficiency (MADD) in a boy with nonketotic hypoglycemia, hepatomegali muscle hypotonia and cardiomyopathy. *Helv. Paediatr. Acta* 38 (1983) 9–26

Packman, S., Sweetman, L., Yoshino, M., Baker, H. and Cowan, M. Biotin-responsive multiple carboxylase deficiency of infantile onset. *J. Pediatr.* 99 (1981) 421–423

Przyrembel, H., Wendel, U., Becker, K., Bremer, H. J., Lieneke, B., Ketting, D. and Wadman, S. K. Glutaric aciduria type II: Report of a previously undescribed metabolic disorder. *Clin. Chim. Acta* 66 (1976) 227–39

Robinson, B. H., Taylor, J. and Sherwood, W. G. Deficiency of dihydro-lipoyl dehydrogenase (a component of the pyruvate and α-keto-glutarate dehydrogenase complexes): a cause of congenital chronic lactic acidosis in infancy. *Pediatr. Res.* 11 (1977) 1198

Robinson, B. H., Sherwood, W. G., Taylor, J., Balfe, J. W. and Mamer, O. A. Acetoacetyl CoA thiolase deficiency: a cause of severe ketoacidosis in infancy simulating salicylism. *J. Pediatr.* 95 (1979) 228–233

Robinson, B. H., Oei, J., Sherwood, W. G., Slyper, A. H., Heininger, J. and Mamer, O. A. Hydroxymethylglutaryl-CoA lyase deficiency: features resembling Reye syndrome. *Neurology* 3 (1980) 714–718

Rosenberg, L. E. Disorders of propionate and methylmalonate metabolism. In Standbury, J. B., Wyngaarden, J. B., Fredrickson, D. S., Goldstein, J. L. and Brown, M. S. (eds.) *The Metabolic Basis of Inherited Disease*, 5th Edn., McGraw-Hill, New York, 1983, pp. 447–497

Sander, J. E., Mallamud, N., Cowan, M. J., Packman, S., Amman, A. J. and Wara, D. W. Intermittent ataxia and immunodeficiency with multiple carboxylase deficiency: a biotin-responsive disorder. *Ann. Neurol.* 8 (1980) 544–547

Sherwood, W. G., Saunders, M., Robinson, B. H., Brewster, T. and Gravel, R. A. Lactic acidosis in biotin-responsive multiple carboxylase deficiency caused by holocarboxylase synthetase deficiency of early and late onset. *J. Pediatr.* 101 (1982) 546–550

Shilkin, R., Wilson, G. and Owles, E. 3-Hydroxy-3-methylglutaryl coenzyme A lyase deficiency. *Acta Paediatr. Scand.* 101 (1982) 546–550

Spence, M. W., Murphy, M. G., Cook, H. W., Ripley, B. A. and Embil, J. A. Succinyl-CoA: 3-ketoacid CoA-transferase deficiency: A 'new' phenotype? *Pediatr. Res.* 7 (1973) 394

Sweetman, L., Nyhan, W. L., Truner, D. A., Merritt, A. and Singh, M. Glutaric aciduria type II. *J. Pediatr.* 96 (1980) 1020–1026

Tanaka, K. and Rosenberg, L. E. Disorders of branched chain amino acid and organic acid metabolism. In Stanbury, J. B., Wyngaarden, J. B., Frederickson, D. S., Goldstein, J. L. and Brown, M. S. (eds.) *The Metabolic Basis of Inherited Disease*, 5th Edn., McGraw-Hill, New York, 1983, pp. 440–473

Tildon, J. T. and Cornblath, M. Succinyl-CoA: 3-ketoacid CoA-transferase deficiency. A cause for ketoacidosis in infancy. *J. Clin. Invest.* 51 (1972) 493

Truscott, R. J. W., Malegan, D., McCairns, E., Burke, D., Hick, L., Sims, P., Hahn, E. A. and Danks, D. M. New metabolites in isovaleric acidemia. *Clin. Chim. Acta* 110 (1981) 187–203

Wadman, S. K., Duran, M., Ketting, D., Bruinvis, L., de Bree, P. K., Camerling, J. P., Gerwig, G. J., Vliegenthart, J. F. G., Przyrembel, H., Becker, K. and Bremer, H. J. D-Glyceric acidemia in a patient with chronic metabolic acidosis. *Clin. Chim. Acta* 71 (1976) 477–84

Williams, H. E. and Smith, L. H. L-Glyceric aciduria: a new genetic variant of primary oxaluria. *N. Engl. J. Med.* 278 (1968) 232

SECTION II: DICARBOXYLIC ACIDURIAS AND ACYL-CoA DEHYDROGENASE DEFICIENCIES

J. Inher. Metab. Dis. 7 Suppl. 1 (1984) 28–32

Fatty Acyl-CoA Dehydrogenase Deficiency: Enzyme Measurement and Studies on Alternative Metabolism

N. GREGERSEN

Research Laboratory for Metabolic Disorders, University Department of Clinical Chemistry, Aarhus Kommunehospital, Aarhus C, Denmark

Fatty acyl-CoA dehydrogenase deficiencies are defined as disorders of the metabolism of straight chain acyl-CoA esters at the level of short chain acyl-CoA, general (medium chain) acyl-CoA and long chain acyl-CoA dehydrogenases. Patients with proven or indicated defects in either general (medium chain) or long chain acyl-CoA dehydrogenase have been reported.

In recent years assays for the enzymatic diagnosis in cells, especially cultured skin fibroblasts, from such patients have been developed. The different methods are reviewed. The urinary excretion profile of organic acids from patients with fatty acyl-CoA dehydrogenase deficiencies are characterized by the presence of different compounds originating from the primary accumulated acyl-CoA ester(s). The most important biochemical processes involved in the formation of these compounds are glycine conjugation and ω/ω-1 oxidation. The biochemistry of these pathways is discussed and the knowledge gained from *in vitro* and *in vivo* studies is used to explain the excretion pattern in some of the patients with general (medium chain) acyl-CoA dehydrogenase deficiency.

The diagnostic power of investigating the urinary excretion pattern of organic acids from patients with fatty acyl-CoA dehydrogenase defects is presently rather low. Due to the lack of precise knowledge about the origin of the dicarboxylic acids and ω-1-hydroxymonocarboxylic acid produced and excreted in substantial amounts in these patients it is not possible to pinpoint exactly the defective acyl-CoA dehydrogenase in fatty acid β-oxidation. The link between the enzyme defects and excretion patterns has further been hampered by the fact that the β-oxidation systems are complicated and that the different parts of them are difficult to measure in cultured fibroblasts.

This communication deals with methods for characterizing fatty acyl-CoA dehydrogenase defects and some of the investigations performed in order to explain the excretion patterns in patients with general (medium chain) acyl-CoA dehydrogenase defect ('non-ketotic dicarboxylic acidurias'). At present (1983) 15–20 cases are published with proven or suggested defect in general (medium chain) acyl-CoA dehydrogenase (Gregersen *et al.*, 1976, 1980; Truscott *et al.*, 1979; Colle *et al.*, 1980, 1983; Mamer *et al.*, 1980; Naylor *et al.*, 1980; Yang *et al.*, 1982; Stanley *et al.*, 1982; Kamerling *et al.*, 1982; Coates *et al.*, 1982; Divry *et al.*, 1983; Rhead *et al.*, 1983) and a few cases with long chain acyl-CoA dehydrogenase defect (Hale *et al.*, 1983; Amendt *et al.*, 1983). The number of reported cases is increasing rapidly.

ENZYMATIC CHARACTERIZATION OF FATTY ACYL-CoA DEHYDROGENASE DEFECTS

The fatty acyl-CoA dehydrogenase defects comprise a subgroup within the broader group designated acyl-CoA dehydrogenation deficiencies, which can be defined as inborn defects in the enzyme systems that catalyse the oxidation of branched chain acyl-CoA, glutaryl CoA and straight chain fatty acyl-CoA esters.

Each enzyme system consists of an acyl-CoA dehydrogenase holoenzyme, which has a specificity towards different acyl-CoA ester substrates (Beinert, 1963; Besrat *et al.*, 1969; Hall and Kamin, 1975; Furuta *et al.*, 1981; Ikeda and Tanaka, 1983; Ikeda *et al.*, 1983), and two electron transporters, which are common to all the acyl-CoA dehydrogenation systems, called respectively electron transfer flavoprotein (ETF) (Hall and Kamin, 1975), and electron transfer flavoprotein dehydrogenase (ETF DH) or iron–sulphur flavoprotein (Ruzicka and Beinert, 1977) (Figure 1).

In the fatty acid β-oxidation pathway three acyl-CoA dehydrogenases exist with overlapping affinities. The short chain acyl-CoA dehydrogenase acts upon C_4–C_{6-8} acyl-CoA esters, the general (medium chain) acyl-CoA dehydrogenase exhibits activity towards C_4–C_{12-16} acyl-CoA esters with peak activity at C_6–C_8 and the long chain acyl-CoA dehydrogenase catalyses

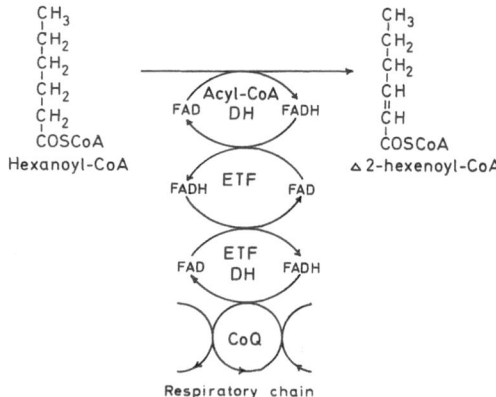

Figure 1 The acyl-CoA dehydrogenation system. The 'enzymes' of the system are: acyl-CoA dehydrogenase (acyl-CoA DH), electron transfer flavoprotein (ETF) and electron transfer flavoprotein dehydrogenase (ETF DH)

28

the dehydrogenation of C_6-C_{22} acyl-CoA esters with peak activity towards the C_{14} ester.

Fatty acyl-CoA dehydrogenase assays

Assays for acyl-CoA dehydrogenases are based on the use of artificial electron acceptors which can accept electrons directly from reduced dehydrogenase ($FADH_2$). The electron transport can thus bypass ETF and ETF DH, making the assay specific for the acyl-CoA dehydrogenase moiety in the acyl-CoA dehydrogenation system (Figure 1).

The conventional spectrophotometric assays are dependent on a secondary electron acceptor dye (Hall, 1981; Furuta *et al.*, 1981) which are not specific for reducing equivalents originating from the acyl-CoA ester substrate. They can be reduced by other reducing substances in the reaction mixture. However, recent advances in methodology have overcome this complication. So far four fundamentally different systems for measurements in human fibroblasts have been developed.

Dye assay

Instead of using crude fibroblast homogenate the enzyme source is the supernatant from sonicated mitochondria isolated from human fibroblasts (Rhead and Tanaka, 1980). This purification procedure eliminates most of the non-specific reduction of the dye and it has been used to measure directly isovaleryl CoA and short chain acyl-CoA dehydrogenases (Rhead and Tanaka, 1980), general (medium chain) acyl-CoA dehydrogenase (Rhead *et al.*, 1983) and long chain acyl-CoA dehydrogenase (Amendt *et al.*, 1983) in patient's fibroblasts.

Tritium release assay

The idea of this assay was to improve the specificity by measuring directly the release of the two hydrogen atoms (^1H) from the acyl-CoA ester substrate (Rhead and Tanaka, 1980; Rhead *et al.*, 1981). In order to detect these hydrogen atoms they were replaced by tritium (^3H) in the substrates. The released tritium was measured in the water phase after binding unreacted 2,3-^3H-acyl-CoA ester onto an ion exchange resin. The method has been used to prove the defect in isovaleryl CoA dehydrogenase deficiency (Rhead and Tanaka, 1980) and to prove a normal activity of short chain acyl-CoA dehydrogenase in patients with glutaric aciduria Type II (Rhead *et al.*, 1980).

Product formation assay

This assay is based on the principle that the primary product of the dehydrogenation, a 2,3-unsaturated acyl-CoA ester is transformed to a 3-hydroxyacyl-CoA ester, in a reaction mixture with added crotonase and phenazinemethosulphate as electron acceptor. After hydrolysis the free 3-hydroxy acid is extracted from the reaction mixture and measured quantitatively by means of selected ion monitoring gas chromatography–mass spectrometry (SIM-GC–MS) (Kølvraa and Gregersen, 1982). This method requires only small amounts of fibroblast enzyme and has so far been useful with hexanoyl CoA, octanoyl CoA and decanoyl CoA as the

substrates. It was used to provide the first evidence of a general (medium chain) acyl-CoA dehydrogenase defect in patients with 'non-ketotic' dicarboxylic aciduria (Kølvraa *et al.*, 1982). The measurements were performed with crude fibroblast homogenate as the enzyme source.

ETF reduction assay

The basis for this assay is the difference in fluorescence between oxidized and reduced ETF. The assay has been used so far to measure acyl-CoA dehydrogenase activity with palmitoyl CoA, octanoyl CoA, butyryl CoA and isovaleryl CoA as substrates in liver, leukocytes and cultured skin fibroblasts from patients with dicarboxylic aciduria (Coates *et al.*, 1982, 1983; Hale *et al.*, 1983).

BIOCHEMICAL EXPLANATIONS OF THE EXCRETION PATTERNS IN PATIENTS WITH GENERAL (MEDIUM CHAIN) ACYL-CoA DEHYDROGENASE DEFECTS

To date, only a few cases of dicarboxylic aciduria exist, where both enzyme measurements and excretion patterns of organic acids have been published. In these cases the excretion pattern of organic acids shows significant differences. In some cases, the compounds excreted in substantial amounts are C_6-C_{10}-dicarboxylic acids, 5-OH-hexanoic acid and hexanoylglycine with only small to insignificant amounts of $C_8-C_{10}-\omega-1$-hydroxymonocarboxylic acids and C_8-C_{10}-acylglycines (Gregersen *et al.*, 1983b; Divry *et al.*, 1983). In other cases the principal compounds were the C_6-C_{10}-$\omega-1$-hydroxymonocarboxylic acids, especially 7-OH-octanoic acid, together with the C_6-C_{10}-dicarboxylic acids (Colle *et al.*, 1983). Despite the differences all these metabolites must reflect the deficiency of medium chain acyl-CoA dehydrogenase.

The relative degree of the consequent accumulation of the acyl-CoA esters of the various chain lengths is not known. It must depend on the relative enzyme activities remaining and consequently on the flow through the β-oxidation pathway at the various levels. Therefore explanations of the origin of the various metabolites must still be somewhat speculative. However, since glycine-N-acylase has been proved to be exclusively a mitochondrial enzyme (Kølvraa, Gregersen and Mortensen, unpublished observations) the hexanoylglycine found in the patient's urine reflects directly the accumulation of hexanoyl CoA inside the mitochondria. In contrast to this is the lack of octanoyl- and decanoylglycines in urine. The K_m values for glycine-N-acylase for octanoyl CoA and decanoyl CoA are in the same order of magnitude as for hexanoyl CoA (Kølvraa, Gregersen and Mortensen, unpublished observations, 1983) and this means that the accumulation of octanoyl CoA and decanoyl CoA must either be lower than that of hexanoyl CoA and/or hitherto unknown pathways must exist which are able to clear octanoyl CoA and decanoyl CoA at rates higher than the clearance rate of hexanoyl CoA from the mitochondria. That this might be the case is indicated by the excretion of another conjugate of octanoic acid in the patients described by Gregersen and co-workers (Gregersen et al., 1983b).

The occurrence of conjugates of octanoic acid is in accordance with the conception that the most serious enzyme block is at the C_8-level, as is evidenced by decreased oxidation in intact cultured skin fibroblasts from the same patient of 1-^{14}C-octanoic acid compared to normal and near normal oxidation of longer and shorter chain length 1-^{14}C-monocarboxylic acids (Kølvraa et al., 1982).

With this background it is difficult to explain why the C_6-dicarboxylic and ω-1-hydroxymonocarboxylic acids (adipic and 5-hydroxyhexanoic acids) are excreted preferentially to the C_8-acids (suberic and 7-hydroxy-octanoic acids) in some of the patients with proved general (medium chain) acyl-CoA dehydrogenase defect. Therefore we performed studies aimed at clarifying to what extent the medium chain fatty acids (C_6–C_{12}) are able to function as substrates for the ω and ω-1 oxidation in man. It was shown that the K_m values for microsomal ω/ω-1 oxidation systems towards hexanoic and octanoic acids were in the millimolar range and therefore most probably of limited biological significance, whereas the K_m values towards decanoic and dodecanoic acids were lower and indicative of a biological role (Gregersen et al., 1983a) (Table 1). It was further shown by in vivo tracer studies in rats that decanoic acid was clearly the best monocarboxylic acid for inducing dicarboxylic aciduria, while the excreted amounts were lower with octanoic and hexanoic acids and with longer chain length monocarboxylic acids (Mortensen and Gregersen, 1981). These investigations make it most probable that the only C_6–C_{16}-acids of biological significance for the ω and ω-1 oxidation pathway are C_{10}-, C_{12}- and possibly C_{14}-mono-carboxylic acids.

The results of these studies show that it is improbable that substantial amounts of adipic acid, suberic acid, 5-OH-hexanoic acid and 7-OH-octanoic acid can be produced by a direct ω/ω-1 oxidation. On the other hand, consistency with the qualitative excretion pattern can be obtained by suggesting that the microsomal ω/ω-1 hydroxylation is involved in the formation of dicarboxylic and ω-1-hydroxymonocarboxylic acids at the C_{10}- and C_{12}-levels and that the C_8–C_6-dicarboxylic and ω-1-hydroxymonocarboxylic acids are formed from

longer chain acids by β-oxidation (Figure 2). Such a β-oxidation pathway for dicarboxylic acid has been proved in rats in vivo and in rat liver homogenates (Mortensen and Gregersen, 1982), but the organelle responsible has not yet been identified. However, some evidence exists that points to a substantial contribution of the peroxisomal β-oxidation system in the production of dicarboxylic and ω-1-hydroxymonocarboxylic acids in patients with general (medium chain) acyl-CoA dehydrogenase deficiency: (1) the first step in the β-oxidation cycle in the peroxisomes is catalysed by an acyl-CoA oxidase which is essentially different from the acyl-CoA dehydrogenases in the mitochondria (Lazarow, 1978; Bronfman et al., 1979), (2) the biochemical evidence obtained by Mortensen and co-workers that peroxisomes in vitro are able to convert dodecanedioic acid (C_{12}) to sebacic, suberic and adipic acids (Mortensen et al., 1982, 1984) and (3) the activity profile of peroxisomal acyl-CoA oxidase towards monocarboxylic acids of different chain lengths shows that the β-oxidation is highly active at medium chain level (C_{10}–C_{12}), whereas the activity is very low at C_6 level (Kindl and Lazarow, 1982). The same has not yet been shown for dicarboxylic acid and ω-1-hydroxy-monocarboxylic acids but if it is so the enzyme-activity profile is paralleled by the relative amounts of dicarboxylic acids excreted in some of the patients.

The peroxisomes may also contribute to monocar-boxylic acid metabolism in the patients. The reason why hexanoyl CoA is accumulated in substantial amounts, as reflected by the excretion of hexanoylglycine despite the fact that this metabolite is located distally to the most serious block in the pathway, may be that hexanoyl CoA is produced in the peroxisomes from medium chain monocarboxylic acids which are channelled to the peroxisomes because of the mitochondrial block. Substantial amounts of hexanoyl CoA from the peroxisomes may then be transported to the mitochon-dria where the metabolism is partially blocked by the enzyme deficiency.

The conception of the biosynthesis of dicarboxylic and ω-1-hydroxymonocarboxylic acids outlined above and the fact that the absence of a conjugate of decanoic acid (Gregersen et al., 1983b) indicates minor accumula-tion of decanoyl CoA, means that the medium chain monocarboxylic acid substrates for the ω/ω-1 oxidation

Table 1 Apparent K_m and V_{max} values of ω and ω-1 hydroxylation systems for hexanoic, octanoic, decanoic and dodecanoic acids in human liver microsomes (the values are the mean of data from two different subjects)

Acid	ω Hydroxylation		ω-1 Hydroxylation	
	K_m μmol/l	V_{max} nmol/min per mg	K_m μmol/l	V_{max} nmol/min per mg
Dodecanoic	95	0.4	110	1.1
Decanoic	390	1.6	1 200	5.7
Octanoic	4400	3.1	3 200	4.2
Hexanoic	8600	6.8	> 20 000	> 20

From: Gregersen et al. (1983a)

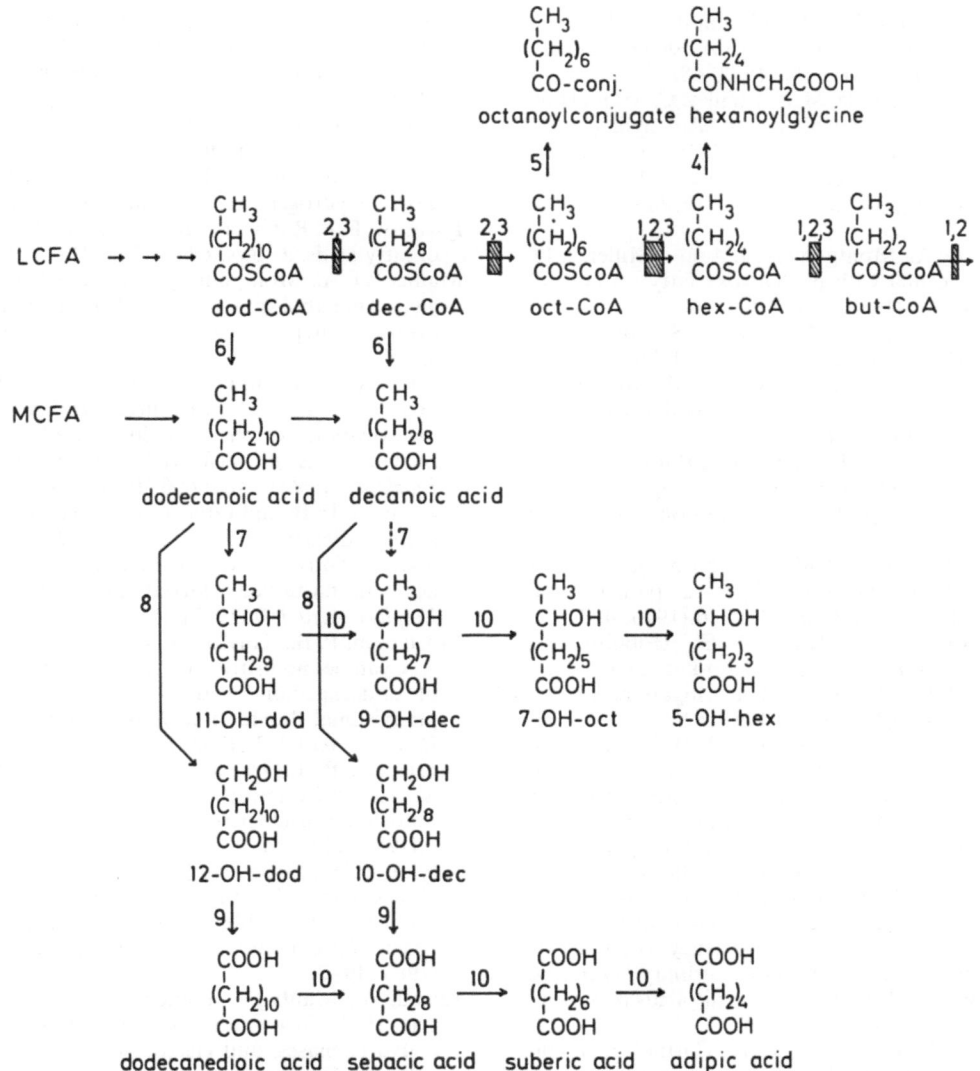

Figure 2 The proposed defective intermediary metabolism in patients with general (medium chain) acyl-CoA dehydrogenase deficiency. The defective steps in the normal pathway of fatty acid β-oxidation are indicated with hatched squares. The enzymes are: (1) short chain acyl-CoA dehydrogenation system, (2) general (medium chain) acyl-CoA dehydrogenation system and (3) long chain acyl-CoA dehydrogenation system. The enzymes proposed to be involved in the production of the compounds found in patient urine are: (4) glycine-*N*-acylase, (5) unknown conjugation mechanism, (6) acyl-CoA hydrolases, (7) ω-1 hydroxylation, (8) ω hydroxylation, (9) alcohol dehydrogenase/aldehyde dehydrogenase and (10) mitochondrial and/or peroxisomal β-oxidation

most probably originate from outside the mitochondria, probably directly liberated from the fat deposits. The consequence of this line of speculation is that the transport of long and medium chain fatty acids is for some still unknown reason partially blocked, leaving these acids to be metabolized in the cytoplasmic reticulum (ω/ω-1 oxidation) and the peroxisomes (β-oxidation). It is also probable that the capacity of the inducible enzyme systems in these organelles to some degree directs the amounts of compounds channelled through the various pathways, thus accounting for the great diversity in the excretion pattern of metabolites in urine from different patients with fatty acyl-CoA dehydrogenase defects.

References

Amendt, B. A., Fritchman, K. N. and Rhead, W. J. Dicarboxylic aciduria due to deficiency of the long-chain acyl-CoA dehydrogenase reversible by addition of flavin adenine dinucleotide. *Pediatr. Res.* 17 (1983) 206A

Beinert, H. Acyl-coenzyme A dehydrogenases. In Boyer, P. D., Lardy, H. and Myrback, K. (eds.) *The Enzymes*, 2nd edn., Academic Press, New York, 1963, pp. 447–466

Besrat, A., Polan, C. E. and Henderson, L. M. Mammalian metabolism of glutaric acid. *J. Biol. Chem.* 244 (1969) 1461–1469

Bronfman, M., Inestrosa, N. C. and Leighton, F. Fatty acid oxidation by human liver peroxisomes. *Biochem. Biophys. Res. Commun.* 88 (1979) 1030–1036

Coates, P. M., Stanley, C. A., Hale, D. E., Corkey, B. E., Hall, C.

L. and Cortner, J. A. Fatty acid oxidation in fibroblasts of patients with medium-chain acyl-CoA dehydrogenase deficiency. *Am. J. Hum. Genet.* 34 (1982) 48A

Coates, P. M., Hale, D. E., Katz, M. R., Stanley, C. A. and Hall, C. L. Detection of medium-chain acyl-CoA dehydrogenase deficiency in leucocytes. *Pediatr. Res.* 17 (1983) 288A

Colle, E., Mamer, O. A. and Montgomery, J. Episodic hypoglycemia with organic aciduria. *Pediatr. Res.* 14 (1980) 570

Colle, E., Mamer, O. A., Montgomery, J. A. and Miller, J. D. Episodic hypoglycemia with psi-hydroxy fatty acid excretion. *Pediatr. Res.* 17 (1983) 171–176

Divry, P., David, M., Gregersen, N., Kølvraa, S., Christensen, E., Collet, J. P., Dellamonica, C. and Cotte, J. Dicarboxylic aciduria due to medium-chain acyl-CoA dehydrogenase defect: A cause of hypoglycemia in childhood. *Acta Paediatr. Scand.* 72 (1983) 943–949

Furuta, S., Miyazawa, S. and Hashimoto, T. Purification and properties of rat liver acyl-CoA dehydrogenases and electron transfer flavoprotein. *J. Biochem.* 90 (1981) 1739–1750

Gregersen, N., Lauritzen, R. and Rasmussen, K. Suberyl-glycine excretion in the urine from a patient with dicarboxylic aciduria. *Clin. Chim. Acta* 70 (1976) 417–425

Gregersen, N., Rosleff, F., Kølvraa, S., Hobolth, N., Rasmussen, K. and Lauritzen, R. Non-ketotic C_6–C_{10}-dicarboxylic aciduria: Biochemical investigations of two cases. *Clin. Chim. Acta* 102 (1980) 179–189

Gregersen, N., Kølvraa, S. and Mortensen, P. B. On the origin of C_6–C_{10}-dicarboxylic and C_6–C_{10}-ω-1-hydroxy mono-carboxylic acids in human and rat with acyl-CoA dehydrogenation deficiencies: *In vitro* studies on the ω- and ω-1-oxidation of medium-chain (C_6–C_{12}) fatty acids in human and rat liver. *Pediatr. Res.* 17 (1983a) 828–834

Gregersen, N., Kølvraa, S., Rasmussen, K., Mortensen, P. B., Divry, P., David, M. and Hobolth, N. General (medium-chain) acyl-CoA dehydrogenase deficiency (non-ketotic dicarboxylic aciduria): Quantitative urinary excretion pattern of 23 biological significant organic acids in 3 cases. *Clin. Chim. Acta* 132 (1983b) 181–191

Hale, D. E., Coates, P. M., Stanley, C. A., Cortner, J. A. and Hall, C. L. Long-chain acyl-CoA dehydrogenase deficiency. *Pediatr. Res.* 17 (1983) 290A

Hall, C. L. Acyl-CoA dehydrogenases from pig liver mitochondria. *Meth. Enzymol.* 71 (1981) 375–385

Hall, C. L. and Kamin, H. The purification and some properties of electron transfer flavoprotein and general fatty acyl coenzyme A dehydrogenase from pig liver mitochondria. *J. Biol. Chem.* 250 (1975) 3476–3486

Ikeda, Y., Dabrowski, C. and Tanaka, K. Separation and properties of five distinct acyl-CoA dehydrogenases from rat liver mitochondria: Identification of a new 2-methyl branched chain acyl-CoA dehydrogenase. *J. Biol. Chem.* 258 (1983) 1066–1076

Ikeda, Y. and Tanaka, K. Purification and characterization of isovaleryl coenzyme A dehydrogenase from rat liver mitochondria. *J. Biol. Chem.* 258 (1983) 1077–1085

Kamerling, J. P., Duran, M., Bruinvis, L., Ketting, D., Wadman, S. K. and Vliegenthart, J. F. G. The absolute configuration of urinary 5-hydroxyhexanoic acid – a product of fatty acid ω-1 oxidation – in patients with non-ketotic dicarboxylic aciduria. *Clin. Chim. Acta* 125 (1982) 247–254

Kindl, H. and Lazarow, P. B. (eds.) Peroxisomes and glyoxysomes. In *Ann. NY Acad. Sci.* 386 (1982)

Kølvraa, S. and Gregersen, N. Methods for the measurement of fatty acid β-oxidation and acyl-CoA dehydrogenase in cultured fibroblasts. *J. Inher. Metab. Dis.* 5, Suppl. 1 (1982) 31–32

Kølvraa, S., Gregersen, N., Christensen, E. and Hobolth, N. *In vitro* fibroblast studies in a patient with C_6–C_{10}-dicarboxylic aciduria: Evidence for a defect in general acyl-CoA dehydrogenase. *Clin. Chim. Acta* 126 (1982) 53–67

Lazarow, P. B. Rat liver peroxisomes catalyze the β-oxidation of fatty acids. *J. Biol. Chem.* 253 (1978) 1522–1528

Mamer, O. A., Montgomery, J. A. and Colle, E. Profiles in altered metabolism III: Ω-1-hydroxyacid excretion in a case of episodic hypoglycemia. *Biochem. Mass Spectrom.* 7 (1980) 53–57

Mortensen, P. B. and Gregersen, N. The biological origin of ketotic dicarboxylic aciduria: *In vivo* and *in vitro* investigations of the ω oxidation of C_6–C_{16}-monocarboxylic acids in unstarved, starved and diabetic rats. *Biochim. Biophys. Acta* 666 (1981) 394–404

Mortensen, P. B. and Gregersen, N. The biological origin of ketotic dicarboxylic aciduria: II. *In vivo* and *in vitro* investigations of the β-oxidation of C_8–C_{16}-dicarboxylic acids in unstarved, starved and diabetic rats. *Biochim. Biophys. Acta* 710 (1982) 477–484

Mortensen, P. B., Kølvraa, S., Gregersen, N. and Rasmussen, K. Cyanide-insensitive and clofibrate enhanced β-oxidation of dodecanedioic acid in rat liver: An indication of peroxisomal β-oxidation of *n*-dicarboxylic acids. *Biochim. Biophys. Acta* 713 (1982) 393–397

Mortensen, P. B., Gregersen, N., Rasmussen, K. and Kølvraa, S. The β-oxidation of dicarboxylic acids in isolated mitochondria and peroxisomes. *J. Inher. Metab. Dis.* 6 Suppl. 2 (1983) 123–124

Naylor, E. W., Mosovich, L. L., Guthrie, R., Evans, J. E. and Tieckelmann, H. Intermittent non-ketotic dicarboxylic aciduria in two siblings with hypoglycemia: An apparent defect in β-oxidation of fatty acids. *J. Inher. Metab. Dis.* 3 (1980) 19–24

Rhead, W., Mantagos, S. and Tanaka, K. Glutaric aciduria type II: *In vitro* studies on substrate oxidation, acyl-CoA dehydrogenases, and electron-transferring flavoprotein in cultured skin fibroblasts. *Pediatr. Res.* 14 (1980) 1339–1342

Rhead, W. and Tanaka, K. Demonstration of a specific mitochondrial isovaleryl-CoA dehydrogenase deficiency in fibroblasts from patients with isovaleric acidemia. *Proc. Natl. Acad. Sci. USA* 77 (1980) 580–583

Rhead, W., Hall, C. L. and Tanaka, K. Novel tritium release assays for isovaleryl-CoA and butyryl-CoA dehydrogenases. *J. Biol. Chem.* 256 (1981) 1616–1624

Rhead, W. J., Amendt, B. A., Fritchman, K. S. and Felts, J. Dicarboxylic aciduria: Deficient 1-^{14}C-octanoate oxidation and medium-chain acyl-CoA dehydrogenase activity in fibroblasts. *Science* 221 (1983) 73–75

Ruzicka, F. J. and Beinert, H. A new iron-sulfur flavoprotein of the respiratory chain. *J. Biol. Chem.* 252 (1977) 8440–8445

Stanley, C. A., Gonzales, E., Yang, W., Kelley, R. I. and Baker, L. Hypoketotic hypoglycemia – Evidence for a new defect in fatty acid oxidation. *Pediatr. Res.* 16 (1982) 264A

Truscott, R. J. W., Hick, L., Pullin, C., Halpern, B., Wilcken, B., Griffiths, H., Silink, M., Kilham, H. and Grunseit, F. Dicarboxylic aciduria: The response to fasting. *Clin. Chim. Acta* 94 (1979) 31–39

Yang, W., Roth, K. S. and Coates, P. M. Hypoglycemic, hypoketotic dicarboxylic aciduria – A possible defect in fatty acid oxidation. *Pediatr. Res.* 16 (1982) 267A

J. Inher. Metab. Dis. 7 Suppl. 1 (1984) 33–37

Glutaric Acidaemia Type II (Multiple Acyl-CoA Dehydrogenation Deficiency)

S. I. GOODMAN

Department of Pediatrics, University of Colorado Health Sciences Center, 4200 East Ninth Avenue, Denver, CO 80262, USA

F. E. FRERMAN

Department of Microbiology, Medical College of Wisconsin, 8701 Watertown Plank Road, Milwaukee, WI 53226, USA

The clinical and biochemical phenotype of glutaric acidaemia type II (GAII) has led to the suggestion that the defect in the disorder affects electron transfer from primary FAD-containing dehydrogenases into the respiratory chain. Two proteins are involved in this process, i.e. electron transfer flavoprotein (ETF) and ETF dehydrogenase, an iron–sulphur flavoprotein with a distinctive EPR signal. Reliable catalytic assays for these proteins are not available, but both proteins have been purified and antisera against them prepared in rabbits.

SDS-PAG electrophoresis of liver mitochondrial membranes from a GAII infant with congenital anomalies, locating ETF dehydrogenase with specific antiserum, showed no cross-reactive material. EPR of the same membranes showed a marked decrease in the ETF dehydrogenase signal. These results suggest that the defect in GAII in some patients is indeed in electron transport, and specifically in ETF dehydrogenase.

INTRODUCTION

Glutaric acidaemia type II is an inborn error of metabolism characterized clinically by non-ketotic hypoglycaemia and metabolic acidosis, pathologically by fatty degeneration of liver parenchymal cells, renal tubular epithelium and myocardium and biochemically by (1) accumulation and excretion of oxidation products of all saturated acyl-CoA esters that are normally metabolized by acyl-CoA dehydrogenases and (2) decreased ability of whole cultured cells and their mitochondria to oxidize compounds metabolized through these esters. In contrast with the apparent deficiency of these enzymes in whole cells and mitochondria, their activities have been normal whenever assayed in disrupted tissues, a discrepancy that might have several causes, including abnormalities in (1) the biosynthesis of FAD (the common coenzyme), (2) the movement of acyl-CoA esters across the inner mitochondrial membrane or (3) the movement of electrons from dehydrogenase flavins into the respiratory chain. The frequent accumulation of sarcosine, whose electrons follow the same path into the respiratory chain as those of the acyl-CoA esters, in patients with glutaric acidaemia type II strongly favours the latter possibility, although some may have other defects.

We shall first describe the considerable clinical and biochemical diversity observed in the condition, then review electron transport in the segment of the respiratory chain that is apparently at fault and finally discuss studies that bear on the hypothesis that the molecular defect indeed lies in this pathway.

CLINICAL AND BIOCHEMICAL FEATURES OF GLUTARIC ACIDAEMIA TYPE II

Patients with glutaric acidaemia type II usually fall into one of three groups, each consistent within a family. We have chosen to designate these groups as (1) neonatal onset GAII with congenital anomalies, (2) neonatal onset GAII without congenital anomalies and (3) later-onset GAII, which in some cases is synonomous with ethylmalonic adipic aciduria. Diagnosis is not difficult and is usually based upon demonstrating the typical organic aciduria in a patient with non-ketotic hypoglycaemia. Three fetal diagnoses have been made, all the affected fetuses showing markedly increased concentrations of glutaric acid in amniotic fluid at 15, 16 and 37 weeks (Goodman *et al.*, unpublished observations; Mitchell *et al.*, 1983; Niederwieser *et al.*, 1983).

Four patients with congenital anomalies and onset of symptoms in the immediate newborn period have been reported (Sweetman *et al.*, 1980; Lehnert *et al.*, 1982; Böhm *et al.*, 1982; Goodman *et al.*, 1983) and several others are known to the authors. All those in the literature have been males but many known to us were girls and none of them were less severely affected than their affected male siblings; all of the pedigrees have been consistent with autosomal recessive inheritance. All four in the literature were born prematurely, all developed symptoms of severe hypoglycaemia and acidosis during the first day of life and all died within the first week. At autopsy, in addition to the typical fatty degeneration of the viscera found in GAII, all had polycystic kidneys and three had a characteristic 'Potter-type' facies as well as anomalies of the abdominal wall and external genitalia.

Journal of Inherited Metabolic Disease. ISSN 0141-8955. Copyright © SSIEM and MTP Press Limited, Queen Square, Lancaster, UK.

Sarcosine was not detected in any of them and, perhaps of significance, two had more than twice normal concentrations of proline and hydroxyproline in plasma. Whole cell oxidation studies have been published on only one such patient (Lehnert *et al.*, 1982) and showed profoundly reduced CO_2 production from compounds metabolized through acyl-CoA dehydrogenases as well as decreased incorporation of radiolabel from these substances into TCA-precipitable material. We do not know of published studies on parents of such patients.

Six patients have been reported who presented in the newborn period but in whom congenital anomalies were not observed and polycystic kidneys not noted at autopsy (Przyrembel *et al.*, 1976; Goodman *et al.*, 1980, 1982; Gregersen *et al.*, 1980; Sweetman *et al.*, 1980; Coudé *et al.*, 1981). Several of them have been girls, again no less severely affected than their affected male siblings, consistent with inheritance as an autosomal recessive trait. In one case, however, the pedigree strongly suggests X-linked inheritance (Coudé *et al.*, 1981), although it is not certain that the four male relatives of the proband who died with what might have been GAII actually had that condition. The patients with this form of the disease all developed symptoms of hypoglycaemia and metabolic acidosis within the first 3 days of life (four of them within the first 24 hours) and death in most occurred shortly thereafter, the two exceptions being cases in which the diagnosis was made early and rather heroic therapeutic efforts instituted (Goodman *et al.*, 1980, 1982). In both of these patients cardiomyopathy was a prominent feature of the terminal illness. In three patients sarcosine was detected in blood and/or urine on at least one occasion (Goodman *et al.*, 1980; Gregersen *et al.*, 1980; Sweetman *et al.*, 1980). Studies on whole fibroblasts (Przyrembel *et al.*, 1976; Saudubray *et al.*, 1982; Rhead *et al.*, 1983) and whole fibroblast mitochondria (Rhead and Amendt, 1982) showed markedly decreased oxidation of substrates metabolized through acyl-CoA dehydrogenases. Further, fibroblasts from the parents of three such patients showed substrate oxidation intermediate between that of the patients and controls, consistent with inheritance as an autosomal recessive trait (Rhead *et al.*, 1983). To our knowledge substrate oxidation studies on cells from the parents or other relatives of the child whose disease was apparently transmitted as an X-linked trait have not been reported. Biosynthesis of FAD from riboflavin was normal in tissue from frozen kidney of one of these patients (Goodman *et al.*, 1980) and that of ubiquinone from (3,4-^{3}H)mevalonic acid and (methyl-^{3}H)methionine was normal in cultured fibroblasts of another (Goodman *et al.*, unpublished data).

At least three patients have been reported with what we would term late-onset glutaric acidaemia type II; we know of one additional patient and have heard of several others. The first patient to be described was a girl with intermittent episodes of vomiting, hypoglycaemia and acidosis that began at 7 weeks of age (Tanaka *et al.*, 1977; Mantagos *et al.*, 1979), another first developed similar episodes at 7 months and died of an apparent cardiomyopathy (Niederwieser *et al.*, 1983), the third developed episodic disease even later, having been totally symptom-free during childhood (Dusheiko *et al.*, 1979). Substrate oxidation studies have shown results similar to those obtained in other forms of the disease but with comparatively less deficiency. Whole cell studies in parents of such patients, like those in parents of children with neonatal onset, have suggested autosomal recessive transmission (Rhead *et al.*, 1983).

The cause(s) of the extensive clinical and biochemical heterogeneity observed in the condition is not yet known. If there is indeed an X-linked form some of the differences can be attributed to differences in the specific genetic loci involved. Genetic heterogeneity does not, however, need to be invoked to explain why sarcosine is not seen in patients with the most severe form of autosomal disease and why it is frequently found in those that are less severely affected. Sarcosine is synthesized and metabolized by dimethylglycine dehydrogenase (DMGDH) and sarcosine dehydrogenase (SDH), both of which pass their electrons to electron transfer flavoprotein (ETF). If glutaric acidaemia type II is indeed due to a defect in this protein or ETF dehydrogenase, sarcosine would not accumulate in total deficiency as its biosynthesis would be curtailed. If the electron carrier were partially active, as it might be in less severe disease, the presence or absence of sarcosine would depend on the relative activities of DMGDH and SDH, and the rates at which they pass electrons to ETF. For example, the apparent K_m of DMGDH and SDH for their substrates, i.e. 0.5×10^{-3} mol/l and 1.0×10^{-3} mol/l respectively (Wittwer and Wagner, 1981), would appear to favour accumulation of sarcosine.

THE ENZYME DEFECT IN GLUTARIC ACIDAEMIA TYPE II

The general scheme of electron transfer in the segment of the respiratory chain thought to be defective in glutaric acidaemia type II is shown in Figure 1. Electrons from the FAD of at least seven dehydrogenases of the mitochondrial matrix, i.e. those specific for sarcosine, dimethylglycine, isovaleryl CoA, isobutyryl CoA and 2-methylbutyryl CoA, short chain fatty acyl-CoAs, medium chain fatty acyl CoAs and long chain fatty acyl CoAs (Ikeda *et al.*, 1983), are passed to ETF, an $\alpha\beta$ dimer whose one flavin becomes reduced to the semiquinone (McKean *et al.*, 1983; Hall and Lambeth, 1980; Beckmann *et al.*, 1981). Although ETF is easily separated from mitochondrial membranes, there is preliminary evidence to suggest that in the physiological state it is ionically bound to ETF dehydrogenase (Beckmann and Frerman, unpublished), the protein of the inner mitochondrial membrane to which reduced ETF passes its electrons (Ruzicka and Beinert, 1977; Beckmann and Frerman, unpublished). It is not certain that ETF is the physiological electron acceptor for glutaryl CoA dehydrogenase, the enzyme that dehydrogenates and decarboxylates glutaryl CoA to crotonyl CoA and which is deficient in glutaric acidaemia (Type I). ETF dehydrogenase contains one flavin and one Fe_4S_4 iron–sulphur cluster per 69 kd monomer, the electrons from ETF probably first reducing the flavin

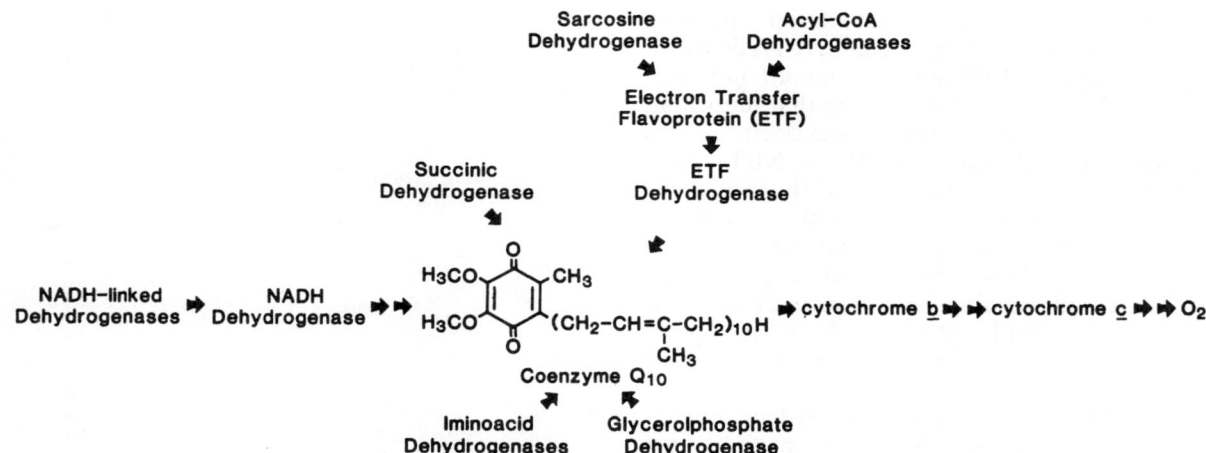

Figure 1 The mitochondrial electron transport chain. The specific site of entry of electrons from imino acids is not known

(to the semiquinone) and then the iron–sulphur cluster. It is by no means certain that electrons from ETF dehydrogenase are passed directly to coenzyme Q, nor is it certain that the latter consists of a single pool. There may, for example, be different pools of coenzyme Q for electrons of different dehydrogenases and some of these differences may relate to a newly described class of mitochondrial coenzyme Q-binding proteins (Gutman, 1980; Yu and Yu, 1981). In any event, the system is extremely complex, and it is no surprise that the primary defect in GAII has remained obscure for so long.

Acyl-CoA dehydrogenases are usually assayed by incubating tissue preparations with an acyl-CoA ester, cycling reduced flavin either with a dye, for example phenazine methosulphate (PMS) or with ETF, measuring the rate of formation of its semiquinone. The advantage of dye reduction assays is that dyes are far easier to obtain than purified ETF; their drawbacks include the high blanks that can be introduced by the presence in tissues of reducing equivalents (e.g. in sulfhydryl groups) and non-specific oxidases which can also pass electrons to PMS. *N*-Ethylmaleimide is often added to such assays to reduce the background but has the unfortunate property of inhibiting some of the dehydrogenases, such as the one specific for isovaleryl CoA (Ikeda and Tanaka, 1983). Assays using ETF are not subject to these difficulties and, now that methods are available to purify the protein in good yield (Husain and Steenkamp, 1983), will probably supplant those dependent on dye reduction. Further, the need for pure mitochondria is obviated when ETF is used and, while this may not be a problem when assaying enzymes in liver and kidney, its advantage in assaying fibroblasts and leukocytes is obvious.

To assay electron transfer flavoprotein one incubates tissue with saturating amounts of substrate, e.g. with octanoyl CoA and ETF-free octanoyl CoA dehydrogenase, reading ETF reduction fluorometrically or by linking it to dichlorophenolindophenol (DCPIP), a dye that will not accept electrons directly from dehydrogenases. One difficulty with such assays lies in obtaining an active preparation of acyl-CoA dehydrogenase(s) that is free of ETF. The dye reduction assays suffer from the possible presence of endogenous reductants, like ascorbic acid; further, transfer of electrons from ETF to DCPIP does not necessarily mean that the ETF site that binds to ETF dehydrogenase is normal. A potential problem with the fluorometric assay is the necessity to remove enough non-ETF fluorescent material from the tissue to be assayed to measure the small changes that attend reduction of ETF to its semiquinone. It may be possible to use purified ETF dehydrogenase as a terminal acceptor in such an assay, measuring its reduction spectrophotometrically and thus obviating the need for extensive sample purification.

It is even more difficult to assay ETF dehydrogenase, the principal problem being to find a terminal electron acceptor that will not oxidize the substrate, i.e. reduced ETF, as well. A catalytic assay has been devised, however, that is based on anaerobically running electrons 'uphill' from menadiol through ETF dehydrogenase to ETF, assaying its rate of reduction (Beckmann and Frerman, unpublished). ETF dehydrogenase is more usually assayed by EPR (electron paramagnetic resonance), reading the extremely characteristic signal of the protein's iron–sulphur cluster before and after reduction with dithionite (Ruzicka and Beinert, 1975).

Rhead *et al.* (1980), using a dye reduction assay, showed ETF activity in fibroblasts from the first patient described with GAII (Przyrembel *et al.*, 1976) to be more than one and a half times normal. Our own studies on cells from a patient with neonatal presentation without congenital anomalies, perhaps with the erroneous assumption that electrons from glutaryl CoA dehydrogenase were passed to ETF, also showed more activity in the mutant cell line than in two controls (Goodman *et al.*, 1982).

Our more recent experience with a histochemical assay for ETF on three cell lines, the two alluded to above and another from a girl with congenital anomalies and neonatal onset, also do not indicate ETF deficiency. In brief, fibroblasts are fixed with glutaraldehyde and are then incubated for 2 hours at 37° in a solution containing 0.2 mmol/l octanoyl CoA, 50 U/l octanoyl CoA dehydrogenase, 50 µmol/l DCPIP and 0.37 mmol/l nitroblue tetrazolium (NBT), the rationale being that mitochondrial ETF (if it survives fixation) will pass electrons from the dehydrogenase through DCPIP to NBT whose reduced form will precipitate directly onto the mitochondria. All relevant blanks in the system are negative; all cell lines examined to date (both normal and GAII) show obvious staining of what appear to be mitochondria and staining is not increased by the addition of 10^{-7} mol/l antimycin A or 10^{-4} mol/l thenoyltrifluoroacetone, an inhibitor of succinic dehydrogenase.

Data on ETF dehydrogenase in GAII have not yet appeared in the literature. We have now studied the tissues of two GAII patients by EPR spectroscopy; the first tissues examined were whole liver and kidney that had been kept at $-20°$ for about 3 years following the death of a child we have already reported (Goodman *et al.*, 1982) and, while the $g_z = 2.08$ signal in the GAII liver was less than 20 per cent of that seen in the control, the prolonged storage interval and the gross increase of fat in the affected tissue made interpretation difficult. We recently had the opportunity to study another patient (a girl with neonatal onset and congenital anomalies), this time using membranes of liver mitochondria that had been isolated about 4 hours after death. As before, the $g_z = 2.08$ signal was far less in the mutant mitochondria than it was in the control, a baby in whom about 12 hours had elapsed between death and autopsy.

We have now electrophoresed these membranes on SDS polyacrylamide gels, locating and staining ETF dehydrogenase with rabbit antiserum and peroxidase-conjugated antirabbit IgG. The result, shown in Figure 2, shows nothing in the patient membranes that cross-reacts with the antiserum, while cross-reacting material is clearly present in the control. Preliminary experiments in cultured fibroblasts appear to confirm these results. We therefore suggest that the primary defect in GAII, at least in this patient, is indeed in electron transport and specifically that it lies in ETF dehydrogenase.

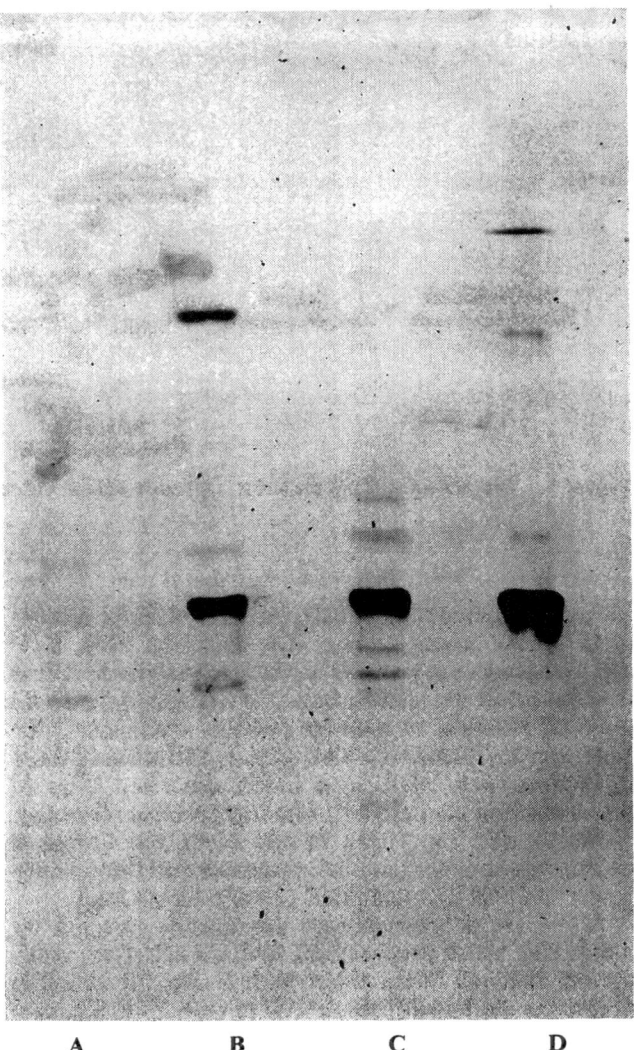

Figure 2 SDS-gel electrophoresis of: **A**, mitochondrial membranes (60 µg) from liver of a GAII patient; **B**, mitochondrial membranes (60 µg) from liver of a control; **C**, pork liver mitochondrial membranes (60 µg); **D**, pure (≥ 97%) pork ETF dehydrogenase. Staining as described in the text

References

Beckmann, J. D., Frerman, F. E. and McKean, M. C. Inhibition of general acyl CoA dehydrogenase by electron transfer flavoprotein semiquinone. *Biochem. Biophys. Res. Commun.* 102 (1981) 1290–1294

Böhm, N., Uy, J., Kiebling, M. and Lehnert, W. Multiple acyl-CoA dehydrogenation deficiency (glutaric aciduria type II), congenital polycystic kidneys, and symmetric warty dysplasia of the cerebral cortex in two newborn brothers. II. Morphology and pathogenesis. *Eur. J. Pediatr.* 139 (1982) 60–65

Coudé, F. X., Ogier, H., Charpentier, C., Thomassin, G., Checoury, A., Amédée-Manesme, O., Saudubray, J. M. and Frézal, J. Neonatal glutaric aciduria type II: An X-linked recessive inherited disorder. *Hum. Genet.* 59 (1981) 263–265

Dusheiko, G., Kew, M. C., Joffe, B. I., Lewin, J. R., Mantagos, S. and Tanaka, K. Recurrent hypoglycemia associated with glutaric aciduria type II in an adult. *N. Engl. J. Med.* 301 (1979) 1405–1409

Goodman, S. I., McCabe, E. R. B., Fennessey, P. V. and Mace, J. W. Multiple acyl-CoA dehydrogenase deficiency (glutaric aciduria type II) with transient hypersarcosinemia and sarcosinuria; possible inherited deficiency of an electron transfer flavoprotein. *Pediatr. Res.* 14 (1980) 12–17

Goodman, S. I., Stene, D. O., McCabe, E. R. B., Norenberg, M. D., Shikes, R. H., Stumpf, D. A. and Blackburn, G. K. Glutaric acidemia type II: Clinical, biochemical, and morphologic considerations. *J. Pediatr.* 100 (1982) 946–950

Goodman, S. I., Reale, M. and Berlow, S. Glutaric acidemia type II: A form with deleterious intrauterine effects. *J. Pediatr.* 102 (1983) 411–413

Gregersen, N., Kølvraa, S., Rasmussen, K., Christensen, E., Brandt, N. J., Ebbesen, F. and Hansen, F. H. Biochemical studies in a patient with defects in the metabolism of acyl-CoA and sarcosine: Another possible case of glutaric aciduria type II. *J. Inher. Metab. Dis.* 3 (1980) 67–72

Gutman, M. Electron flux through the mitochondrial ubiquinone. *Biochim. Biophys. Acta* 595 (1980) 53–84

Hall, C. L. and Lambeth, J. D. Studies on electron transfer from general acyl-CoA dehydrogenase to electron transfer flavoprotein. *J. Biol. Chem.* 255 (1980) 3591–3595

Husain, M. and Steenkamp, D. J. Electron transfer flavoprotein from pig liver mitochondria: A simple purification and re-evaluation of some of the molecular properties. *Biochem. J.* 209 (1983) 541–545

Ikeda, Y., Dabrowski, C. and Tanaka, K. Separation and properties of five distinct acyl-CoA dehydrogenases from rat liver mitochondria: Identification of a new 2-methyl branched chain acyl-CoA dehydrogenase. *J. Biol. Chem.* 258 (1983) 1066–1076

Ikeda, Y. and Tanaka, K. Purification and characterization of isovaleryl-CoA dehydrogenase from rat liver mitochondria. *J. Biol. Chem.* 258 (1983) 1077–1085

Lehnert, W., Wendel, U., Lindenmaier, S. and Böhm, N. Multiple acyl-CoA dehydrogenation deficiency (glutaric aciduria type II), congenital polycystic kidneys, and symmetric warty dysplasia of the cerebral cortex in two brothers. I. Clinical, metabolical and biochemical findings. *Eur. J. Pediatr.* 139 (1982) 56–59

Mantagos, S., Genel, M. and Tanaka, K. Ethylmalonic-adipic aciduria: *In vivo* and *in vitro* studies indicating deficiency of activities of multiple acyl-CoA dehydrogenases. *J. Clin. Invest.* 64 (1979) 1580–1589

McKean, M. C., Beckmann, J. D. and Frerman, F. E. Subunit structure of electron transfer flavoprotein. *J. Biol. Chem.* 258 (1983) 1866–1870

Mitchell, G., Saudubray, J. M., Benoit, Y., Rocchiccioli, F., Charpentier, C., Ogier, H. and Boue, J. Antenatal diagnosis of glutaric aciduria type II. *Lancet* 1 (1983) 1099

Niederwieser, A., Steinmann, B., Exner, U., Neuheiser, F., Redwik, U., Wang, M., Rampini, S. and Wendel, U. Multiple acyl-CoA dehydrogenation deficiency (MADD) in a boy with nonketotic hypoglycemia, hepatomegaly, muscle hypotonia and cardiomyopathy: Detection of *N*-isovalerylglutamic acid and its monoamide. *Helv. Paediatr. Acta* 38 (1983) 9–26

Przyrembel, H., Wendel, U., Becker, K., Bremer, H. J., Bruinvis, L., Ketting, D. and Wadman, S. K. Glutaric aciduria type II: Report on a previously undescribed metabolic disorder. *Clin. Chim. Acta* 66 (1976) 277–239

Rhead, W., Mantagos, S. and Tanaka, K. Glutaric aciduria type II: *In vitro* studies on substrate oxidation, acyl-CoA dehydrogenases, and electron-transferring flavoprotein in cultured skin fibroblasts. *Pediatr. Res.* 14 (1980) 1339–1342

Rhead, W. J. and Amendt, B. A. Oxidation of (1-^{14}C)palmitoyl-CoA and (1-^{14}C)-isovaleric acid by fibroblast mitochondria from individuals with glutaric aciduria type II. *Pediatr. Res.* 16 (1982) 263A (Abstr.)

Rhead, W. J., Fritchman, K. N. and Grundmeyer, P. A. Evidence supporting autosomal recessive inheritance of glutaric aciduria type II. *Pediatr. Res.* 17 (1983) 218A (Abstr.)

Ruzicka, F. J. and Beinert, H. A new membrane iron sulfur flavoprotein of the mitochondrial electron transfer system: The entrance point of the fatty acyl dehydrogenation pathway? *Biochem. Biophys. Res. Commun.* 66 (1975) 622–631

Ruzicka, F. J. and Beinert, H. A new iron-sulfur flavoprotein of the respiratory chain: A component of the fatty acid β oxidation pathway. *J. Biol. Chem.* 252 (1977) 8440–8445

Saudubray, J. M., Coudé, F. X., Demaugre, F., Johnson, C., Gibson, K. M. and Nyhan, W. L. Oxidation of fatty acids in cultured fibroblasts: A model system for the detection and study of defects in oxidation. *Pediatr. Res.* 16 (1982) 877–881

Sweetman, L., Nyhan, W. L., Trauner, D. A., Merritt, T. A. and Singh, M. Glutaric aciduria type II. *J. Pediatr.* 96 (1980) 1020–1026

Tanaka, K., Mantagos, S., Genel, M., Seashore, M. R., Billings, B. A. and Baretz, B. H. New defect in fatty-acid metabolism with hypoglycaemia and organic aciduria. *Lancet* 2 (1977) 968–987

Wittwer, A. J. and Wagner, C. Identification of the folate-binding proteins of rat liver mitochondria as dimethylglycine dehydrogenase and sarcosine dehydrogenase: Flavoprotein nature and enzymatic properties of the purified proteins. *J. Biol. Chem.* 256 (1981) 4109–4115

Yu, C. A. and Yu, L. Ubiquinone-binding proteins. *Biochim. Biophys. Acta* 639 (1981) 99–128

J. Inher. Metab. Dis. 7 Suppl. 1 (1984) 38–43

Carnitine Metabolism and Inborn Errors

A. G. ENGEL and C. J. REBOUCHE

Neuromuscular Research Laboratory, Department of Neurology, Mayo Clinic and Mayo Foundation, Rochester, MN 55905, USA

Current knowledge of the metabolic role, biosynthesis, cellular uptake, excretion and turnover of carnitine is reviewed. The clinical spectrum and possible aetiology of the primary muscle and primary systemic carnitine deficiency syndromes are considered and the various genetic defects of intermediary metabolism which can give rise to secondary carnitine deficiency are indicated.

CARNITINE METABOLISM

L-Carnitine, β-hydroxy-γ-N-trimethylammonium butyrate, is ubiquitous in cells of higher animals. The primary function of the molecule is to transfer long chain fatty acids across the inner mitochondrial membrane (Fritz, 1968). Cytosolic long chain fatty acids are activated to their coenzyme A (CoA) esters by fatty acyl-CoA synthetase (EC 6.2.1.3). The activated long chain fatty acids thus formed are transesterified to L-carnitine by carnitine palmitoyltransferase I (EC 2.3.1.21), an enzyme located on the external surface of the inner mitochondrial membrane (Hoppel, 1982). Transfer of the long chain fatty acylcarnitine esters across the inner mitochondrial membrane is mediated by acylcarnitine translocase (Pande and Parvin, 1976). Subsequently, long chain fatty acyl-CoA is regenerated by the action of carnitine palmitoyltransferase II on the matrix side of the inner mitochondrial membrane (Hoppel, 1982). The fatty acyl-CoA undergoes β-oxidation, and carnitine returns to the cytosol.

Carnitine may also function in other metabolic processes (Bieber *et al.*, 1982). These include (1) facilitation of branched chain α-keto acid oxidation, (2) shuttling of acyl moieties chain-shortened by β-oxidation out of hepatic peroxisomes and (3) modulation of the acyl-CoA/CoASH ratio in mammalian cells.

L-Carnitine is synthesized endogenously from lysine and methionine (Tanphaichitr and Broquist, 1973; Wolf and Berger, 1961) via the intermediates ε-N-trimethyllysine (Tanphaichitr and Broquist, 1973), β-hydroxy-ε-N-trimethyllysine (Henderson *et al.*, 1982), ε-trimethylaminobutyraldehyde (Henderson *et al.*, 1982), and γ-butyrobetaine (Bremer, 1962). In humans, the final reaction, hydroxylation of γ-butyrobetaine, occurs in liver, kidney and brain but not in cardiac or skeletal muscle (Rebouche and Engel, 1980a, b). In mammalian systems, the initial step in synthesis involves methylation of protein-bound lysine to ε-N-trimethyllysine which becomes available for carnitine synthesis on proteolysis (LaBadie *et al.*, 1976). The biosynthetic enzymes are cytosolic except ε-N-trimethyllysine hydroxylase which is mitochondrial. Ascorbate, Fe^{2+}, O_2 and α-ketoglutarate are required for optimal activity of ε-N-trimethyllysine hydroxylase (Henderson *et al.*, 1982) and γ-butyrobetaine hydroxylase (EC 1.14.11.1) (Lindstedt and Lindstedt, 1970). Pyridoxine is a cofactor for the aldolase which cleaves ε-N-trimethyllysine into γ-trimethylaminobutyraldehyde and glycine (Dunn *et al.*, 1982).

In addition to endogenous synthesis, dietary intake of carnitine can serve to maintain tissue stores. Meat products, particularly red meats and dairy products, are important dietary sources of L-carnitine (Rudman *et al.*, 1977). The relative contributions of endogenously synthesized and dietary carnitine in maintaining tissue stores in clinically normal and abnormal states have not been established to date. An adequate supply of dietary carnitine is probably important in early infancy as the capacity for carnitine biosynthesis at that time may be limited by the relatively low tissue levels of γ-butyrobetaine hydroxylase (Rebouche and Engel, 1980a). Total parenteral nutrition in newborn infants results in low serum and tissue carnitine levels (Penn *et al.*, 1981) but in children from age 1 to 10 only the serum level falls below normal (Paturneau-Jouas *et al.*, 1982).

Carnitine uptake into many cell types is against a concentration gradient by a saturable active transport process. This has been demonstrated in cultured human heart cells (Bohmer *et al.*, 1977), swine hearts (Liedtke *et al.*, 1982), perfused adult rat hearts (Vary and Neely, 1983), rat skeletal muscle (Rebouche, 1977), cultured human muscle cells and fibroblasts (Rebouche and Engel, 1982), rat kidney cortex slices (Huth and Shug, 1980), renal brush border membranes (Rebouche and Mack, 1983), isolated liver cells (Christiansen and Bremer, 1976) and rat small intestine (Shaw *et al.*, 1983). A carnitine binding protein has been isolated from rat heart plasma membrane (Cantrell and Borum, 1982) which resembles the carrier system in heart cells in specific and saturable binding of carnitine, competitive inhibition of this binding by carnitine analogues, and sensitivity to sulfhydryl reagents.

In a 70 kg adult the total body carnitine store is close to 100 mmol. Ninety-eight per cent of this is in muscle, 0.6% in extracellular fluid and only 1.6% in liver and kidney. Despite earlier reports, an intracellular pathway of carnitine degradation has not been identified. Carnitine is lost from the body via stool and urine but the faecal loss usually accounts for less than 1% of the total (Rebouche and Engel, 1984). In normal subjects the renal plasma excretory threshold for both free and total carnitine is close to the serum carnitine level (about 50 μmol/l) (Engel *et al.*, 1981) suggesting that this threshold can regulate the serum carnitine level. Kinetic

Journal of Inherited Metabolic Disease. ISSN 0141-8955. Copyright © SSIEM and MTP Press Limited, Queen Square, Lancaster, UK.

compartment analysis of carnitine metabolism in dogs indicates that the turnover time for carnitine is 0.4 h in extracellular fluid, 232 h in muscle, and 63 days for the whole body (Rebouche and Engel, 1983). Comparable values were recently obtained by us in normal human subjects (Rebouche and Engel, 1984).

In tissues and physiologic fluids, L-carnitine is present in free form and in esterified form as short chain and long chain fatty acids. The predominant short chain acylcarnitine ester is water-soluble acetyl-L-carnitine. Substantial amounts of propionyl, butyryl- isobutyryl- and isovaleryl-L-carnitine were found in rat tissues (Choi *et al.*, 1977). Trace amounts of methacrylyl-, tiglyl- and caproyl-L-carnitine were also identified (Choi *et al.*, 1977). Many of these compounds are also found in human serum and/or urine (Valkner and Bieber, 1982). Relative amounts of specific long chain fatty acylcarnitine esters have not been quantitated, but fatty acyl chains in these esters presumably reflect the composition of the free and triglyceride-bound long chain fatty acid pool within the cell. In normal humans, acylcarnitine esters account for 9–42 % (mean, 22 %) of total carnitine in serum or plasma and about 4–33 % (mean, 13 %) of total carnitine in muscle and liver. Acylcarnitine esters may constitute as much as 50–60 % of total carnitine in urine. These proportions may vary considerably with nutritional condition, exercise, and disease states (Bieber *et al.*, 1982).

CLINICAL SYNDROMES

Considerable interest in carnitine metabolism has been kindled by reports of cases of primary genetic carnitine deficiency and clinical states associated with secondary carnitine deficiency. The primary autosomal recessive carnitine deficiency syndromes include a myopathic form (MCD) and a systemic form (SCD). Carnitine deficiency secondary to a variety of genetic defects of intermediary metabolism or other disorders has been recognized.

PRIMARY MUSCLE CARNITINE DEFICIENCY

The first patient was described a decade ago (Engel and Angelini, 1973). This was a young woman who had progressive muscle weakness and lipid excess in muscle. Without added carnitine, the oxidation of [1-^{14}C]-labelled long chain fatty acids by homogenates of the patient's muscle was impaired. The oxidation of [3-^{14}C]-DL-β-hydroxybutyrate, [2-^{14}C]-pyruvate and of [1,4-^{14}C]-succinate was in the normal range. Direct assays revealed a deficiency of carnitine in muscle but not in liver or serum.

Since 1973, 18 additional cases of the more restricted myopathic form of carnitine deficiency have been reported (for references see Engel, 1980; Engel and Rebouche, 1982; Cornelio *et al.*, 1979; Carrier and Berthillier, 1980; Brucher *et al.*, 1981). Ten of the patients were male and nine were female. The age of onset of symptoms ranged from 18 months to 44 years. Seventeen patients had muscle weakness. Exertional

weakness and myalgias were found in 2/19; myocardio-pathy occurred in 5/19; myoglobinuria complicated the illness in 2/16. In two of three patients who became pregnant, the disease was worsened by pregnancy. The oldest patient in the series developed a peripheral neuropathy but she was also diabetic. Lipid excess was found in muscle in all cases, in leukocytes in one case and in Schwann cells in two cases.

The muscle carnitine level was reduced in all cases. The serum carnitine was normal in 15/19 but was decreased in 4/19 patients. In one of the patients the decrease was noted after pregnancy. Liver carnitine content was determined in the first case only, and was normal. Improvement with prednisone therapy was observed in 3/5 cases. One patient did not respond to prednisone alone but improved clinically when propranolol was also administered. Carnitine replacement therapy was tried in 11 patients; 7/11 improved clinically. Muscle carnitine content was not significantly altered by replacement therapy.

Primary MCD was thought to arise from defective transport of carnitine into muscle (Engel and Angelini, 1973; Engel *et al.*, 1974). To date, few studies have addressed this issue. Recently, however, we demonstrated by kinetic compartmental analysis that the rate of carnitine entry into muscle in a patient with primary MCD was reduced compared with that in control subjects, a result that is consistent with the above hypothesis (Rebouche and Engel, 1984).

PRIMARY SYSTEMIC CARNITINE DEFICIENCY

The clinical spectrum

The first patient was described by Karpati *et al.*, in 1975. This was an 11-year-old boy who was always weak and clumsy. He had acute episodes of encephalopathy at 3.5 and 9 years of age associated with hepatic enlargement and dysfunction. Hypoglycaemia was observed during the first episode. Muscle weakness became progressive at age 11. At this time, muscle, serum and liver carnitine levels were markedly depressed. There was lipid excess in muscle but not in liver. Forearm perfusion studies revealed impaired oxidation of long chain fatty acids and a sixfold increase of glucose utilization. There was also short chain dicarboxylic aciduria (adipic and suberic acids), presumably due to increased ω-oxidation of long chain fatty acids. The patient's weakness responded to carnitine therapy. The serum carnitine level returned to normal but the muscle and liver carnitine contents remained unchanged.

Since 1975, 21 additional cases have been reported (for references see Engel, 1980; Scarlato *et al.*, 1979; Cornelio *et al.*, 1979; Scholte *et al.*, 1979; Chapoy *et al.*, 1980; Engel *et al.*, 1981; DiDonato *et al.*, 1981; Tripp *et al.*, 1981; Waber *et al.*, 1982), and autosomal recessive inheritance has been demonstrated (Engel *et al.*, 1981; DiDonato *et al.*, 1981; Tripp *et al.*, 1981). The hallmarks of the syndrome are recurrent episodes of acute encephalopathy (17/22), progressive muscle weakness (17/22) and lipid excess in muscle (22/22) and other tissues at one stage of illness or at death. Carnitine levels were reduced in muscle (22/22), serum (16/18), heart (5/5) and liver (13/14). The kidney carnitine levels were normal in the two patients in whom this was measured. In four patients investigated by us the serum carnitine fluctuated from very low to low normal values on repeated determinations over a period of days to weeks.

The age at onset of symptoms ranged from 3 months to 38 years. In 14 patients the disease presented with encephalopathy; in three patients the weakness preceded the encephalopathy. Five of 22 patients had cardiomyopathy. In some patients the cardiomyopathy dominates the clinical picture and there are no encephalopathic attacks (Tripp *et al.*, 1981; Waber *et al.*, 1982). The disease was fatal in 11/22 cases.

Some patients have shown subjective and objective improvement with carnitine replacement therapy. In particular, treatment with L-carnitine resulted in reduced cardiomegaly and improved myocardial function in three patients who presented with cardiomyopathy. In two of these patients therapy increased the carnitine concentration in skeletal muscles, but only slightly, even after several months of treatment.

The acute attacks

The encephalopathic episodes of SCD resemble attacks of Reye's syndrome and also the Reye's syndrome-like attacks which occur in some of the organic acidurias. Conversely, some of the organic acidurias are associated with secondary carnitine deficiency (see below). In SCD the attacks are typically triggered by caloric deprivation. The initial symptom is usually vomiting followed by deepening stupor, confusion and coma. Other features of the acute attacks are hepatomegaly (16/17), increased plasma alanine or aspartate aminotransferase (10/10), hypoglycaemia (13/15), hyperammonaemia (6/7), metabolic acidosis (11/17) and hypoprothrombinaemia (2/5). Elevated urinary short chain dicarboxylic acids (adipic and/or suberic) were observed in four cases (Karpati *et al.*, 1975; Glasgow *et al.*, 1980; Engel and Rebouche, unpublished data).

The mechanism of the hypoglycaemia is of special interest. Fasting calls for increased utilization of fatty acids and increased gluconeogenesis. Fatty acid utilization is limited by the carnitine deficiency and hepatic gluconeogenesis is probably inadequate because it requires energy derived from the oxidation of fatty acids. The already higher than normal utilization of glucose by peripheral tissues, the impaired gluconeogenesis and the lack of dietary carbohydrate probably lead to rapid depletion of available glycogen stores and hypoglycaemia.

Accelerated utilization of branched chain amino acids is also likely to occur (Felig, 1975). These give rise to branched chain keto acids which, in turn, may require carnitine for their complete oxidation (Bieber *et al.*, 1982; Van Hinsbergh, 1978). Accumulation of these compounds, and also of dicarboxylic acids derived from ω-oxidation of fatty acids and of lactic acid from accelerated glycogenolysis could result in metabolic acidosis. The encephalopathy could be a consequence of the hypoglycaemia, the metabolic acidosis, the abnormal accumulation of a toxic metabolite or a combination of these factors.

Aetiology of primary SCD

Hypothetically, SCD could arise from (1) a defect in carnitine biosynthesis, (2) abnormal renal handling of carnitine, (3) alteration in cellular mechanisms for carnitine transport affecting uptake or release (or both of carnitine from tissues), (4) excessive degradation of carnitine or (5) defective intestinal absorption of carnitine.

Carnitine biosynthesis from ε-*N*-trimethyl-lysine was normal in two patients with SCD who were studied in our laboratory (Rebouche and Engel, 1981). Furthermore, in three patients with SCD studied by us, activities of hepatic enzymes subserving carnitine biosynthesis from ε-*N*-trimethyl-lysine were not decreased (Rebouche and Engel, 1980c).

We demonstrated a renal carnitine leak in four patients with SCD but found normal renal handling of carnitine in MCD (Engel *et al.*, 1981). The apparent threshold for carnitine excretion, the maximal value for tubular reabsorption and the fractional reabsorption of carnitine were lower in these subjects than in nine of ten normals. One control subject (with no clinical symptoms of SCD and normal carnitine concentration in muscle), however, also had a renal carnitine leak. Thus the renal carnitine leak alone could not account for the low carnitine levels in tissue in SCD, but this factor may act in combination with other defects of carnitine transport through cellular membranes. A recent independent study (Waber *et al.*, 1982) of a single case of SCD confirmed our finding of abnormal renal carnitine reabsorption in SCD.

Kinetic measurements of carnitine transport into cultured muscle cells and skin fibroblasts of patients with SCD did not differ from those of control subjects (Rebouche and Engel, 1982). Furthermore, carnitine fluxes (measured *in vivo*, by kinetic compartmental analysis) across the muscle plasma membrane were directly correlated with carnitine concentrations in plasma in both patients with SCD and control subjects (Rebouche and Engel, 1984) indicating that no intrinsic abnormality existed in the transport process.

Radioactive metabolites (other than acylcarnitine esters) of L-carnitine were not found in urine of patients with SCD or normal subjects between 1 and 28 days after intravenous administration of the isotope (Rebouche and Engel, 1984).

To date, intestinal absorption of L-carnitine has not been studied in SCD.

SECONDARY CARNITINE DEFICIENCY SYNDROMES

Table 1 lists the carnitine deficiency syndromes secondary to a variety of genetic defects of intermediary metabolism or other disorders. Some of these defects involve the mitochondrial utilization of lipids and low-molecular-weight organic acids, and these defects are often associated with organic aciduria. The putative mechanism of the carnitine deficiency in these syndromes

Table 1 **Secondary carnitine deficiency syndromes**

	Reference
Secondary to genetic defects of intermediary metabolism	
Methylmalonyl-CoA apomutase mutation	Seccombe *et al.*, 1982; Coudé *et al.*, 1982
Methylenetetrahydrofolate reductase deficiency*	Allen *et al.*, 1980, 1982
Propionyl-CoA carboxylase deficiency*	Allen *et al.*, 1982; Roe and Bohan, 1982
Mitochondrial respiratory chain block at NADH-ubiquinone reductase	Busch *et al.*, 1981
Cytochrome c oxidase deficiency	Müller-Höcker *et al.*, 1983
Fatty acyl-CoA dehydrogenase deficiencies	
Long chain acyl-CoA dehydrogenase deficiency	Hale *et al.*, 1983
Medium chain acyl-CoA dehydrogenase deficiency	Stanley *et al.*, 1982
Multiple acyl-CoA dehydrogenase deficiency associated with	
ornithine transcarbamylase deficiency†	Krieger *et al.*, 1983
Isovaleric acidaemia	Stanley *et al.*, 1983
Glutaric aciduria	Dusheiko *et al.*, 1979
Kearns–Sayre syndrome‡	Allen *et al.*, 1983
Carnitine octanoyltransferase deficiency	Sansaricq *et al.*, 1983
Mitochondrial ATPase deficiency	Hayes *et al.*, 1982
Secondary to other disorders	
Chronic renal failure treated by haemodialysis	Bohmer *et al.*, 1978
Cirrhosis with cachexia	Rudman *et al.*, 1977
Chronic severe myopathies	Borum *et al.*, 1977
Renal Fanconi syndrome	Netzloff *et al.*, 1981
Total parenteral nutrition of premature infants	Penn *et al.*, 1980, 1981
Kwashiorkor†	Khan *et al.*, 1977
Hyperammonaemia associated with valproic acid therapy†	Ohtani *et al.*, 1982
Valproate-induced Reye syndrome*†	Böhles *et al.*, 1982
Myxedema, hypopituitarism and adrenal insufficiency†	Maebashi *et al.*, 1977 a, b
Pregnancy†	Angelini *et al.*, 1978; Scholte *et al.*, 1978

* In these cases, only free carnitine was measured and found to be reduced in tissues or fluids. Total carnitine was not reported. Thus, there is no evidence that these syndromes were associated with total carnitine deficiency
† L-Carnitine was measured only in serum or plasma and was reduced. Tissue levels were not determined
‡ Multiple partial mitochondrial enzyme deficiencies were observed in one case of this syndrome. The syndrome probably is biochemically heterogenous

is as follows. Organic acids that undergo chain-shortening intramitochondrially accumulate at the point of the metabolic defect and thus create an abnormally high intramitochondrial acyl-CoA/CoASH ratio. Carnitine may relieve this pressure by accepting the acyl moieties from coenzyme A. Excess acylcarnitine esters may then be transported out of the mitochondrion and out of the cell; if they are preferentially excreted, a relative deficiency of carnitine is created.

Secondary carnitine deficiency may manifest with symptoms that are usually observed in the primary carnitine deficiency syndromes. For example, a patient with mitochondrial adenosine triphosphatase deficiency had recurrent episodes of vomiting, muscle weakness, and fatigue (Hayes *et al.*, 1982). Severe myopathy and lipid excess in muscle fibres occurred in a patient who had methylmalonic acidaemia and carnitine deficiency in muscle and serum (Coudé *et al.*, 1982). An infant with methylenetetrahydrofolate reductase deficiency and reduced free carnitine in serum and muscle had a lipid storage myopathy (Allen *et al.*, 1980). Reye's syndrome-like episodes associated with secondary carnitine deficiency have been observed in glutaric aciduria type II (Dusheiko *et al.*, 1979), in isovaleric acidaemia (Stanley *et al.*, 1983), in ornithine transcarbamylase deficiency (Krieger *et al.*, 1983), in a case of long chain acyl-CoA dehydrogenase deficiency (Hale *et al.*, 1983), in C_6–C_{10}

dicarboxylic aciduria (Kølvraa *et al.*, 1982), and in a case of carnitine octanoyltransferase deficiency (Sansaricq *et al.*, 1983). A child with severe Fanconi syndrome had reduced carnitine levels in plasma, muscle and liver, muscle weakness, excessive lipids in type 1 fibres and hypoglycaemic episodes (Netzloff *et al.*, 1981). It is likely that these symptoms probably develop in response to decreased carnitine levels in tissue. In some of these diseases, a decrease in the carnitine concentration in plasma may be an early marker for impending carnitine deficiency in tissue and may be useful in diagnosis. Although the carnitine deficiency is secondary in these diseases, it may contribute to the disability caused by the primary disorder; thus, treatment of the carnitine deficiency may be warranted. Secondary carnitine deficiency should respond to carnitine therapy; indeed, clinical improvement with oral carnitine supplementation has been confirmed in several of the aforementioned diseases (Allen *et al.*, 1980; Roe and Bohan, 1982; Hayes *et al.*, 1982; Ohtani *et al.*, 1982; Seccombe *et al.*, 1982).

An additional implication of the carnitine deficiency syndromes occurring in association with defects in organic acid metabolism is that some of those patients presumed to suffer from primary SCD may eventually be shown to have an underlying defect in organic acid intermediary metabolism.

References

Allen, R. J., DiMauro, S. and Coulter, D. L. Kearns–Sayre syndrome (KSS): a possible disorder of folate and carnitine metabolism (abstract). *Pediatr. Res.* 17 (1983) 286A

Allen, R. J., Hansch, D. B. and Wu, H. L. Hypocarnitinaemia in disorders of organic acid metabolism (letter to the editor). *Lancet* 2 (1982) 500–501

Allen, R. J., Wong, P., Rothenberg, S. P., DiMauro, S. and Headington, J. T. Progressive neonatal leukoencephalomyopathy due to absent methylenetetrahydrofolate reductase, responsive to treatment. *Ann. Neurol.* 8 (1980) 211 (Abstr.)

Angelini, C., Govoni, E., Bragaglia, M. M. and Vergani, L. Carnitine deficiency: acute postpartum crisis. *Ann. Neurol.* 4 (1978) 558–561

Bieber, L. L., Emaus, R., Valkner, K. and Farrell, S. Possible functions of short-chain and medium-chain carnitine acyltransferases. *Fed. Proc.* 41 (1982) 2858–2862

Böhles, H., Richter, K., Wagner-Thiessen, E. and Schäfer, H. Decreased serum carnitine in valproate induced Reye syndrome. *Eur. J. Pediatr.* 139 (1982) 185–186

Bohmer, T., Bergrem, H. and Eiklid, K. Carnitine deficiency induced during intermittent haemodialysis for renal failure. *Lancet* 1 (1978) 126–128

Bohmer, T., Eiklid, K. and Jonsen, J. Carnitine uptake into human heart cells in culture. *Biochim. Biophys. Acta* 465 (1977) 627–633

Borum, P. R., Broquist, H. P. and Roelofs, R. I. Muscle carnitine levels in neuromuscular disease. *J. Neurol. Sci.* 34 (1977) 279–286

Bremer, J. Carnitine precursors in the rat. *Biochim. Biophys. Acta* 57 (1962) 327–335

Brucher, J. M., Tassin, S., Walter, G. F., Scholte, H. B. and deBarsy, Th. Myopathic carnitine deficiency. Clinical, morphologic and biochemical findings in three cases. In Busch, H. F. M., Jennekens, F. G. I. and Scholte, H. R. (eds.) *Mitochondria and Muscle Disease*, Beetsterzwaag, The Netherlands, 1981, pp. 199–205

Busch, H. F. M., Scholte, H. R., Arts, W. F. and Luyt-Houwen, I. E. M. A mitochondrial myopathy with a respiratory chain defect and carnitine deficiency. In Busch, H. F. M., Jennekens, F. G. I. and Scholte, H. R. (eds.) *Mitochondria and Muscle Disease*, Beetsterzwaag, The Netherlands, 1981, pp. 207–211

Cantrell, C. R. and Borum, P. R. Identification of a cardiac carnitine binding protein. *J. Biol. Chem.* 257 (1982) 10599–10604

Carrier, H. N. and Berthillier, G. Carnitine levels in normal children and adults and in patients with diseased muscle. *Muscle Nerve* 3 (1980) 326–324

Chapoy, P. R., Angelini, C., Brown, W. J., Stiff, J. E., Shug, A. L. and Cederbaum, S. D. Systemic carnitine deficiency – a treatable inherited lipid-storage disease presenting as Reye's syndrome. *N. Engl. J. Med.* 303 (1980) 1389–1394

Choi, Y. R., Fogle, P. J., Clarke, P. R. H. and Bieber, L. L. Quantitation of water-soluble acylcarnitines and carnitine acyltransferases in rat tissues. *J. Biol. Chem.* 252 (1977) 7930–7931

Christiansen, R. Z. and Bremer, J. Active transport of butyrobetaine and carnitine into isolated liver cells. *Biochim. Biophys. Acta* 448 (1976) 562–577

Cornelio, F., DiDonato, S., Peluchetti, D., Rimoldi, M., Daniel, S., Testa, D. and Mora, M. Heterogeneity of carnitine deficiency. Clinicopathologic aspects of eight cases. *Perspect. Inher. Metab. Dis.* 3 (1979) 129–150

Coudé, F. X., Ogier, H., Carrier, H., Berthillier, G., Charpentier, C., Pham Dinh, D., Aicardi, J. and Saudubray, J. M. Myopathy in methylmalonic acidemia: a new secondary carnitine deficiency syndrome (abstract). In *Abstracts of Free Communications, Fifth International Congress on Neuromuscular Diseases*, 1982

DiDonato, S., Rimoldi, M., Cornelio, F., Botacchi, E. and Giunta, A. Evidence for autosomal recessive inheritance in systemic carnitine deficiency. *Ann. Neurol.* 11 (1981) 190–192

Dunn, W. A., Aronson, N. N. Jr. and England, S. The effects of 1-amino-D-proline on the production of carnitine from exogenous protein-bound trimethyllysine by the perfused rat liver. *J. Biol. Chem.* 257 (1982) 7948–7951

Dusheiko, G., Kew, M. C., Joffe, B. I., Lewin, J. R., Mantagos, S. and Tanaka, K. Recurrent hypoglycemia associated with glutaric aciduria type II in an adult. *N. Engl. J. Med.* 301 (1979) 1405–1409

Engel, A. G. Possible causes and effects of carnitine deficiency in man. In Frenkel, R. A. and McGarry, J. D. (eds.) *Carnitine Biosynthesis, Metabolism, and Functions*, Academic Press, New York, 1980, pp. 271–285

Engel, A. G. and Angelini, C. Carnitine deficiency of human skeletal muscle with associated lipid storage myopathy: a new syndrome. *Science* 179 (1973) 899–902

Engel, A. G., Angelini, C. and Nelson, R. A. Identification of carnitine deficiency as a cause of human lipid storage myopathy. *Excerpta Medica International Congress Series* No. 333 (1974) 601–617

Engel, A. G. and Rebouche, C. J. Pathogenetic mechanisms in human carnitine deficiency syndromes. In Schotland, D. L. (ed.) *Disorders of the Motor Unit*, Wiley, New York, 1982, pp. 643–656

Engel, A. G., Rebouche, C. J., Wilson, D. M., Glasgow, A. M., Romshe, C. A. and Cruse, R. P. Primary systemic carnitine deficiency. II Renal handling of carnitine. *Neurology (NY)* 31 (1981) 819–825

Felig, P. Amino acid metabolism in man. *Ann. Rev. Biochem.* 44 (1975) 933–955

Fritz, I. B. The metabolic consequences of the effects of carnitine on long-chain fatty acid oxidation. In Gran, F. C. (ed.) *Cellular Compartmentalization and Control of Fatty Acid Metabolism*, Academic Press, New York, 1968, pp. 39–63

Glasgow, A. M., Eng, G. and Engel, A. G. Systemic carnitine deficiency simulating recurrent Reye syndrome. *J. Pediatr.* 92 (1980) 889–891

Hale, D. E., Coates, P. M., Stanley, C. A., Cortner, J. A. and Hall, C. L. Long-chain acyl CoA dehydrogenase deficiency. *Pediatr. Res.* 17 (1983) 290A (Abstr.)

Hayes, D. J., Summers, B. A., Morgan-Hughes, J. A. and Clark, J. B. A combined deficiency of muscle carnitine and mitochondrial ATPase activity in a patient with multisystem disease partially responsive to oral carnitine (abstract). In *Abstracts of Free Communications, Fifth International Congress on Neuromuscular Diseases*, 1982

Henderson, L. M., Nelson, P. J. and Henderson, L. Mammalian enzymes of trimethyllysine conversion to trimethylaminobutyrate. *Fed. Proc.* 41 (1982) 2843–2847

Hoppel, C. L. Carnitine and carnitine palmitoyltransferase in fatty acid oxidation and ketosis. *Fed. Proc.* 41 (1982) 2853–2857

Huth, P. J. and Shug, A. L. Properties of carnitine transport in rat kidney cortex slices. *Biochim. Biophys. Acta* 602 (1980) 621–634

Karpati, G., Carpenter, S., Engel, A. G., Watters, G., Allen, J., Rothman, S., Klassen, G. and Mammer, O. A. The syndrome of systemic carnitine deficiency: clinical, morphologic, biochemical, and pathophysiologic features. *Neurology (Minneap.)* 25 (1975) 16–24

Khan, L. and Bamji, M. S. Plasma carnitine level in children with protein-calorie malnutrition before and after rehabilitation. *Clin. Chim. Acta* 75 (1977) 163–166

Kølvraa, S., Gregersen, N., Christensen, E. and Hobolth, N. *In vitro* fibroblast studies in a patient with C_6–C_{10}-dicarboxylic aciduria: evidence for a defect in general CoA dehydrogenase. *Clin. Chim. Acta* 126 (1982) 53–67

Krieger, I., Taqi, Q., Sweeley, C. C. and Snodgrass, P. J. Ornithine transcarbamylase (OTC) deficiency in intermittent Reye's syndrome due to multiple acyl-CoA dehydrogenase defect. *Pediatr. Res.* 17 (1983) 292A (Abstr.)

LaBadie, J., Dunn, W. A. and Aronson, N. N. Jr. Hepatic synthesis of carnitine from protein-bound trimethyllysine. Lysosomal digestion of methyllysine-labeled asialo-fetuin. *Biochem. J.* 160 (1976) 85–95

Liedtke, A. J., Vary, T. C., Nellis, S. H. and Fultz, C. W. Properties of carnitine incorporation in working swine hearts. Effects of coronary flow, ischemia, and excess of fatty acids. *Circ. Res.* 50 (1982) 767–774

Lindstedt, G. and Lindstedt, S. Cofactor requirements of γ-butyrobetaine hydroxylase from rat liver. *J. Biol. Chem.* 245 (1970) 4178–4186

Maebashi, M., Kawamura, N., Sato, M., Imamura, A., Yoshinaga, K. and Suzuki, M. Urinary excretion of carnitine in patients with hyperthyroidism and hypothyroidism: augmentation by thyroid hormone. *Metabolism* 26 (1977a) 351–356

Maebashi, M., Kawamura, N., Sato, M., Imamura, A., Yoshinaga, K. and Suzuki, M. Urinary excretion of carnitine and serum concentrations of carnitine and lipids in patients with hypofunctional endocrine diseases: involvement of adrenocorticoid and thyroid hormones in ACTH-induced augmentation of carnitine and lipids metabolism. *Metabolism* 26 (1977b) 357–361

Müller-Höcker, J., Pongratz, D., Deufel, T., Trijbels, J. M. F., Endres, W. and Hübner, G. Fatal lipid storage myopathy with deficiency of cytochrome-c-oxidase and carnitine: a contribution to the combined cytochemical–fine structural identification of cytochrome-c-oxidase in long term frozen muscle. *Virchows Arch. (Pathol. Anat.)* 399 (1983) 11–23

Netzloff, M. L., Kohrman, A. F., Jones, M. Z., Emaus, R. K., Bieber, L. L. and DiMauro, S. Carnitine deficiency associated with renal Fanconi syndrome. *J. Neuropathol. Exp. Neurol.* 40 (1981) 351 (Abstr.)

Ohtani, Y., Endo, F. and Matsuda, I. Carnitine deficiency and hyperammonemia associated with valproic acid therapy. *J. Pediatr.* 101 (1982) 782–785

Pande, S. V. and Parvin, R. Characterization of carnitine acylcarnitine translocase system of heart mitochondria. *J. Biol. Chem.* 251 (1976) 6683–6691

Paturneau-Jouas, M., Amédée-Manesme, O., Bresson, J. L., Masson, M., Bourra, J. M. and Ricour, C. Carnitine levels during long-term total parenteral nutrition (TPN). *Abstracts of Free Communications, Fifth International Congress on Neuromuscular Diseases*, 1982

Penn, D., Schmidt-Sommerfeld, E. and Pascu, F. Decreased tissue carnitine concentrations in newborn infants receiving total parenteral nutrition. *J. Pediatr.* 98 (1981) 976–978

Penn, D., Schmidt-Sommerfeld, E. and Wolf, H. Carnitine deficiency in premature infants receiving total parenteral nutrition. *Early Hum. Dev.* 4 (1980) 23–24

Rebouche, C. J. Carnitine movement across muscle cell membranes. Studies in isolated rat muscle. *Biochim. Biophys. Acta* 471 (1977) 145–155

Rebouche, C. J. and Engel, A. G. Tissue distribution of carnitine biosynthetic enzymes in man. *Biochim. Biophys. Acta* 630 (1980a) 22–29

Rebouche, C. J. and Engel, A. G. Significance of renal γ-butyrobetaine hydroxylase for carnitine biosynthesis in man. *J. Biol. Chem.* 255 (1980b) 8700–8705

Rebouche, C. J. and Engel, A. G. *In vitro* analysis of hepatic carnitine biosynthesis in human systemic carnitine deficiency. *Clin. Chim. Acta* 106 (1980c) 295–300

Rebouche, C. J. and Engel, A. G. Primary systemic carnitine deficiency. I. Carnitine biosynthesis. *Neurology (NY)* 31 (1981) 813–818

Rebouche, C. J. and Engel, A. G. Carnitine transport in cultured muscle cells and skin fibroblasts from patients with primary systemic carnitine deficiency. *In Vitro* 18 (1982) 495–500

Rebouche, C. J. and Engel, A. G. Kinetic compartmental analysis of carnitine metabolism in the dog. *Arch. Biochem. Biophys.* 220 (1983) 60–70

Rebouche, C. J. and Engel, A. G. Kinetic compartmental analysis of carnitine metabolism in the human carnitine deficiency syndromes: evidence for alterations in tissue carnitine transport. *J. Clin. Invest.* 73 (1984) 857–867

Rebouche, C. J. and Mack, D. Carnitine transport across rat renal bushborder membranes (abstract). *Fed. Proc.* 42 (1983) 1053

Roe, C. R. and Bohan, T. P. L-Carnitine therapy in propionicacidaemia (letter to the editor). *Lancet* 1 (1982) 1411–1412

Rudman, D., Sewell, C. W. and Ansley, J. D. Deficiency of carnitine in cachectic cirrhotic patients. *J. Clin. Invest.* 60 (1977) 716–723

Sansaricq, C., Kaufmann, R., DiMauro, S., Schacht, R. G., Greco, A., Goldstein, F., Naylor, E. W., Bazaz, G. and Snyderman, S. E. Mixed form of carnitine deficiency with dicarboxylic-aciduria unresponsive to carnitine. *Pediatr. Res.* 17 (1983) 295A (Abstr.)

Scarlato, G., Pellegrini, G., Moggio, M., Meola, G. and Frattola, L. Carnitine deficiency and lipid storage myopathy in three patients: analysis of some differential features. *Perspect. Inher. Metab. Dis.* 3 (1979) 109–128

Scholte, H. R., Meijer, A. E. F. H. and Van Wijngaarden, G. K. *et al.* Familial carnitine deficiency. A fatal case and subclinical state in a sister. *J. Neurol. Sci.* 42 (1979) 87–101

Scholte, H. R., Stinis, J. T. and Jennekens, F. G. I. Low carnitine levels in serum of pregnant women (letter to the editor). *N. Engl. J. Med.* 299 (1978) 1079–1080

Seccombe, D. W., Snyder, F. and Parsons, H. G. L-Carnitine for methylmalonicaciduria (letter to the editor). *Lancet* 2 (1982) 1401

Shaw, R. D., Shug, A. L. and Olsen, W. A. Studies of carnitine transport by rat small intestine. *Pediatr. Res.* 17 (1983) 194A

Stanley, C. A., Gonzales, E., Kelley, R. L. and Yang, W. Reduced tissue carnitine associated with a defect in fatty acid beta-oxidation. *Diabetes* 31, Suppl. 2 (1982) 165A (Abstr.)

Stanley, C. A., Hale, D. E., Whiteman, D. E. H., Coates, P. M., Yudkoff, M., Berry, G. T. and Segal, S. Systemic carnitine (carn) deficiency in isovaleric acidemia (IVA). *Pediatr. Res.* 17 (1983) 296A (Abstr.)

Tanphaichitr, V. and Broquist, H. P. Role of lysine and ε-N-trimethyllysine in carnitine biosynthesis. II. Studies in the rat. *J. Biol. Chem.* 248 (1973) 2176–2181

Tripp, M. E., Katcher, M. L., Peters, H. A., Gilbert, E. F., Arya, S., Hodach, R. J. and Shug, A. L. Systemic carnitine deficiency presenting as familial endocardial fibroelastosis: a treatable cardiomyopathy. *N. Engl. J. Med.* 305 (1981) 385–390

Van Hinsbergh, W. V., Veerkamp, J. H., Engelen, P. J. M. *et al.* Effect of L-carnitine on the oxidation of leucine and valine by rat skeletal muscle. *Biochem. Med.* 20 (1978) 115–124

Valkner, K. J. and Bieber, L. L. Short-chain acylcarnitines of human blood and urine. *Biochem. Med.* 28 (1982) 197–302

Vary, T. C. and Neely, J. R. Sodium dependence of carnitine transport in isolated perfused adult rat hearts. *Heart Circ. Physiol.* 13 (1983) H247–252

Waber, L. J., Valle, D., Neill, C., DiMauro, S. and Shug, A. Carnitine deficiency presenting as familial cardiomyopathy: a treatable defect in carnitine transport. *J. Pediatr.* 101 (1982) 700–705

Wolf, G. and Berger, C. R. A. Studies on the biosynthesis and turnover of carnitine. *Arch. Biochem. Biophys.* 92 (1961) 360–365

J. Inher. Metab. Dis. 7 Suppl. 1 (1984) 44–47

Gas Chromatography–Mass Spectrometry (GC–MS) Diagnosis of Two Cases of Medium Chain Acyl-CoA Dehydrogenase Deficiency

P. Divry, C. Vianey-Liaud and J. Cotte
Laboratoire de Biochimie, Hôpital Debrousse, 29, rue Soeur Bouvier, 69322 Lyon Cédex 05, France

Two patients with hypoketotic hypoglycaemia and dicarboxylic aciduria are described. Studies of their urinary organic acids by gas chromatography–mass spectrometry (GC–MS) showed an excretion of dicarboxylic acids (adipic suberic and sebacic acids), unsaturated dicarboxylic acids (*cis*-octenedioic and decenedioic acids), 5-hydroxyhexanoic acid, hexanoyl-glycine and suberylglycine. Deficiency of the medium chain acyl-CoA dehydrogenase (MCAD) in fibroblasts was documented for both children. Despite a similar presentation (hypoglycaemic coma), organic acid profile (dicarboxylic aciduria and suberylglycine excretion) and enzyme deficiency (MCAD), they did not respond similarly to glucose infusion.

Since the first case of non-ketotic dicarboxylic aciduria (Gregersen *et al.*, 1976), 15 cases have been published with proven or indicated defect in medium chain fatty acyl-CoA dehydrogenase (MCAD). The number of reported cases is increasing rapidly and most of them have been described very recently (Yang *et al.*, 1982; Stanley *et al.*, 1982; Colle *et al.*, 1983; Divry *et al.*, 1983; Duran *et al.*, 1983, 1984). All these patients exhibit the same clinical history of single or recurrent severe episodes of hypoglycaemia with mild or absent ketonuria. A number of different defects of β-oxidation can lead to similar symptoms and to dicarboxylic aciduria. These include systemic carnitine deficiency, carnitine palmitoyl transferase deficiency and long chain acyl-CoA dehydrogenase deficiency. As demonstrated recently (Duran *et al.*, 1984), it seems that among the other β-oxidation disorders, MCAD deficiency may exhibit a rather characteristic urinary profile. This organic acid profile reflects the C_6–C_8 acyl-CoA accumulation (hexanoyl-CoA, octanoyl-CoA) with excretion of unusual metabolites: octanoyl carnitine, suberylglycine and hexanoylglycine.

We report here the GC–MS studies of two unrelated MCAD deficient patients.

CASE HISTORIES

Case 1

S.G. This patient has recently been reported (Divry *et al.*, 1983). She is the second child of unrelated parents. The eldest child died when he was 4 years old on the second day of a febrile illness with vomiting. She was first admitted to the hospital when she was 14 months old in a severe hypoglycaemic coma following 48 hours' history of vomiting and gastroenteritis. She recovered after intravenous glucose infusion. During extensive metabolic investigation, a 24 h fast and a protein loading test

were tolerated without any abnormal clinical or biochemical effects. Conversely, she developed a severe and dramatic hypoglycaemia (0.2 mmol/l) 23 hours after beginning a ketogenic diet. She recovered after intravenous infusion of glucose. At 5 years of age she has normal psychomotor development. Analysis of urine (collected during the attack) for organic acids revealed a massive dicarboxylic aciduria. Systemic carnitine deficiency was excluded by a normal free plasma carnitine value (28 μmol/l). Deficiency of medium chain acyl-CoA dehydrogenase has been demonstrated in her fibroblasts (Saudubray *et al.*, 1982; Divry *et al.*, 1983; Rhead *et al.*, 1983).

Case 2

X.D., a boy born in 1978 from healthy unrelated parents, was first referred to the hospital in September 1982 with a 48 h history of vomiting and progressive lethargy. (He has four sibs, one of them died suddenly when he was 22 months old.) On admission he was comatose. Routine biochemical analysis revealed a severe hypoglycaemia (0.3 mmol/l) and hyperammonaemia (268 μmol/l). Blood ketones were elevated (3.5 mmol/l) and ketonuria was noticed (Acetest + +). Blood glucose was promptly corrected by intravenous glucose infusion but the child remained comatose for 48 h with progressive elevation of transaminases and some enlargement of the liver. Free carnitine in plasma was low (19 μmol/l). A urine sample was collected the day after the hypoglycaemic attack. His second hospital admission occurred in January 1983. He had been vomiting from the morning and the parents observed a mild lethargy. On admission the same afternoon he was slightly sleepy, with normal blood glucose (4.5 mmol/l), normal blood ammonia (34 μmol/l), no liver enlargement and serum transaminase values in the normal range. The boy recovered rapidly and was discharged the next morning. Studies of β-oxidation in fibroblasts were strongly suggestive of MCAD deficiency.

Journal of Inherited Metabolic Disease. ISSN 0141–8955. Copyright © SSIEM and MTP Press Limited, Queen Square, Lancaster, UK.

METHODS

Plasma carnitine was measured according to Ramsay and Tubbs (1975). Urinary organic acids were extracted with solvents and analysed using gas chromatography–mass spectrometry (GC–MS) as their methyl esters formed with diazomethane. The presence of hydroxy fatty acids (5-hydroxyhexanoic) was checked by analysis of trimethylsilyl derivatives.

RESULTS

S.G. Urinary organic acid profile of a urine sample collected 3 hours after the hypoglycaemic attack showed massive dicarboxylic aciduria and peaks of hexanoylglycine, suberylglycine and 5-hydroxyhexanoic acid. Suberylglycine was first identified after acid hydrolysis of the urine leading to disappearance of the suberylglycine peak and an increase of the suberic acid peak. Absolute identification was performed by GC–MS. A urine sample was collected later on, when the girl was in good clinical condition. The organic acid profile was virtually normal although suberylglycine and hexanoylglycine were still excreted in small amounts (Table 1).

X.D. A urine sample collected 20 hours after the metabolic attack showed a mild dicarboxylic aciduria. Excretion of dicarboxylic acids and 5-hydrohexanoic acid was not correlated with the clinical status (child remaining in deep coma despite a normal plasma glucose value). However, the presence of small peaks of suberylglycine and hexanoylglycine suggested impairment of fatty acid β-oxidation, possibly at MCAD. Conversely, the urine sample collected during the second hospital admission was more characteristic. The GC–MS profile (Figure 1) exhibited massive dicarboxylic aciduria with excretion of large quantities of 5-hydroxyhexanoic acid, hexanoylglycine and suberylglycine. The use of a capillary column allowed a good

separation of unsaturated dicarboxylic acids (*cis*-4-octenedioic acid and decenedioic acid).

DISCUSSION

High concentrations of urinary dicarboxylic acids produced by increased ω-oxidation are frequently noted in situations in which fatty acid oxidation is considerably increased, e.g. ketotic episodes (Pettersen *et al.*, 1972) and triglyceride loads (Shigematsu *et al.*, 1981). The latter is easy to recognize even from the organic acid profile as the sebacic acid excretion is greater than that of adipic acid. Massive dicarboxylic aciduria with 5-hydroxyhexanoic acid excretion may be seen in acute episodes of ketonuria but suberylglycine has never been documented in this situation (Table 1).

On the other hand, discrimination from other conditions associated with decreased β-oxidation of fatty acids has not yet been achieved. MCAD deficient patients often have plasma carnitine values in the low to low normal range. The diagnostic value of urinary metabolites varies between authors. Some authors (Colle *et al.*, 1983) indicate that 7-hydroxyoctanoic and other ω-1-hydroxy fatty acids seem to be good indicators of MCAD deficiency. However, 7-hydroxyoctanoic acid has been measured in our first patient and two patients of Gregersen (Gregersen *et al.*, 1983) and was not elevated as much.

Suberylglycine excretion was the striking metabolite in the first patient described (Gregersen *et al.*, 1976). It seems to be with hexanoylglycine a very important compound in MCAD deficiency. Including the five patients described by Duran *et al.* (1984) and both our patients, suberylglycine excretion has been demonstrated in ten patients out of 15 (Truscott *et al.*, 1979; Gregersen *et al.*, 1983). In one child, Naylor *et al.* (1980) using methyl esters for special investigation did not find

Table 1 Excretion of dicarboxylic acids and related metabolites (quantities in mmol/mol creatinine)

	Adipic acid	Suberic acid	Sebacic acid	5-OH-hexanoic	Hexanoyl-glycine	Suberyl-glycine
S.G.						
hypoglycaemia	950	332	45	+	40	140
normoglycaemia	7	17	8	(+)	10	12
X.D.						
20 h after the						
hypoglycaemic attack	36	60	NM	+	+	80
attack without						
hypoglycaemia	180	146	124	+	+	200
Ketotic patients (*n* = 10)	6–300	5–50	1–18	(+)	ND	ND
MCT treated children (*n* = 3)	23–420	58–663	247–1294	+	ND	ND
Controls 1 day–15 years (*n* = 70)	1–15	1—5	1–5	ND	ND	ND

NM: not measured, overlapping peak in the area; ND: not detectable

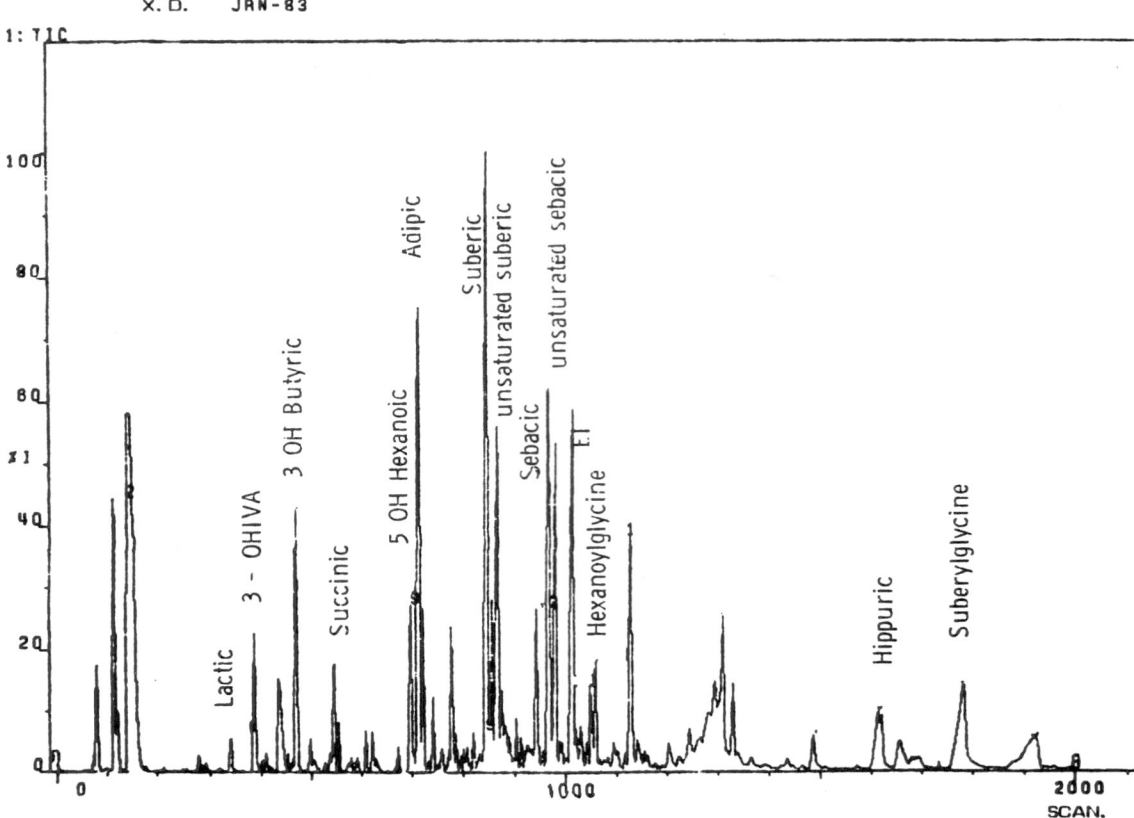

Figure 1 Capillary GC–MS profile of methylated urinary organic acids from X.D.

any suberylglycine. In the extensive work on two patients reported by Mamer *et al.* (1980) and Colle *et al.* (1983) it is not mentioned.

Another recently discovered metabolite, octanoyl carnitine (Duran *et al.*, 1983) seems to reflect the accumulation of octanoyl-CoA in MCAD deficiency. Octanoyl carnitine has not been measured in our patients. However, in our first case the urinary carnitine values are indicative of a very high excretion of carnitine ester (free carnitine: 164 µmol/l; total carnitine: 1500 µmol/l). On the same urine sample, analysis of octanoic acid before and after hydrolysis of urine (Gregersen *et al.*, 1983) revealed an increase of octanoic acid value from 44 to 1082 µmol/l. These results, in favour of octanoyl carnitine excretion, have been observed in both acute and normal clinical conditions.

In the study of our second patient, a discrepancy was observed between the urinary profile and the plasma glucose level. The first analysis, with subnormal dicarboxylic excretion, related to a normal blood glucose as a consequence of i.v. glucose therapy in a 'post-hypoglycaemic state'. The second analysis, with massive dicarboxylic aciduria and characteristic profile, related also to a normal blood glucose without extra glucose in possibly a 'pre-hypoglycaemic state'. This is not a unique feature and has been described (Duran *et al.*, 1984) in a patient who exhibited a urinary profile consistent with MCAD deficiency at the end of a fasting

test in spite of normal blood glucose value. As most of the biochemical studies have been performed during hypoglycaemic attacks or more frequently during the following 24–48 hours, one can speculate that the dicarboxylic aciduria may precede the hypoglycaemia. It is known that, in fasted rats, adipic, suberic and sebacic acids appear in urine 1 day before the ketone bodies (Mortensen, 1980).

Another discrepancy can be observed between the biochemical results and the clinical status. Despite a similar urinary organic acid profile and the same symptomatic treatment, one child emerged from coma and was alert soon after the i.v. glucose infusion, while the other one remained comatose for 48 hours in spite of a normalized blood glucose value. Both children, after recovery, have had a normal development.

Elevated values of plasma octanoate have been involved in brain dysfunction (Staeffen *et al.*, 1979). This metabolite has not been measured in our cases. Whether plasma octanoate is one of the factors responsible for the prolonged coma or whether there are other unknown compounds is a question that emphasizes the need for extensive studies of these patients, including analysis of plasma and urinary metabolites and determination of the enzyme deficiency in leukocytes (Coates *et al.*, 1983), fibroblasts (Kølvraa and Gregersen, 1982) and the mitochondrial fraction of fibroblasts (Rhead *et al.*, 1983).

We thank Professor M. David and Dr Floret for referring samples from the patients and the Centre de Spectrometrie de Masse, Solaize, France for allowing us to use their mass spectrometer.

References

Coates, P. M., Hale, D. E., Katz, M. R., Stanley, C. A. and Hall, C. L. Detection of medium-chain acyl-CoA dehydrogenase deficiency in leucocytes. *Pediatr. Res.* 17 (1983) 288A

Colle, E., Mamer, O. A., Montgomery, J. A. and Miller, J. D. Episodic hypoglycemia with psi-hydroxy fatty acid excretion. *Pediatr. Res.* 17 (1983) 171–176

Divry, P., David, M., Gregersen, N., Kølvraa, S., Christensen, E., Collet, J. P., Dellamonica, C. and Cotte, J. Dicarboxylic aciduria due to medium-chain acyl-CoA dehydrogenase defect: A cause of hypoglycemia in childhood. *Acta Paediatr. Scand.* 72 (1983) 943–949

Duran, M., De Klerk, J. B. C., Van Pelt, J., Wadman, S. K., Scholte, H. R., Beekman, R. P. and Jennekens, F. G. The analysis of plasma and urinary organic acids during prolonged fasting differentiates between systemic carnitine deficiency and a defect of fatty acid oxidation. *J. Inher. Metab. Dis.* 6, Suppl. 2 (1983) 121–122

Duran, M., De Klerk, J. B. C., Wadman, S. K., Bruinvis, L. and Ketting, D. The differential diagnosis of dicarboxylic aciduria. *J. Inher. Metab. Dis.* 7 Suppl. 1 (1984) 48–51

Gregersen, N., Lauritzen, R. and Rasmussen, L. Suberylglycine excretion in the urine from a patient with dicarboxylic aciduria. *Clin. Chim. Acta* 70 (1976) 417–425

Gregersen, N., Kølvraa, S., Rasmussen, K., Mortensen, P. B., Divry, P., David, M. and Hobolth, N. General (medium-chain) acyl-CoA dehydrogenase deficiency (non-ketotic dicarboxylic aciduria): quantitative urinary excretion pattern of 23 biological significant organic acids in 3 cases. *Clin. Chim. Acta.* 132 (1983) 181–191

Kølvraa, S. and Gregersen, N. Methods for the measurement of fatty acid β-oxidation and acyl-CoA dehydrogenase in cultured fibroblasts. *J. Inher. Metab. Dis.* 5, Suppl. 1 (1982) 31–32

Mamer, O. A., Montgomery, J. A. and Colle, E. Profile in altered metabolism III: Ω-1-hydroxy-acid excretion in a case of episodic hypoglycemia. *Biochem. Mass Spect.* 7 (1980) 53–57

Mortensen, P. B. The possible antiketogenic and gluconeogenic effect of the ω oxidation of fatty acids in rat. *Biochim. Biophys. Acta* 620 (1980) 177–185

Naylor, E. W., Mosovich, L. L., Guthrie, R., Evans, J. E. and Tieckelmann, H. Intermittent non-ketotic dicarboxylic aciduria in two siblings with hypoglycaemia: an apparent defect in β-oxidation of fatty acids. *J. Inher. Metab. Dis.* 3 (1980) 19–24

Pettersen, J. E., Jellum, E. and Eljarn, L. The occurrence of adipic and suberic acid in urine from ketotic patients. *Clin. Chim. Acta* 38 (1972) 17–24

Ramsay, R. R. and Tubbs, P. K. The mechanism of fatty acids uptake by heart mitochondria: an acylcarnitine–carnitine exchange. *FEBS Lett.* 54 (1975) 21–25

Rhead, W. J., Amendt, B. A., Fritchman, K. S. and Felts, J. Dicarboxylic aciduria: deficient 1-^{14}C-octanoate oxidation and medium-chain acyl-CoA dehydrogenase activity in fibroblasts. *Science* 221 (1983) 73–75

Saudubray, J. M., Coude, F. X., Demaugre, F., Johnson, C., Gibson, K. M. and Nyhan, W. L. Oxidation of fatty acids in cultured fibroblast. A model system for the detection and study of defects in β-oxidation. *Pediatr. Res.* 16 (1982) 877–881

Shigematsu, Y., Momoi, T., Sudo, M. and Sozuki, Y. (ω-1) Hydroxymonocarboxylic acids in urine of infants fed medium chain triglycerides. *Clin. Chem.* 27/10 (1981) 1661–1664

Staeffen, J., Rabinowitz, J. L., Aumonier, P., Ballen, P., Ferrer, J., Terme, R., Series, C. and Meyerson, R. M. Hyperoctanoatemia and the hepatic encephalopathy of cirrhosis. *Nouv. Presse Med.* 8 (1979) 1663–1666

Stanley, C. A., Gonzales, E., Yang, W., Kelley, R. E. and Baker, L. Hypoketotic hypoglycemia. Evidence for a new defect in fatty acid oxidation. *Pediatr. Res.* 16 (1982) 264A

Truscott, R. J., Hick, L., Pullin, C., Halpern, B., Wilcken, B., Griffiths, H., Silink, M., Kilham, H. and Grunseit, F. Dicarboxylic aciduria: the response to fasting. *Clin. Chim. Acta* 94 (1979) 31–39

Yang, W., Roth, K. S. and Coates, P. B. Hypoglycemic, hypoketotic dicarboxylic aciduria. A possible defect in fatty acid oxidation. *Pediatr. Res.* 16 (1982) 267A

J. Inher. Metab. Dis. 7 Suppl. 1 (1984) 48–51

The Differential Diagnosis of Dicarboxylic Aciduria

M. DURAN, J. B. C. DE KLERK, S. K. WADMAN, L. BRUINVIS and D. KETTING
University Children's Hospital 'Het Wilhelmina Kinderziekenhuis', Nieuwe Gracht 137, Utrecht, The Netherlands

Various types of dicarboxylic aciduria are known, most of them are accompanied by non-ketotic hypoglycaemia. For the differential diagnosis of these conditions several methods of investigation have been used: (1) analysis of urinary organic acids in both native and hydrolysed samples, (2) analysis of free and esterified carnitine, the latter by means of chromatographic separation and identification of acyl moieties, (3) analysis of plasma organic acids, including the so-called free fatty acids, (4) a prolonged fasting test with serial measurements of the aforementioned parameters and close monitoring of the blood glucose and (5) an oral loading test with medium chain triglycerides accompanied by the same measurements as those named in item (4).

So far differentiation has been made between patients with a metabolite profile most probably characteristic of medium chain acyl-CoA dehydrogenase deficiency and other dicarboxylic acidurias, among the latter systemic carnitine deficiency. Patients belonging to the first group accumulate octanoate, decanoate and *cis*-4-decenoate in their plasma; they excrete hexanoylglycine, octanoylcarnitine and suberylglycine in addition to the usual C_6–C_{10} dicarboxylic acids. There was a high prevalence of an increased plasma free fatty acid/3-hydroxybutyrate ratio.

INTRODUCTION

The number of reports of patients with non-ketotic hypoglycaemia due to a defect of fatty acid oxidation is steadily growing, as more and more paediatricians begin to recognize the clinical entity. In the past the limited availability of organic acid analysis by means of gas chromatography/mass spectrometry in the paediatric clinical laboratory did not allow an exact diagnosis in many instances.

As a consequence, children with episodic hypoglycaemia leading to (sub)coma were often given inadequate follow-up treatment and counselling. The pioneering work of Gregersen (1976) and the discovery of systemic carnitine deficiency as one of the factors causing this complex of symptoms (Karpati *et al.*, 1975) has been followed by the discovery of a number of different defects of fatty acid oxidation, virtually all leading to similar symptoms. To date the following defects have been proposed or have been proven: (1) systemic carnitine deficiency, (2) long chain acyl-CoA dehydrogenase deficiency, (3) medium chain acyl-CoA dehydrogenase deficiency, (4) short chain acyl-CoA dehydrogenase deficiency (ethylmalonic/adipic aciduria?), (5) hepatic carnitine palmitoyltransferase deficiency, (6) multiple acyl-CoA dehydrogenase deficiency (glutaric aciduria type II) and (7) riboflavin-responsive C_6–C_{10} dicarboxylic aciduria. Still other possibilities, such as palmitoyl-CoA synthetase deficiency and acylcarnitine translocase deficiency may be expected to come to light.

In this paper we describe the various excretion patterns of dicarboxylic acids that have been observed during acute attacks of illness in ten patients with various defects of fatty acid oxidation and the results of clinical tests such as a prolonged fasting test and a loading test with medium chain triglycerides.

MATERIALS AND METHODS

Urinary and plasma organic acids were analysed by gas-liquid chromatography/mass spectrometry of their trimethylsilyl derivatives after extraction with ethyl acetate (Dorland *et al.*, 1983). The presence of acylglycines was checked by analysis of the corresponding methyl esters, which were formed with diazomethane. For a quantitative analysis of glycine conjugates the urine samples were subjected to alkaline hydrolysis (5.5 mol/l NaOH, 100°, 3 h), followed by the usual analytical procedure. 'Total plasma-free fatty acids' (FFA) was calculated by addition of the concentrations of the individual C_{12}–C_{18} fatty acids. Carnitine was measured by an enzymatic method (Pearson *et al.*, 1969). Octanoylcarnitine was identified by a previously described method (Duran *et al.*, 1983) using paper chromatographic separation of the carnitine esters. All other determinations were done by routine clinical chemical methods.

RESULTS AND DISCUSSION

Ten patients were included in this study, with ages ranging from 4 days to 14 years. The clinical history of the patients will be published elsewhere. In summary the symptoms were variable from mild hypotonia to diarrhoea and vomiting with lowered consciousness or deep coma and a rapid death. Six patients died and one of the surviving children had severe brain damage (Table 1). The age of onset of the symptoms did not vary widely,

Journal of Inherited Metabolic Disease. ISSN 0141–8955. Copyright © SSIEM and MTP Press Limited, Queen Square, Lancaster, UK.

Table 1 Clinical findings in dicarboxylic aciduria

Patient no.	'Diagnosis'	Age of 1st attack	Symptoms	Outcome
1	MCAD	19/12	Hypoglycaemia, coma, convulsions	Died
2	MCAD	7/12	(Sub)coma, hypotonia, diarrhoea	Healthy
3	Syst. carnitine deficiency	9/12	'Reye-like syndrome'	Healthy
4*	Dicarboxylic aciduria	2 days	Hypoglycaemia, cardiogenic shock	Died
5*	Dicarboxylic aciduria	3/12	Hypotonia, hepatomegaly, feeding diff.	Died
6	'Riboflavin type?'	14 9/12¦	Hypotonia, coma, rhabdomyolysis	Died
7	MCAD	12/12	Hypoglycaemia, coma	Severe brain damage
8	Dicarboxylic aciduria	9/12	Hypoglycaemia, hypotonia, cardiomyopathy	Died
9	MCAD	1 5/12	Hypoglycaemia, vomiting, coma	Died
10	MCAD	9/12	Hypoglycaemia, coma, 'Reye-like'	Healthy

* Siblings

with two exceptions: the siblings numbers 4 and 5 started having problems very early in life, and patient 6 was already in her teens. The patients were selected for further investigation because dicarboxylic aciduria was found in the urine sample referred for diagnosis. At least five of the present patients showed a virtually normal organic acid pattern when they were in a good clinical condition and fed regularly.

For comparison of the metabolic profiles of the various patients a characteristic urine from each patient was chosen (Table 2). These urine samples were all but one (patient 7) collected during a period of metabolic decompensation. The urine from patient 7 was obtained at the end of a prolonged fasting test. The patients divide into three categories. Five patients had a metabolic profile which included the metabolites hexanoylglycine, suberylglycine and octanoylcarnitine, suggestive of medium chain acyl-CoA dehydrogenase deficiency (MCAD) (numbers 1, 2, 7, 9 and 10, to be denoted ('MCAD-patients'). Octanoylcarnitine cannot be analysed directly. However, the octanoate moiety can be measured easily after alkaline hydrolysis of the urine

sample. Patient 6 had a different profile, with large amounts of glutaric acid (6.28 mmol/g creatinine) and 3-hydroxybutyric acid (3.70 mmol/g creatinine) and small quantities of isobutyrylglycine, isovalerylglycine, hexanoylglycine and suberylglycine. The excretion pattern in this patient resembled that of the riboflavin-responsive dicarboxylic aciduria, as described by Gregersen *et al.* (1982). Patient 6 was moribund at the time of urine collection; no therapeutic trials could be made. The remaining patients 3, 4, 5 and 8 showed only C_6–C_{10} dicarboxylic aciduria (Table 2).

The excretion of 7-hydroxyoctanoic acid seemed to be variable: the highest values were found among the 'MCAD patients'. Patient 7 excreted small amounts of 5-hydroxyhexanoic acid, (684 µmol/g creatinine) and suberic acid (374 µmol/g creatinine) exclusively when he was admitted in coma, but he had already been on i.v. glucose for 1 day. At the end of a prolonged fasting test, however, this boy displayed the full spectrum of MCAD-metabolites in spite of normal blood glucose.

The non-conjugated dicarboxylic acids and (ω-1)-hydroxy fatty acids were excreted by all patients and

Table 2 Urinary excretion of main fatty acid oxidation products in patients with dicarboxylic aciduria (amounts in µmol/g creatinine)

Compound	Patient									
	1	2	3	4	5	6	7	8	9	10
3-OH-butyric acid	1715	844	488	1562	239	3695	490	1406	1286	14455
Adipic acid	5449	563	6024	16672	11229	6462	465	2040	6916	42082
5-OH-hexanoic acid	757	1793	508	1128	160	92	417	230	1440	3400
Hexanoylglycine	1534	tr.	—	—	—	71	1322	—	1626	tr.
Suberic acid	1942	711	624	2373	1578	401	719	562	1787	2571
Suberylglycine	3262	867	—	—	—	602	2848	—	6933	6448
Cis-4-octenedioic acid	406	412	1242	3278	4609	1282	135	527	596	2317
Octanoylcarnitine	3705	126	—	—	—	—	2695	—	1156	993
7-OH-octanoic acid	1153	444	tr.	tr.	—	—	656	192	356	1380
Sebacic acid	6781	tr.	—	745	tr.	87	610	214	1910	7448
Decenedioic acid	3703	192	2512	3445	789	493	427	588	1510	6772
3-OH-sebacic acid	1017	94	377	650	2686	128	269	1141	676	2731

tr. = trace

their concentrations as such do not seem to have a clear discriminative power with respect to the exact diagnosis of the underlying defect. Nevertheless, some interesting observations could be made. Patients 4 and 5 (sibs who died very early in life) had a remarkably high adipic acid excretion, whereas the other acids were rather low. The patients who did not belong to the 'MCAD-group' all excreted saturated and unsaturated hydroxy C_{10} and C_{12} dicarboxylic acids and patient 8 even excreted the hydroxylated C_{14} dicarboxylic acid. However, these acids could also be detected in the 'MCAD-group'; thus their presence does not seem to have discriminative power. There was a significantly lower ratio of unsaturated suberic acid excretion vs. suberic acid excretion in the 'MCAD-group' ($p < 0.05$) compared with the other patients. The analysis of plasma organic acids in these ten patients, either during an attack or after fasting, showed marked differences: octanoic, decanoic and *cis*-4-decenoic acid were only present in samples of the 'MCAD-patients'. The latter compound, unsaturated decanoic acid, is an intermediate of linoleic acid breakdown and its finding supports the hypothesis that linoleic acid degradation involves medium chain acyl-CoA dehydrogenase. The ratio of plasma free fatty acid to 3-hydroxybutyric acid concentrations was increased in all but one patient with dicarboxylic aciduria (Figure 1). Patient 6 had a relatively high plasma 3-hydroxybutyric level of 6.0 mmol/l.

A fasting test was performed in patients 2, 3, 7, 8 and 10, with ages ranging from 8 to 27 months. The test was started on day one after their evening meal and was continued for a maximum time span of 24 h or until hypoglycaemia occurred. Urine samples were collected in three portions: the first sample from the start until the next morning at 8:00, the second from 8:00 to 12:00, and the last one from 12:00 to the end of the test. Venous blood samples were taken at the end of each period of urine collection. Patient 8 was the only one who was definitely hypoglycaemic at the end of the test (blood glucose 2.0 mmol/l). All patients showed excessive mobilization of fatty acids without ketosis (Figure 1). There was an enormous increase of the dicarboxylic acid excretion in all patients.

An oral loading test with medium chain triglycerides (1 g/kg body weight; Liquigen, Scientific Hospital Supplies) was performed in patient 10. Plasma organic acids were analysed at 0, 1, 2 and 3 h and urinary organic acids in samples collected 0–3 and 3–6 h after loading. The patient's plasma 3-hydroxybutyrate level did not exceed 0.5 mmol/l (control 1.6 mmol/l), while the octanoate concentration reached 1.0 mmol/l (control 0.4 mmol/l). The sum of the urinary excretions of suberate, suberylglycine, 7-hydroxyoctanoate and octanoylcarnitine was increased sixfold over the control value. There were no adverse clinical effects during this test. Similar loading tests may be hazardous to 'MCAD-patients' who are not in an excellent clinical condition. Free carnitine and total carnitine was measured in plasma and urine. The results of the plasma determinations are shown in Table 3. The levels of free carnitine were low in all samples. On the other hand the acylcarnitine concentrations were increased in most of

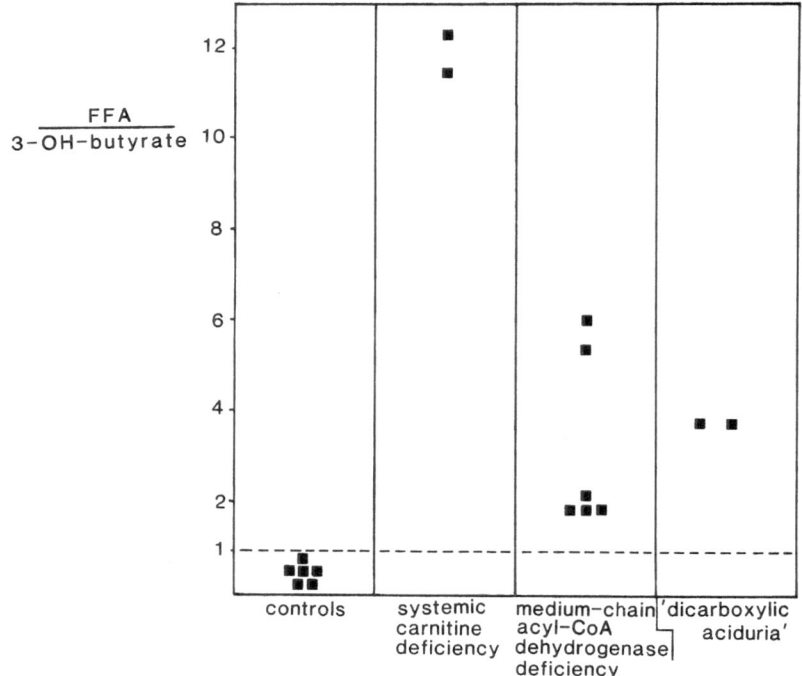

Figure 1   Ratio of plasma-free fatty acid concentrations to 3-hydroxybutyrate concentration. Blood samples were taken either at the end of a prolonged fasting test or on admission of the patient during an attack. The data obtained in patient 6 (possibly riboflavin-responsive type of dicarboxylic aciduria; normal FFA/3-hydroxybutyric ratio) are not shown

Table 3 **Plasma carnitine in dicarboxylic aciduria (μmol/l)**

					Patient					
	1	2	3	4	5	6	7	8	9	10
Free carnitine	13	13	2	14	n.a.	3	18	8	n.a.	1
Acylcarnitine	38	17	3	13		12	6	18		35

n.a. = not analysed
Controls: free carnitine 25–60 μmol/l; acylcarnitine < 5 μmol/l

the patients. This was also reflected in the urinary acylcarnitine excretion (data not shown). The only exception in this series was patient 3, whose total carnitine level was extremely low. Subsequent analysis of his liver and muscle carnitine (H. R. Scholte, Erasmus University, Rotterdam) showed him to have systemic carnitine deficiency. At present no exact diagnosis could be made in patients 4, 5 and 8. The urinary organic acid profile in the latter patients did not differ very much from that observed in systemic carnitine deficiency. Possibly the detailed enzymatic study of the fatty acid oxidizing system in tissues from these patients will give a clue to the nature of their disease.

The inborn errors of fatty acid oxidation leading to dicarboxylic aciduria described here were lethal in most of our cases. It remains to be seen whether a more rapid diagnosis and aggressive treatment will lead to an improvement. The immediate collection of a blood sample and a urine sample at the time of an acute attack is an absolute necessity for a chromatographic

diagnosis. After symptomatic treatment, for even a few days, the excretion of abnormal metabolites may have ceased almost completely. Consequently the diagnosis may be missed when only a sample collected after treatment is analysed.

References

Dorland, L., Duran, M., Wadman, S. K., Niederwieser, A., Bruinvis, L. and Ketting, D. Isovalerylglucuronide, a new metabolite in isovaleric acidemia. Identification problems due to rearrangement reactions. *Clin. Chim. Acta* 13 (1983) 77–83

Duran, M., de Klerk, J. B. C., van Pelt, J., Wadman, S. K., Scholte, H. R., Beekman, R. P. and Jennekens, F. G. I. The analysis of plasma and urinary organic acids during prolonged fasting differentiates between systemic carnitine deficiency and a defect of fatty acid oxidation. *J. Inher. Metab. Dis.* 6, Suppl. 2 (1983) 121–122

Gregersen, N., Lauritzen, R. and Rasmussen, K. Suberylglycine excretion in the urine from a patient with dicarboxylic aciduria. *Clin. Chim. Acta* 70 (1976) 417–425

Gregersen, N., Wintzensen, H., Kølvraa, S., Christensen, E., Christensen, M. F., Brandt, N. J. and Rasmussen, K. C_6–C_{10}-Dicarboxylic aciduria: investigations of a patient with riboflavin responsive multiple acyl-CoA dehydrogenation defects. *Pediatr. Res.* 16 (1982) 861–868

Karpati, G., Carpenter, S., Engel, A. G., Watters, G., Alan, J., Rothman, S., Klassen, G. and Mamer, O. A. The syndrome of systemic carnitine deficiency. Clinical, morphological, biochemical, and pathophysiologic features. *Neurology (Minneap.)* 25 (1975) 16–24

Pearson, D. J., Tubbs, P. K. and Chase, J. F. A. Carnitine and acylcarnitines. *Meth. Enzymol.* 14 (1969) 1758–1771

NOTE ADDED IN PROOF

Enzymological data in cultured fibroblasts from patients 2, 7 and 10 (Dr G. Mitchell, Hôpital Necker des Enfants Malades, Paris, France) suggest that the excretion pattern observed in these patients is due to a deficiency of medium-chain acyl-CoA dehydrogenase and will be the subject of another paper. This should provide the necessary evidence for the next stage in the interpretation of our profiles.

J. Inher. Metab. Dis. 7 Suppl. 1 (1984) 52–56

Animal Models for Dicarboxylic Aciduria

H. S. A. SHERRATT and R. K. VEITCH
Department of Pharmacological Sciences, Medical School, University of Newcastle upon Tyne, Newcastle upon Tyne NE1 7RU, UK

Four compounds, 2[5(4-chlorophenyl)pentyl] oxirane-2-carboxylate (POCA), pent-4-enoate, hypoglycin and valproate, which are hypoglycaemic in fasted animals and form unusual acyl-CoA esters *in vivo*, inhibit mitochondrial β-oxidation by different mechanisms. POCA, hypoglycin and valproate are known to cause dicarboxylic aciduria. Saturated dicarboxylic acids are thought to be derived from long chain fatty acids by peroxisomal β-oxidation when mitochondrial β-oxidation is severely impaired. The use of these inhibitors provides animal models of dicarboxylic aciduria found in some inborn errors of metabolism.

Dicarboxylic aciduria may occur in man in metabolic states where there is excessive fatty acid oxidation, or when β-oxidation is impaired. In these conditions it appears that the supply of fatty acids to the liver is greater than the capacity for β-oxidation and for esterification into complex lipids. It is supposed that some of the excess fatty acids undergo ω-oxidation in a one stage process to give long chain dicarboxylic acids which are then converted to medium chain dicarboxylic acids by β-oxidation. It is difficult to estimate the rates of competing pathways for the disposal of fatty acids in man, and animal models of dicarboxylic aciduria may be useful.

Apart from experimental diabetes with ketoacidosis and the provision of excess dietary medium chain triacylglycerols, dicarboxylic aciduria may be induced by inhibition of mitochondrial β-oxidation. However, there are relatively few selective inhibitors of β-oxidation known, and we have investigated four of these in some detail: 2[5(4-chlorophenyl)pentyl]xoirane-2-carboxylate (POCA), pent-4-enoate, hypoglycin and valproate (Figure 1), although not from the point of view of dicarboxylic aciduria (see Sherratt and Osmundsen, 1976; Sherratt, 1981; Sherratt *et al.*, 1984 for references).

These all act at different sites of β-oxidation (Figure 2). None of these compounds is a clean inhibitor and information about their effects is still incomplete. Further, the pharmacological effects of these compounds differ dramatically depending on whether the animals are fed or fasted. They inhibit fatty acid oxidation and gluconeogenesis in various *in vitro* systems and are hypoglycaemic in fasted animals. POCA and valproate are strongly hypoketonaemic, while by contrast, pent-4-enoate and hypoglycin are hyperketonaemic. Three of these compounds are known to cause dicarboxylic aciduria but pent-4-enoate has not been investigated in this respect. The complex effects of these four compounds on β-oxidation will be outlined and compared. Another model for dicarboxylic aciduria is the severely riboflavin deficient rat (Gregersen and Kølvraa, 1982).

MECHANISM OF FORMATION OF MEDIUM CHAIN DICARBOXYLIC ACIDS

Free long chain and medium chain fatty acids may undergo ω-oxidation by enzymes associated with the endoplasmic reticulum in hepatocytes, which convert the ω-methyl group to a carboxylic acid group. The

Inhibitor	Structure	Clinical implications
POCA	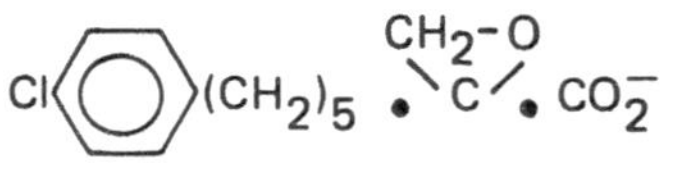	Candidate hypoglycaemic drug
Hypoglycin		Toxin of Jamaican Ackee fruit
Pent-4-enoate	$CH_2{=}CH.CH_2CH_2CO_2^-$	Supposed analogue of hypoglycin
Valproate		Proven antiepileptic drug

Figure 1 Four hypoglycaemic inhibitors of β-oxidation

Journal of Inherited Metabolic Disease. ISSN 0141-8955. Copyright © SSIEM and MTP Press Limited, Queen Square, Lancaster, UK.

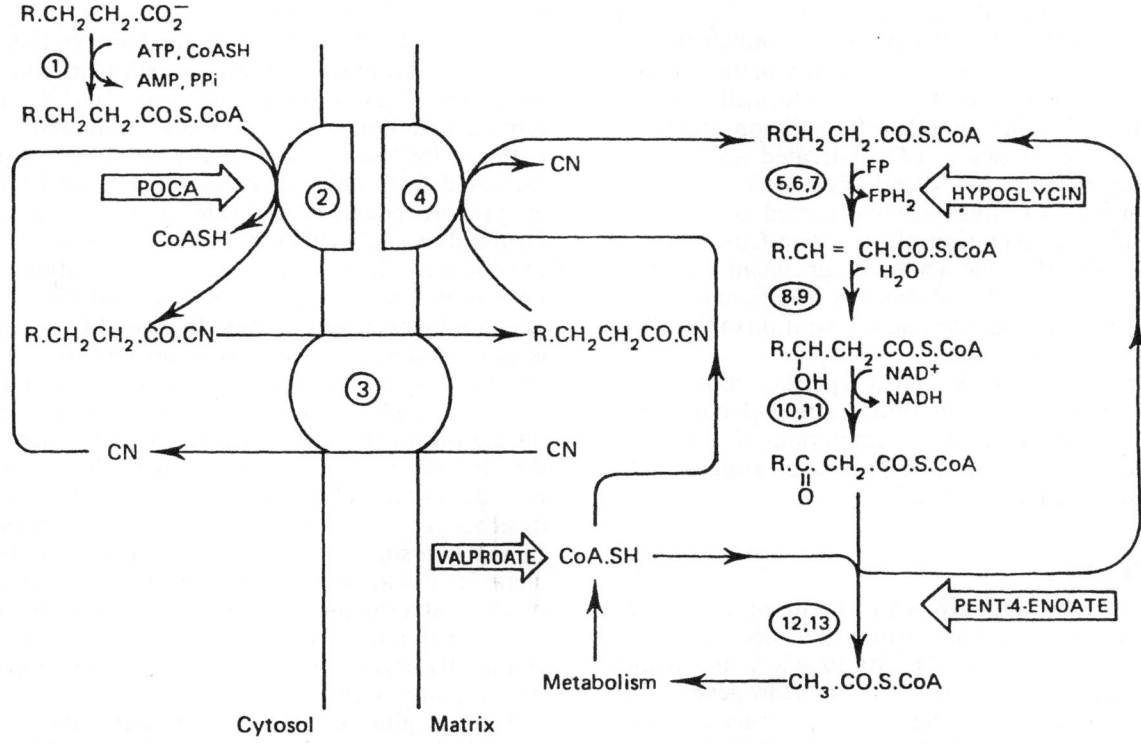

Figure 2 Sites of inhibition of mitochondrial β-oxidation by metabolites of POCA, hypoglycin, pent-4-enoate and valproate. Inhibition is indicated by large arrows. CN, L-carnitine. Enzymes involved in β-oxidation: (1) long chain acyl-CoA synthase; (2) carnitine palmitoyltransferase I; (3) carnitine/acyl-carnitine exchange carrier; (4) carnitine palmitoyltransferase II; (5, 6, 7) palmitoyl CoA, general acyl-CoA and butyryl CoA dehydrogenases; (8, 9) long chain enoyl CoA hydratase and crotonyl CoA hydratase; (10, 11) 3-hydroxyacyl CoA and 3-hydroxybutyryl CoA dehydrogenases; (12, 13) 3-oxoacyl CoA and acetoacetyl CoA thiolases. POCA-CoA inhibits (2), MCPA-CoA inhibits (6, 7), 3-oxopent-4-enoyl CoA inhibits (12, 13), and the formation of valproyl CoA increases the acyl-CoA/CoASH ratio in the mitochondrial matrix, and valproyl CoA presumably competitively inhibits weakly some enzymes with binding sites for acyl-CoA esters

mono-CoA esters of long chain dicarboxylic acids are formed outside the mitochondrial matrix by the action of palmitoyl CoA synthase (Pettersen and Ass, 1973). It is generally assumed that these esters are then subjected to partial β-oxidation in the mitochondrial matrix to the mono-CoA esters of medium chain dicarboxylic acids which are deacylated to the corresponding free acids (sebacic, suberic and adipic acids). This pathway requires the conversion of mono-CoA esters of long chain dicarboxylic acids to their monocarnitine esters by carnitine palmitoyltransferase I (CPT I) located on the outer surface of the inner mitochondrial membrane, which then enter the matrix to reform the mono-CoA esters prior to partial β-oxidation. However, we can find no convincing evidence that mitochondrial β-oxidation of mono-CoA esters of dicarboxylic acids actually occurs. The mono-CoA esters of dicarboxylic acids are poor substrates for CPT I compared with palmitoyl CoA (Pettersen, 1973). When there is an excess of free long chain fatty acids it is unlikely that significant amounts of long chain monocarnitine esters would enter the mitochondrial matrix because of competition by the CoA esters of long chain monocarboxylic acids. Further, there is significant dicarboxylic aciduria in hereditary carnitine deficiency with hepatic involvement, where low cell carnitine concentrations limit

mitochondrial β-oxidation and there is no ketogenic response to fasting (Karpati *et al.*, 1975).

It was shown by Lazarow and de Duve in 1976 that partial β-oxidation of the CoA esters of long chain monocarboxylic acids occurs in peroxisomes. Mortensen *et al.* (1982) have recently provided convincing evidence that β-oxidation of mono-CoA esters of long chain dicarboxylic acids also occurs in hepatic peroxisomes. Therefore, the CoA esters of both long chain and mono- and dicarboxylic acids which accumulate outside the matrix when mitochondrial β-oxidation is impaired would be substrates for peroxisomal β-oxidation.

POCA

The CoA ester of POCA, a candidate antidiabetic drug, is formed *in vivo* and is a powerful inhibitor of long chain β-oxidation at the stage of CPT I. POCA-CoA at low concentrations (< 1 µmol/l) strongly inhibits the oxidation of palmitoyl-CoA plus carnitine, but not of palmitoyl carnitine, by mitochondrial fractions. POCA has little apparent effect on intermediary metabolism in fed animals, by contrast with its powerful hypoketonaemic and hypoglycaemic effects in fasted animals, even though liver CPT I is less sensitive to inhibition by

POCA-CoA in fasted than in fed animals. In this respect, inhibition of CPT I by POCA-CoA resembles that by malonyl CoA which is also most effective in the fed state. Nevertheless, enough POCA-CoA is formed in fasted animals to inhibit mitochondrial β-oxidation, and hence gluconeogenesis strongly. POCA-treated animals are interesting models for dicarboxylic aciduria since inhibition of CPT I would also be expected to inhibit any mitochondrial β-oxidation of the mono-CoA esters of long chain dicarboxylic acids. In agreement with this, saturated dicarboxylic acids (mainly sebacic and suberic acids) are excreted following administration of POCA to fasted, but not to fed, rats.

So far POCA is the most specific inhibitor of mitochondrial β-oxidation studied, although it has a few other effects including some inhibition of fatty acid biosynthesis. POCA may also provide an animal model for hereditary CPT deficiency.

HYPOGLYCIN

Hypoglycin, the hypoglycaemic toxin of the unripe ackee fruit, is converted *in vivo* to methylenecyclopropylacetyl CoA (MCPA-CoA). MCPA-CoA inactivates several, but not all, acyl-CoA dehydrogenases by forming an adduct with their FAD prosthetic groups. This causes severe disturbances of metabolism: (1) mitochondrial glutaryl CoA dehydrogenase is inhibited causing an accumulation of glutaryl CoA derived from the catabolism of lysine and tryptophane and hence glutaric aciduria, (2) inhibition of branched chain acyl-CoA dehydrogenases interferes with the metabolism of leucine and isoleucine causing isovaleric and 2-methylbutyric acidaemia and aciduria and (3) general acyl-CoA and butyryl CoA dehydrogenases are inactivated, but not palmitoyl CoA dehydrogenase, so that mitochondrial β-oxidation of long chain acyl-CoA esters only proceeds as far as butyryl CoA. Butyryl CoA is then deacylated with recycling of CoA, for example

$$\text{palmitoyl-CoA} + 60_2 \rightarrow \text{3-acetoacetate}$$
$$+ \text{ butyrate} + \text{CoASH}.$$

With mitochondrial fractions from liver, the maximum possible rate of generation of acetyl-groups is about 50% of the maximum uninhibited rate. The extent of inhibition may be less *in vivo* with conditions where β-oxidation is not maximal. Ethylmalonic and methylsuccinic acids are excreted in hypoglycin poisoning. Ethylmalonic acid is derived from carboxylation of accumulated butyryl CoA by propionyl CoA carboxylase to ethylmalonyl CoA followed by deacylation, and methylsuccinic acid by isomerization of ethylmalonyl CoA to methylsuccinyl CoA catalysed by methylmalonyl CoA isomerase followed by deacylation.

There is a massive dicarboxylic aciduria in hypoglycin poisoning although there are species differences in response. Large amounts of *cis*-decene-1,10-dioic and *cis*-octene-1,8-dioic acids, but relatively small amounts of sebacic, suberic and adipic acids are excreted by poisoned rats (Tanaka, 1972). In two cases of human hypoglycin poisoning large amounts of adipic acid were excreted together with both saturated and unsaturated

C_{10} and C_8 dicarboxylic acids (Tanaka *et al.*, 1976). Kunau and Lauterbach (1978) have shown that in rats [14C]-labelled unsaturated dicarboxylic acids are derived from [U-14C]linoleate, but not from [U-14C]stearate. Kunau and Dommes (1978) suggested that a major pathway for the mitochondrial β-oxidation of polyunsaturated fatty acids involves the NADPH-linked 4-enoyl-CoA reductase, and this has been supported by Osmundsen *et al.* (1982). By contrast with the formation of saturated dicarboxylic acids, the formation of these unsaturated dicarboxylic aids in hypoglycin-poisoning may not involve peroxisomes. If 4-enoyl-CoA reductase is also inhibited the oxidation of linoleate may only proceed as far as *cis*-4-deceneoyl-CoA and *cis*-4-octeneoyl-CoA which are deacylated and the free acids diffuse out of the matrix where they are converted to dicarboxylic acids by ω-oxidation in the endoplasmic reticulum. The relatively small amounts of saturated dicarboxylic acids excreted by rats poisoned with hypoglycin suggest that β-oxidation of saturated long chain fatty acids may not necessarily be impaired to the extent that a significant saturated dicarboxylic aciduria occurs. This is further evidence that the transport of long chain fatty acyl-groups into the matrix is unimpaired in hypoglycin poisoning.

Type II glutaric aciduria has many similarities to hypoglycin poisoning with a general loss of all acyl-CoA dehydrogenase activities, probably at the level of the electron transferring flavoprotein (Przyrembel *et al.*, 1976). In both conditions there is a large excretion of a similar range of organic acids.

PENT-4-ENOATE

Pent-4-enoate, a hypoglycaemic toxin often wrongly thought to be an analogue of hypoglycin, is rapidly metabolized by many tissues (see Sherratt, 1981). Pent-4-enoyl CoA formed in the mitochondrial matrix is first dehydrogenated to penta-2,4-dienoyl CoA by butyryl CoA dehydrogenase. This is reduced to pent-2-enoyl CoA by the NADPH-linked 4-enoyl CoA reductase. Pent-2-enoyl CoA is then converted to propionyl CoA and acetyl CoA by β-oxidation. Only when this pathway is overloaded by high pent-4-enoate concentrations is some penta-2,4-dienoyl CoA converted to 3-oxopent-4-enoyl CoA which inhibits mitochondrial β-oxidation, apparently by inactivating mitochondrial thiolases. Hepatic mitochondrial β-oxidation remains inactive for 3–4 hours after fasted rats have recovered from the hypoglycaemic effects of pent-4-enoate, so it will be interesting to determine whether dicarboxylic acids are excreted during this time.

RIBOFLAVIN DEFICIENCY

Riboflavin deficiency has many of the characteristics of Type II glutaric aciduria with a massive dicarboxylic aciduria in fasted rats (Gregersen and Kølvraa, 1982). There is a much greater loss of acyl-CoA dehydrogenase activities, particularly butyryl CoA dehydrogenase, than of succinate or NADH dehydrogenases, all of which have flavin prosthetic groups. This results in up to 85%

loss of the capacity for mitochondrial β-oxidation with little effect on the oxidation of succinate or of glutamate (Hoppel *et al.*, 1979), an observation which we have confirmed.

VALPROATE

Valproate (valproic acid, dipropylacetate) is an effective and widely used antiepileptic drug which has on rare occasions been implicated in cases of fatal hepatotoxicity. In therapeutic doses it is hypoketonaemic in fasted rats and normal humans (Turnbull *et al.*, 1983 and unpublished work) and causes dicarboxylic aciduria in these species, particularly during fasting (Mortensen *et al.*, 1980). Valproyl CoA, formed in the mitochondrial matrix, is a weak inhibitor of mitochondrial β-oxidation. This is probably due to an increase in the acyl-CoA/CoASH ratio, and by weak competitive inhibition of various enzymes of β-oxidation. Valproyl CoA only undergoes partial metabolism and it is our impression that most of its metabolites are not very reactive chemically so that enzymes concerned with β-oxidation are not strongly inhibited or inactivated, by contrast with the effects of metabolites of POCA, hypoglycin and pent-4-enoate.

INHIBITION OF β-OXIDATION

The different mechanisms of inhibition of β-oxidation by four compounds outlined here which are converted *in vivo* to unusual CoA esters are summarized in Figure 2. There is also extensive acylation of CoA secondary to the primary inhibitions in hypoglycin and pent-4-enoate poisoning, although this is not complete. It is very unlikely that intermediary metabolism is severely impaired by simple sequestration of CoASH. Metabolic disturbances are probably caused by inhibition or inactivation of specific enzymes by unusual acyl-CoA esters. Indeed, with conditions in which liver mitochondria oxidize palmitoyl carnitine at maximum rates as much as 95 % of the total matrix CoA content may be acylated. The mitochondrial matrix contains up to 5 mmol/l total CoA and there are non-specific acyl-CoA hydrolases with high K_m values for most acyl-CoA esters which oppose *total* acylation of the CoA. Finally, the K_m values for enzymes acting on acyl-CoA esters involved in normal metabolism are usually in the micromolar range. (See Sherratt and Osmundsen (1976), Billington *et al.* (1978) and Sherratt (1981), for further discussion.)

MODELS FOR INBORN ERRORS OF METABOLISM IN MAN

There are many analogies between the effects of inhibitors of β-oxidation in animals and the metabolic consequences of some inherited enzyme deficiencies, particularly those found in the organic acidaemias. These disorders are characterized by the excretion of simple aliphatic acids including mono- or dicarboxylic acids and their metabolites (glycine conjugates, carnitine esters). In most of these disorders the substrate of the defective enzyme is an acyl-CoA ester. The accumulation of abnormal amounts of these esters often causes the resultant metabolic disturbances. It is not surprising, therefore, that the effects of drugs and toxins which are converted to unusual CoA esters have many similarities.

Animals treated with inhibitors of β-oxidation provide models for the study of those inborn errors in man which cause dicarboxylic acidurias, which will be useful both because of the rarity of the inborn errors and the lack of strains of animals with similar defined genetic defects. However, it must be stressed that these models only approximately resemble human disorders. It is usually very difficult to interpret the effects of inhibitors (Sherratt and Osmundsen, 1976) and extrapolation to the understanding of human disease has many pitfalls. Nevertheless, careful studies with these and other inhibitors of β-oxidation will provide valuable information about the perturbation of intermediary metabolism caused by genetic defects.

We thank the Wellcome Trust for support.

References

Billington, D., Osmundsen, H. and Sherratt, H. S. A. Mechanism of the metabolic disturbances caused by hypoglycin and by pent-4-enoic acid. *In vitro* studies. *Biochem. Pharmacol.* 27 (1978) 2879–2890

Gregersen, N. and Kølvraa, S. The occurrence of C_6–C_{10}-dicarboxylic acids, ethylmalonic acid, 5-hydroxycaproic acid, butyrylglycine, isovalerylglycine, isobutyrylglycine, 2-methylbutyrylglycine and glutaric acid in the urine of riboflavin deficient rats. *J. Inher. Metab. Dis.* 5, Suppl. 1 (1982) 17–18

Hoppel, C., DiMarco, J. P. and Tandler, B. Riboflavin and rat hepatic cell structure and function. Mitochondrial oxidative metabolism in deficiency states. *J. Biol. Chem.* 254 (1979) 4164–4170

Karpati, G., Carpenter, S., Engel, A. W., Watters, G., Allen, J., Rothman, S., Klassen, G. and Mamer, O. The syndrome of systemic carnitine deficiency. Clinical, morphologic, biochemical, and pathophysiological features. *Neurology* 25 (1975) 16–24

Kunau, W.-H. and Dommes, P. Degradation of unsaturated fatty acids. Identification of intermediates in the degradation of *cis*-decenoyl-CoA by extracts of beef-liver mitochondria. *Eur. J. Biochem.* 91 (1978) 533–544

Kunau, W.-H. and Lauterbach, F. Inhibition of linoleic acid degradation by hypoglycin A. *FEBS Lett.* 94 (1978) 120–124

Lazarow, P. and de Duve, C. A fatty acyl-CoA oxidising system in rat liver peroxisomes; enhancement by clofibrate. *Proc. Natl. Acad. Sci. USA* 73 (1976) 2043–2046

Mortensen, P. B., Gregersen, N., Kølvraa, S. and Christensen, E. The occurrence of C_6–C_{10}-dicarboxylic acids in urine from patients and rats treated with dipropylacetate. *Biochem. Med.* 24 (1980) 153–161

Mortensen, P. B., Kølvraa, S., Gregersen, N. and Rasmussen, K. Cyanide-insensitive and clofibrate enhanced β-oxidation of dodecanedioic acid in rat liver. An indication of peroxisomal β-oxidation of N-dicarboxylic acids. *Biochim. Biophys. Acta* 713 (1982) 393–397

Osmundsen, H., Cervenka, J. and Bremer, J. A role for 2,4-enoyl-CoA reductase in mitochondrial β-oxidation of polyunsaturated fatty acids. *Biochem. J.* 208 (1982) 749–757

Pettersen, J. E. *In vitro* studies on the metabolism of hexadecandioic acids and its mono-L-carnitine ester. *Biochim. Biophys. Acta* 306 (1973) 1–14

Pettersen, J. E. and Ass, M. ATP-dependent activation of dicarboxylic acids in rat liver. *Biochim. Biophys. Acta* 326 (1973) 305–313

Przyrembel, H., Wendel, U., Becker, K., Bremer, H. J., Bruinvis, L., Ketting, D. and Wadman, S. K. Glutaric aciduria Type II: Report on a previously undescribed metabolic disorder. *Clin. Chem. Acta* 66 (1976) 227–239

Sakurai, T., Miazawa, S., Furuta, S. and Hashimoto, T. Riboflavin deficiency and β-oxidation systems in rat liver. *Lipids* 17 (1982) 598–604

Sherratt, H. S. A. The inhibition of gluconeogenesis by nonhormonal hypoglycaemic compounds. In Hue, L. and van de Werve, G. (eds.) *Short-term Regulation of Liver Metabolism*, Elsevier, Amsterdam, 1981, pp. 199–227

Sherratt, H. S. A. and Osmundsen, H. On the mechanism of some pharmacological actions of the hypoglycaemic toxins hypoglycin and pent-4-enoate. A way out of the present confusion. *Biochem. Pharmacol.* 25 (1976) 743–750

Sherratt, H. S. A., Bartlett, K. and Turnbull, D. M. Four compounds that inhibit β-oxidation: 2[5(4-chlorophenyl)-pentyl]ozirane-2-carboxylate (POCA), hypoglycin, pent-4-enoate and valproate. A comparison of their mechanisms of action. In Kabara, J. (ed.) *The Pharmacological Role of Lipids*, a Monograph of the American Oil Association, 1984 (In press)

Tanaka, K. On the mode of action of hypoglycin A. III. Isolation and identification of *cis*-4-decene-1,10-dioic, *cis*, *cis*-4,7-decadiene-1-10-dioic, *cis*-4-octene-1,8-dioic, glutaric and adipic, *N*(methylenecyclopropyl)acetylclycine, and *N*-isovalerylglycine, and *N*-isovalerylglycine from urine of hypoglycin A treated rats. *J. Biol. Chem.* 247 (1972) 7465–7478

Tanaka, K., Kean, E. A. and Johnson, B. Jamaican vomiting sickness. Biochemical investigations of two cases. *N. Engl. J. Med.* 295 (1976) 461–467

Turnbull, D. M., Bone, A. J., Bartlett, K., Koundakjian, P. P. and Sherratt, H. S. A. The effects of valproate on intermediary metabolism in isolated rat hepatocytes and intact rats. *Biochem. Pharmacol.* 32 (1983) 1887–1892

SECTION III: DISORDERS OF THE RESPIRATORY CHAIN AND THE LACTIC ACIDAEMIAS

J. Inher. Metab. Dis. 7 Suppl. 1 (1984) 57–61

Mitochondrial Oxidative Phosphorylation and Respiratory Chain: Review

D. C. GAUTHERON

Université Claude Bernard de Lyon, Laboratoire de Biologie et Technologie des Membranes du C.N.R.S., 43 Boulevard du 11 Novembre 1918, 69622 Villeurbanne Cedex, France

Basic events concerning oxidative phosphorylation, i.e. the synthesis of ATP at the expense of respired oxygen at the level of mitochondria are described. Our knowledge concerning the functioning of respiratory chain, its structure, organization and topology inside the inner membrane of mitochondria has considerably improved in recent years. A central question – how does the respiratory chain cooperate with ATP-synthetase, also embedded in the inner membrane, to bring about the oxidative phosphorylation of ADP to ATP – has been one of the most challenging and difficult problems in biochemical research. The chemiosmotic hypothesis proposed by the British biochemist Peter Mitchell appears best in describing the basic events of the recovery of the redox energy liberated along the respiratory chain to synthesize ATP through a membrane process. Moreover the chemiosmotic hypothesis is not restricted to mitochondrial oxidative phosphorylation but appears to provide a general explanation to the synthesis of ATP in all transducing membranes: inner mitochondrial membrane, bacterial plasma membrane, thylakoid membranes in chloroplasts of green plants.

Oxidative phosphorylation concerns the synthesis of ATP at the expense of respired oxygen. In aerobic cells much more energy can be recovered for ATP synthesis during oxidation at the expense of molecular oxygen than from anaerobic processes:

Complete aerobic oxidation of glucose
$$C_6H_{12}O_6 + 6O_2 \rightarrow 6CO_2 + 6H_2O \; \Delta G' = -686 \, kcal$$
Production of 38 ATP

Partial anaerobic oxidation of glucose (or glucosyl)
$$C_6H_{12}O_6 \rightarrow 2 \; pyruvate \; \Delta G' = -57 \, kcal$$
Production of 2 to 3 ATP

Respiration essentially refers to the oxygen oxidizing the respiratory chain located in mitochondria and that consumes 90–97% of respired oxygen according to the type of cells.

DISCOVERY OF OXIDATIVE PHOSPHORYLATION

Our modern concept of oxidative phosphorylation really comes from Belitzer and Tsibakova (1939). Cell respiration occurs in three major stages. In the first stage organic molecules – carbohydrates, fatty acids and some amino acids – are partially oxidized to yield 2C-fragments in the form of acetyl coenzyme A. In the second stage acetyl groups are progressively degraded via the Krebs citric acid cycle to yield CO_2 and energy-rich hydrogen atoms which are transferred to electron carriers NAD, FMN, FAD. In the third stage the hydrogen atoms loaded on the carriers are separated into protons (H^+) and energy-rich electrons which are finally oxidized by the respiratory chain with oxygen to yield H_2O.

With the first model of Krebs tricarboxylic acid cycle (Krebs and Johnson, 1937) it was obvious that no phosphorylated intermediate was involved and therefore could not serve as precursor to make ATP. Much later, when the β-oxidation cycle of fatty acid was described by Lynen no phosphorylated derivatives appeared either.

The important contribution of Belitzer and Tsibakova was the hypothesis that the phosphorylation of ADP into ATP occurred during the oxidation of H^+ and electron carriers by the respiratory chain at the expense of molecular oxygen. After 44 years all experimental data prove that they were right. To measure the efficiency of oxidative phosphorylation they introduced the P/O ratio that defined the number of moles ATP synthesized for each atom of oxygen respired:

P/O = number of inorganic phosphate moles used to synthesize ATP/number of oxygen atoms respired to reoxidize H^+ and electrons.

It soon became evident that:

NAD(P) linked substrates had a P/O ratio of 3;
FMN or FAD linked substrates had a P/O ratio of 2;
Oxidation of reduced cytochrome c had a P/O ratio of 1.

CENTRAL ROLE OF THE ATP–ADP SYSTEM

ATP is the major supplier of energy in living cells and, in most cases, with the cleavage of its γ-terminal phosphoryl, with or without phosphorylation of a metabolite:

$$ATP + H_2O \rightarrow ADP + Pi + nH^+$$
$$\Delta G' \simeq -7.3\text{–}8 \, kcl/mol$$
around pH 7 at physiological temperature.

Journal of Inherited Metabolic Disease. ISSN 0141-8955. Copyright © SSIEM and MTP Press Limited, Queen Square, Lancaster, UK.

ATP must be immediately resynthesized to reconstitute our energy stores according to the reverse global reaction, the energy required for this synthesis being essentially supplied by coupling to a redox reaction. The coupled redox reaction can be an individual one as with the 3-phosphoglyceraldehyde dehydrogenase. But in respiring cells, about 95 % of ATP is synthesized by coupling to the reoxidation of electron carriers of respiratory chain.

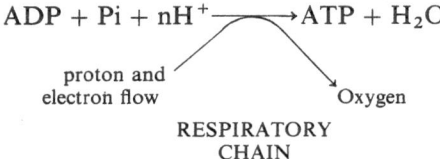

$$ADP + Pi + nH^+ \longrightarrow ATP + H_2O$$

proton and
electron flow   Oxygen

RESPIRATORY
CHAIN

This coupling means that both O_2 consumption and ATP synthesis proceed at the same rate; when energy is needed, ATP is cleaved, the level of ADP becomes high and the rate of oxidation is rapid and the state 3 as defined by Chance and Williams (1956) is reached. In contrast when the cell does not require much energy ATP is high, almost no ADP is available and the rate of oxygen consumption is very slow. This is the 'resting' respiration or state 4 of Chance and Williams (1956), therefore the amount of ADP available per unit of time controls the rate of the respiratory chain, the rate of the respiration. The process is quantitatively very important since an adult human being consumes and resynthesizes every day from 55 to 70 kg of ATP.

LOCATION OF OXIDATIVE PHOSPHORYLATION

In eukaryotic cells the process takes place in mitochondria. Mitochondria have two membranes (Figure 1). The outer membrane is smooth and surrounds the organelle. The inner membrane is the

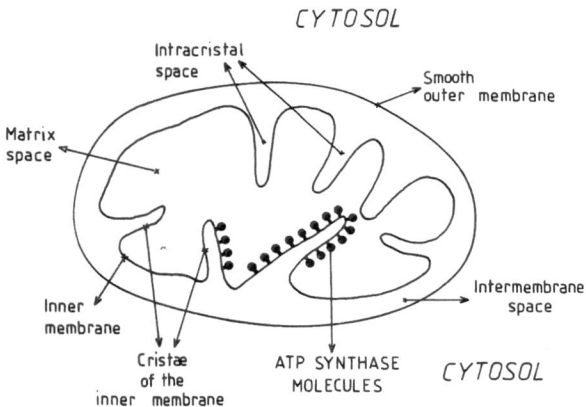

Figure 1 A mitochondrial section showing the various mitochondrial compartments. The intermembrane space contains adenylate kinase and creatine kinase when present (brain, heart mitochondria). ATP-synthase molecules are asymmetrically embedded and the pointing knobs represent the F_1-ATPase part of the synthase that faces the matrix

'transducing membrane' responsible for oxidative phosphorylation; it has a much greater surface area than the outer membrane since it has infoldings called cristae. The intensity of respiration and ATP synthesis is directly related to the number of mitochondria and to the number of cristae. The respiratory chain and the 'ATP-synthase' that makes ATP from ADP and inorganic phosphate are embedded in the inner membrane. Most of the specific dehydrogenases for the oxidation of pyruvate, substrates of the Krebs citric acid cycle and of the β-oxidation cycle, are located in the internal compartment of mitochondria or matrix, very close to the inner membrane or inside the membrane itself.

The outer membrane appears freely permeable to molecules of molecular weight $\leqslant 10\,000$. In contrast, the inner membrane is very selective and impermeable not only to many metabolites but also to small ions like H^+, OH^-, K^+, etc. Since most important events take place inside the inner membrane or in the matrix, special membrane transport systems in the inner membrane promote the entry of pyruvate and other metabolites coming from the cytosol, the entry of phosphate and ADP and the exit of ATP during oxidative phosphorylation.

COMPARTMENTATION AND FUNCTIONAL ASYMMETRY OF THE INNER MEMBRANE

The two membranes create several distinct compartments, as shown in Figure 1. Moreover, complex lipids and enzyme systems are specifically distributed in the compartments, in the membranes, on the various faces of the membranes. This creates a functional asymmetry, as will be described further.

UNCOUPLING AGENTS AND INHIBITORS

Oxidative phosphorylation can be prevented by uncouplers, for example 2,4-dinitrophenol. They allow the electron transport to occur but prevent the phosphorylation of ADP to ATP. This separation of the two processes stimulates oxygen consumption. Uncouplers increase the permeability of the inner membrane to H^+ and therefore prevent formation of proton gradients across the membrane. Such H^+-conducting uncouplers are also called protonophores. Oligomycin and similar toxic antibiotics inhibit the phosphorylation when binding to the F_O part of the ATP-synthase (see Figure 4). Some ionophores, which are lipid-soluble, bind and carry specific cations through the membrane and therefore prevent oxidative phosphorylation. For example the toxic antibiotic valinomycin forms a lipid-soluble complex with K^+ which readily passes through the inner membrane, thus collapsing the membrane potential.

Specific inhibitors of electrons transporters inhibit the respiratory chain at various levels (Figure 2). Many scientists contributed to the discovery and study of the electron transporters of respiratory chain (see review by Keilin, 1966).

SPECIFIC SEQUENCE OF RESPIRATORY CHAIN – SITES OF PHOSPHORYLATION

The sequence of the electron transport chain is shown in Figure 2. When a pair of e^- and H^+ are transported along the respiratory chain from NAD to O_2, three molecules of ATP are synthesized:

$$NADH + H^+ + 1/2 O_2 + 3 ADP + 3 Pi$$
$$\rightarrow NAD^+ + ATP + 4H_2O.$$

Therefore three sites of phosphorylation must be present along the respiratory chain. In addition to the transporters shown in Figure 2, the respiratory chain includes iron–sulphur centres (Fe–S) or non-heme iron (NHI) (Figure 3). Fe–S centres are powerful redox systems which are required for good electron transfer.

THE RESPIRATORY COMPLEXES – RECONSTITUTION

Our knowledge of the organization of the respiratory chain improved tremendously in the 1960s when Hatefi and co-workers succeeded in purifying four respiratory complexes from mitochondria (Figure 3) that appeared to be natural segments of the respiratory chain (Hatefi, 1976). These complexes can reassociate and in the presence of coenzyme Q and cytochrome c reconstitute the electron pathway of the respiratory chain. More and more data have increased our knowledge of the arrangement of proteins in the mitochondrial inner membrane (Capaldi, 1982).

The concentrations of the complexes that are integral protein components of inner membrane have been estimated and are more or less in the same range as the ATP synthase. Minimum molecular weights of the complexes are: 700 000 for I, 200 000 for II, 300 000 for III and 160 000 for IV (cytochrome oxidase) eight. These enormous complexes are made by the association of prosthetic groups and series of different polypeptides: complex I, 26 peptides, complex II, five, complex III, ten and complex IV (cytochrome oxidase) eight. The organization of the complexes and their asymmetry and topology in the inner membrane are known in varying levels of detail, with complex I the least well known and complex IV (cytochrome oxidase) the best characterized.

The arrangement of the eight subunits of cytochrome oxidase is known, as well as the structural model of the monomer and the transmembrane arrangement of the

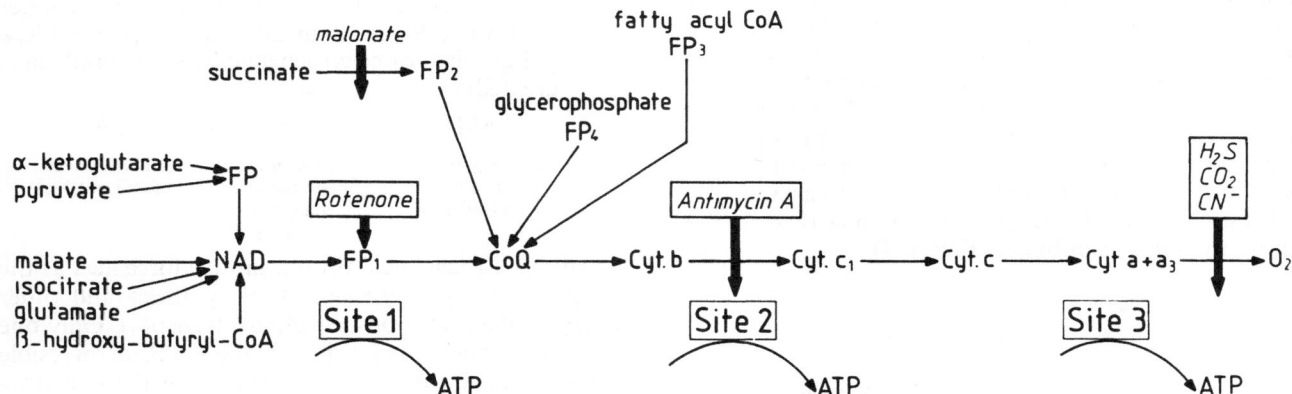

Figure 2 Specific sequence of respiratory chain of eukaryotic cells, sites of phosphorylation and sites of action of inhibitors. FP = Flavoprotein; CoQ = coenzyme Q (for quinone) or ubiquinone; Cyt. = cytochromes. Mammalian mitochondria contain at least three spectrally resolvable species of cytochrome b, viz. b_K or b_{562}, b_T or b_{566}, b_{558}

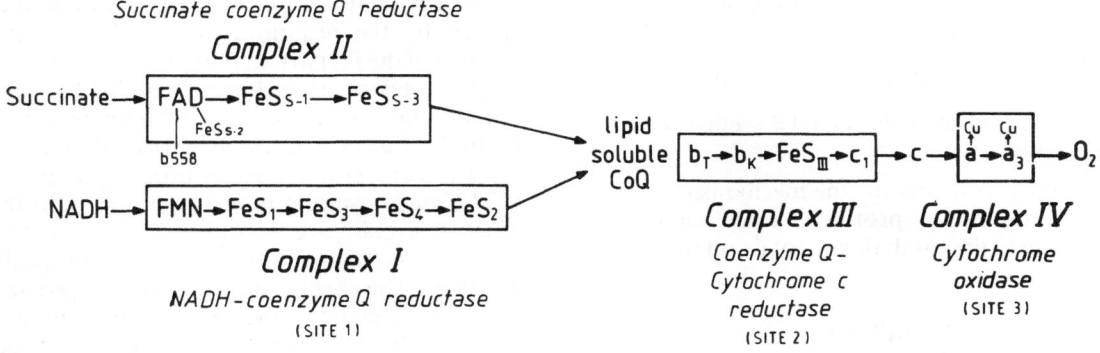

Figure 3 The respiratory complexes. Fe–S: Iron–sulphur centres – b, c_1, c, a, a_3: cytochromes – b_T, b_K: cytochromes b, Transducer and Keilin respectively

dimer. The cytosolic and matrix domains and the location of the copper atoms have been determined. The high affinity site of binding of cytochrome c is on subunit 1 of cytochrome oxidase on the cytosolic domain and on the cytochrome c_1 subunit 4 of complex III, also on the C-side of the membrane. In contrast the oxygen binding site of cytochrome oxidase is not yet clearly understood. NADH and succinate bind to the matrix-side of complexes I and II respectively.

ATP-SYNTHASE

The ATP-synthesizing enzyme system is also a transmembrane complex of the inner membrane, complex V according to Hatefi and coworkers (1976) or $F_O–F_1$-ATPase,. Indeed it has two major components, the factors F_O and F_1. *In situ* F_1 resembles a knob protruding on the matrix side of inner membrane (Figure 1). It is linked to F_O by a stalk. F_O is the very hydrophobic part deeply embedded in the inner membrane and extends across it. The letter O of F_O denotes that this part of the ATP synthase binds the antibiotic oligomycin, an inhibitor of oxidative phosporylation. F_1 was first extracted and purified by Racker (see Racker, 1976). Purified F_1 cannot synthesize ATP but can hydrolyze it to ADP + Pi, thus it is called F_1-ATPase. If F_1 is carefully extracted from inverted vesicles of inner membrane, the vesicles still catalyse electron transport but since the F_1-knobs have disappeared, they no longer make ATP. When purified F_1 is reassociated to the F_1-depleted inner membrane, the knobs are reconstituted and ATP synthesis is restored. This shows that F_1 contains the catalytic sites that make ATP. The $F_1–F_O$ ATP synthase complex is now fairly well understood as well as the asymmetric distribution of its 11–12 protein subunits (five in F_1) across the inner membrane (Figure 4).

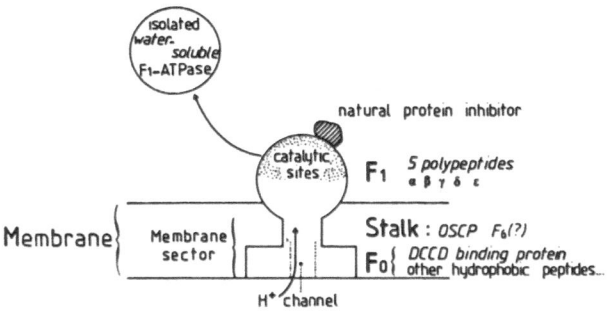

$F_O–F_1$ ATPase –ATPsynthase complex

Figure 4 Arrangement of the $F_1–F_O$-ATP synthase complex in inner membrane

This asymmetry is essential for the mechanism of ATP synthesis. F_O contains a proton channel on the C-domain opposite to the catalytic sites of F_1 on the matrix domain.

MECHANISM OF OXIDATIVE PHOSPHORYLATION

The question that now arises is: how is the transmembrane respiratory chain coupled to the ATP-

synthase to make ATP from ADP and phosphate? Three types of mechanisms have been proposed.

(1) Chemical coupling based on the mechanism of the 3-phosphoglyceraldehyde dehydrogenase and involving high-energy intermediates formed during electron transport was first suggested. All attempts to detect these hypothetical intermediates have failed. Besides, this hypothesis does not take into account inner membrane, and we know that oxidative phosphorylation requires intact inner membrane and impermeable vesicles to take place.

(2) The conformational hypothesis proposed that the transfer of electrons along the respiratory chain produces conformational changes of the $F_1–F_O$-ATP synthase, thus energizing it. Relaxation of the energized conformation provides energy for the synthesis and release of ATP.

(3) The chemiosmotic hypothesis proposed and developed by Mitchell (Mitchell, 1961, 1979) requires a membrane with a low conductivity and impermeable to ionic species including protonated water. The components of the respiratory chain are organized in the inner membrane in such a way that there is an asymmetric translocation of electrons and protons across the membrane. Protons are ejected on the outer face of inner membrane. Since the membrane is impermeable, a pH gradient or electrochemical proton gradient is created:

$$\Delta\tilde{\mu}H = \Delta\psi - Z\,\Delta pH$$

Electrochemical proton gradient	Membrane potential (negative inside)	pH gradient (acid outside).

This electrochemical proton motive force acts as the primary energy source for ATP synthesis and other energy-linked reactions, e.g. active transport. Only one enzyme system is needed to make ATP, a reversible proton-translocating ATPase located in the impermeable inner membrane which can either use the proton motive force created by the electron transport and the proton ejection to make ATP or alternatively hydrolyses ATP and thus creates a proton gradient.

The $F_O–F_1$-ATP synthase system (Figure 5) makes use of the proton motive force. It pumps the protons ejected by the respiratory chain through the proton channel of the F_O part on the cytosolic side to drive them to the catalytic sites located in the F_1 part on the opposite matrix side, where ATP is made from ADP and Pi. In this way both electron carriers of the chain and the $F_O–F_1$-ATP synthase act as proton pumps.

The chemiosmotic model appears to be the best in describing oxidative phosphorylation and to fit many experimental data although it leaves some problems still unsolved. The chemiosmotic model is a general one and is widely accepted as the basic mechanism for coupling ATP synthesis to electron transfer in mitochondria, bacteria and chloroplasts, which all contain transducing membranes with $F_O–F_1$-ATP synthases. Provided there exists some system that can release protons on one side

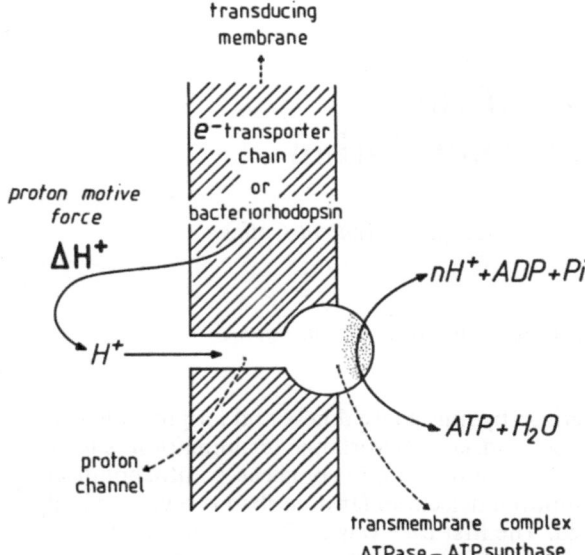

Figure 5 A transmembrane ATP synthase making use of the electrochemical proton motive force to synthesize ATP via the pumping of protons through its proton channel

of an impermeable membrane, the electrochemical potential produced will drive protons through specific channels to the ATP-synthase leading to ATP synthesis on the other side of the membrane. The protons can be produced by respiratory or photosynthetic chains or even by a single photosensitive protein capable of asymmetric proton capture or release under a photochemical event as in the purple membrane of halobacteria.

SPECIFIC TRANSPORT SYSTEMS OF INNER MEMBRANE

As the inner membrane is very impermeable to ionic species, in fact and according to the chemiosmotic model and, since all important events take place in the inner membrane or on its matrix side, the mitochondrial inner membrane (or any transducing membrane) must have the necessary transport systems.

(1) Adenine nucleotide translocase which specifically transports one ADP^{3-} inward in exchange for one newly synthesized ATP^{4-} coming out. It is very specifically inhibited by atractyloside and bong-krekic acid.

(2) Phosphate carrier which is responsible for the cotransport of $H_2PO_4^-$ from the outside together with a H^+ to the site of oxidative phosphorylation.

(3) Other specific transporters are present in the inner membrane, for pyruvate, dicarboxylates (malate, succinate, etc.) tricarboxylates (citrate, isocitrate, etc.), aspartate, glutamate, α-ketoglutarate, etc.

(4) Shuttle systems. Mitochondria are very impermeable to cytosolic NADH, which can however be reoxidized at the expense of respiratory chain due to the existence of special shuttle systems, e.g. the malate–aspartate shuttle. The reducing equivalents of cytosolic NADH are first transferred to oxaloacetate to yield malate catalysed by cytosolic malate dehydrogenase. The malate thus formed

carries the protons and electrons from the cytosolic NADH and passes through the inner membrane on the dicarboxylate carrier. On the matrix side malate is oxidized by the mito-chondrial malate dehydrogenase reducing matrix NAD^+ to $NADH + H^+$ which is finally re-oxidized by the respiratory chain yielding three molecules of ATP generated by oxidative phosphorylation. In brain, skeletal muscle and in insects, the glycerophosphate shuttle occurs.

CONCLUSION

In recent years our knowledge of oxidative phosphory-lation and the respiratory chain has greatly progressed. However, by no means are these simple processes or structures. Obviously many questions on the mechanisms involved in ATP synthesis and the electron pathway in the respiratory chain remain to be answered. Also we do not know as yet whether protons ejected along the respiratory chain are delocalized in the two phases on each side of the inner membrane or localized in special circuits linked to the F_1–F_O-ATP synthase system.

Since this report is included in a Symposium on Inborn Errors of Metabolism, we must stress that the complexity of the systems described here offers many sites or targets where mitochondrial deficiencies might appear. If the deficiencies are too severe, they become lethal.

References

Belitzer, V. A. and Tsibakova, E. T. The mechanism of phosphorylation associated with respiration. *Biokimiia* 4 (1939) 516–526

Capaldi, R. A. Arrangement of proteins in the mitochondrial inner membrane. *Biochim. Biophys. Acta* 694 (1982) 291–306

Chance, B. and Williams, G. R. The respiratory chain and oxidative phosphorylation. *Adv. Enzymol.* 17 (1956) 65–134

Hatefi, Y. The enzymes and the enzyme complexes of the mitochondrial oxidative phosphorylation system. In Martonosi, A. (ed.) *The Enzymes of Biological Membranes*, Plenum Press, New York, 1976, Vol. 4, pp. 3–41

Keilin, D. *The History of Cell Respiration and Cytochromes*, Cambridge University Press, London, 1966

Krebs, H. A. and Johnson, W. A. The role of citric acid in intermediary metabolism in animal tissue. *Enzymologia* 4 (1937) 148

Mitchell, P. Coupling of phosphorylation to electron and hydrogen transfer by a chemiosmotic type of mechanism. *Nature (London)* 191 (1961) 105

Mitchell, P. Keilin's respiratory chain concept and its chemiosmotic consequences. Nobel Lecture. *Science* 206 (1979) 1148–1159

Racker, E. *A New Look at Mechanisms in Bioenergetics*, Academic Press, New York, 1976.

Books and General Reviews

Boyer, P. D., Chance, B., Ernster, L., Mitchell, P., Racker, E. and Slater, E. C. Oxidative phosphorylation and photo-phosphorylation. *Ann. Rev. Biochem.* 46 (1977) 955–1026

Lehninger, A. L. *The Mitochondrion: Molecular Basis of Structure and Function*, Benjamin, 1965, New York

Lehninger, A. L. Mitochondria and biological mineralization processes: an exploration. In E. Quagliariello, F. Palmieri and T. Singer, eds. *Horizons in Biochemistry and Biophysics*, vol. 4 (1977) pp. 1–30, Addison-Wesley, Reading, Mass

Tzagoloff, A. *Mitochondria*, 1982, Plenum Press, New York.

J. Inher. Metab. Dis. 7 Suppl. 1 (1984) 62–68

Mitochondrial Myopathies: Disorders of the Respiratory Chain and Oxidative Phosphorylation

J. B. CLARK* and D. J. HAYES*†
* *Department of Biochemistry, University of London, St Bartholomew's Hospital Medical College, Charterhouse Square, London EC1M 6BQ, UK*

J. A. MORGAN-HUGHES† and E. BYRNE†
† *Department of Clinical Neurology, University of London, Institute of Neurology, Queen Square, London WC1 3BG, UK*

Mitochondrial myopathies are a clinical condition characterized by muscle weakness and fatigue in which the primary defect is localized at the level of the mitochondria. Microscopic examination shows accumulations of mitochondria at the fibre periphery (ragged red fibres) and in some cases mitochondrial paracrystalline inclusions. The spectrum of different mitochondrial defects so far described is reviewed and data from cases investigated in this laboratory are described. The first case was a 17-year-old boy with a multisystem disorder whose muscle mitochondria showed low respiratory activity with all substrates, which doubled in the presence of uncoupler. Further investigation showed that the mitochondrial ATPase activity was only 6% of normal. The next cases were a mother and daughter who showed a typical lipid storage myopathy. The latter was treated successfully with oral carnitine but the myopathy persisted. Mitochondrial investigations indicated a low respiratory activity with NAD-linked substrates but normal activity with succinate and ascorbate + TMPD. A defect in the NADH-CoQ reductase section of the respiratory chain was pinpointed possibly at an iron–sulphur centre. The fourth and fifth cases were two sisters who exhibited no lipid storage myopathy but whose mitochondrial activity was low with NAD-linked substrates but normal with succinate. Again a defect in the NADH-CoQ reductase (complex I) of the respiratory chain was determined. They were also investigated using ^{31}P-NMR. It was found after exercise that their muscle creatine phosphate levels took seven times longer to return to pre-exercise concentrations than control subjects.

These results are discussed with respect to the synthesis of mitochondrial proteins and the influence that both the mitochondrial and nuclear DNA have on this process.

In several human myopathies, the underlying biochemical error has now been defined (for reviews see DiMauro, 1979; Morgan-Hughes, 1982, 1983). Some disorders are associated with an apparent deficiency in the activity of a single enzyme, e.g. myophosphorylase (EC 2.4.1.1), phosphofructokinase (EC 2.7.1.11), carnitine palmitoyl transferase (EC 2.3.1.21). In others, a low level of muscle carnitine has been implicated as the primary defect thus limiting the availability of fatty acids for oxidative energy production. In a third group of disorders, which include multisystem diseases as well as myopathies, defects in mitochondrial oxidative phosphorylation itself rather than in substrate supply have been demonstrated (for reviews see Land and Clark, 1979; Morgan-Hughes, 1982, 1983; Morgan-Hughes *et al.*, 1982; Hayes *et al.*, 1982; Morgan Hughes *et al.*, 1984). In this third group, however, the defect is often less well defined in terms of the specificity of the defective protein. This paper describes the spectrum of defects which have been reported in skeletal muscle mitochondria associated with muscle disease and considers possible underlying genetic factors.

A major clinical presentation in many cases is one of muscle weakness and fatigue. A lactic acidosis usually ensues after very mild exercise (Morgan-Hughes *et al.*, 1977, 1979); some cases present with a systemic lactic acidosis generally in the neonatal period (Van Biervliet *et al.*, 1977; DiMauro *et al.*, 1980; Heiman-Patterson *et al.*, 1982; Stansbie *et al.*, 1982), and in this situation the disease is often fatal. Others, however, present as complex multisystem diseases without detectable myopathy, but on subsequent analysis of the isolated muscle mitochondrial fraction show a defective respiratory chain (see Morgan-Hughes *et al.*, 1982). This may be related to the proportion of affected organelles or cells in any one tissue, and whether this proportion has a discernible clinical effect on the function of the said tissue.

The morphological findings have been similar in most cases reported. With the Gomori trichrome stain (Figure 1a) a varying percentage (10–70%) of muscle fibres have a 'ragged red' appearance (Olson *et al.*, 1972) and stain intensely for some (but not all) mitochondrially located enzymes, e.g. succinic dehydrogenase (EC 1.3.99.1) (Figure 1b). On electron microscopic examination the fibres contain abnormal looking mitochondria, some with paracrystalline inclusions (Figure 2).

Table 1 lists the range of reported mitochondrial defects and is divided into three sections: (1) defects in the utilization of substrate, (2) defects in the respiratory chain and (3) defects in the production of energy. There

Journal of Inherited Metabolic Disease. ISSN 0141-8955. Copyright © SSIEM and MTP Press Limited, Queen Square, Lancaster, UK.

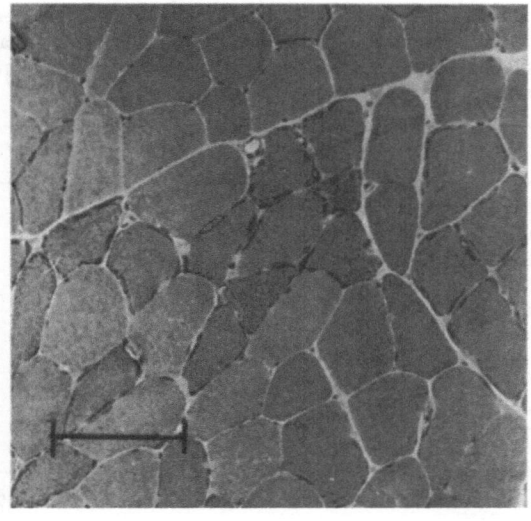

a

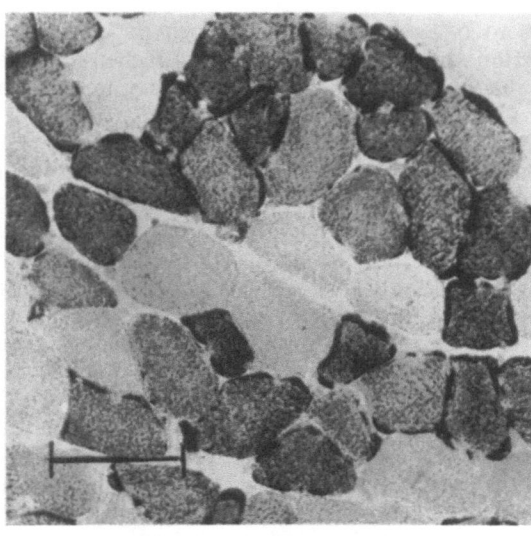

b

Figure 1 Typical histological appearance of skeletal muscle as seen in the mitochondrial myopathies. Muscle biopsy sections from two different patients were stained by the following histological techniques: (a) Gomori's trichrome; (b) succinic dehydrogenase reaction. The ragged red fibres are the fibres which show intense staining at their periphery, about 10 % in (a) and about 50 % in (b). Scale bar = 100 μm

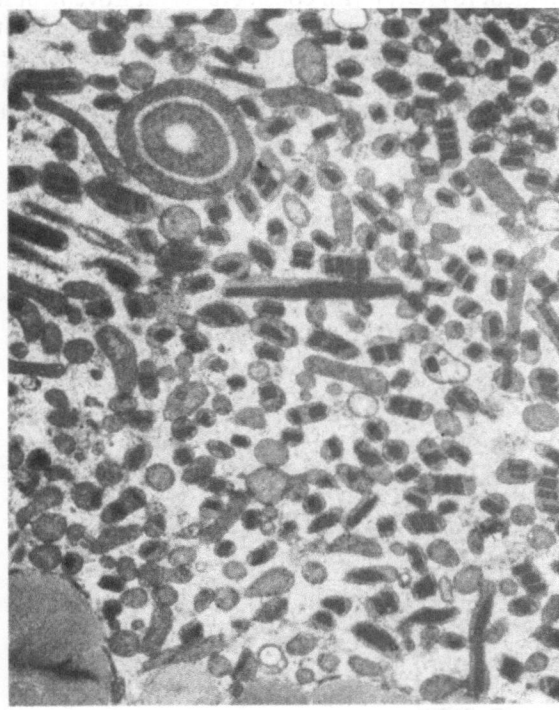

Figure 2 Typical electron microscopic appearance of skeletal muscle seen in the mitochondrial myopathies. The EM shows the accumulation of abnormal and normal mitochondria at the periphery of a muscle fibre. Some mitochondria contain paracrystalline inclusions and others have concentric cristae. × 7500

Table 1   A classification of the mitochondrial myopathies[a]

Defect	References
(1) *Defects in the utilization of substrate*	
Locus	
(a) Monocarboxylate translocase	DiMauro *et al.*, 1973; Kark *et al.*, 1978
(b) Pyruvate dehydrogenase complex	Blass *et al.*, 1970; Robinson and Sherwood, 1975; Robinson *et al.*, 1977; Prick *et al.*, 1981
(c) Carnitine including carnitine-palmitoyl transferase	DiMauro *et al.*, 1973; Engel and Angelini, 1973; Karpati *et al.*, 1975; DiDonato *et al.*, 1978, 1981; Layzer *et al.*, 1980; Cerri *et al.*, 1981
(2) *Defects in the respiratory chain*	
Locus	
(a) NADH-CoQ reductase	Morgan-Hughes *et al.*, 1979; Land *et al.*, 1981
(b) Cytochromes	Spiro *et al.*, 1970; Morgan-Hughes *et al.*, 1977
(3) *Defects in the production of energy*	
Locus	
(a) Coupling mechanism	Luft *et al.*, 1962; DiMauro *et al.*, 1972
(b) ATPase	Schotland *et al.*, 1976; Hayes *et al.*, 1982

[a] With selected references: for a more comprehensive list see Morgan-Hughes, 1982

appears to be no correlation between the site of the dysfunction and the clinical features. Biochemical data will be presented on a patient with multisystem disease and two families with myopathy only.

The multisystem disease patient was a 17-year-old boy who presented at 10 years with muscle carnitine deficiency (Smyth *et al.*, 1975) which responded to oral carnitine therapy (Hosking *et al.*, 1977; Hayes *et al.*, 1982). Although muscle strength improved he went on to develop dementia, ataxia, retinopathy and peripheral neuropathy. At 17 years of age, *in vitro* studies on skeletal muscle mitochondria revealed moderate but coupled respiration with NAD- and FAD-linked substrates (see Figure 3 and Table 2). However, respiration rates were almost doubled (to that of state 3) by the addition of an uncoupler, carbonyl cyanide *p*-triffuormethoxyphenylhydrazone (FCCP), or calcium ions (Table 2). This situation is not normally encountered, i.e. state 3 and uncoupled rates are usually comparable (see Schotland *et al.*, 1976). The cytochrome spectrum and concentrations were within the normal range as were the activities of several key enzymes. Since the uncoupled and the calcium stimulated rates were much greater than that of the state 3 rates, the defect must be distal to the respiratory chain. This may be at the level of the adenine nucleotide translocase or the endogenous ATPase (ATP synthase). Measurement of the mitochondrial ATPase activity showed it to be 6 % of control values (patient's activity 105, controls 1800 ± 480 [SD, $n = 3$] nmol inorganic phosphate/min per mg mitochondrial protein). It would thus seem likely that in this case the rate limiting step was at the level of mitochondrial ATPase (ATP synthase).

Studies have also been carried out on two families; the prepositus in the first family was a 24-year-old housewife

Table 2 Respiratory activities at 25°C of human skeletal muscle mitochondria from a patient with multisystem disease and mitochondrial myopathy (expressed as natmsO/min per mg mitochondrial protein)

Substrate	State 3[a]	RCR[b]	+FCCP[c]	+Ca^{2+} [d]
Pyruvate + malate	36	2.1	71	ND
Glutamate + malate	45	1.9	ND	79
Succinate	61	2.4	110	ND
Palmitoyl carnitine (+ malate)	40	2.4	66	ND
Ascorbate + TMPD[e]	—	—	129	ND

Mitochondrial respiration was studied as detailed by Morgan-Hughes *et al.*, 1977 and 1982 at 25 °C
[a] State 3 = respiration in the presence of ADP
[b] RCR = respiratory control ratio, i.e. respiration in the presence of ADP/respiration in the absence of ADP
[c] Respiration in the presence of uncoupler FCCP (carbonyl cyanide *p*-triffuormethoxyphenylhydrazone)
[d] Respiration in the presence of calcium ions
[e] Tetramethylphenylenediamine

who presented with progressive muscle weakness during her second pregnancy. Muscle biopsy showed a typical lipid storage myopathy (Figure 4). Muscle and plasma carnitine levels were 12 % and 27 % of the mean control values respectively. She was started on oral DL-carnitine supplement (6 g/day) with considerable improvement in muscle strength. 14 months after starting treatment, plasma carnitine was 190 % of the mean control value (36 ± 4.9 [SD, $n = 5$] nmol/ml) and muscle carnitine had been restored to 62 % of the mean control value

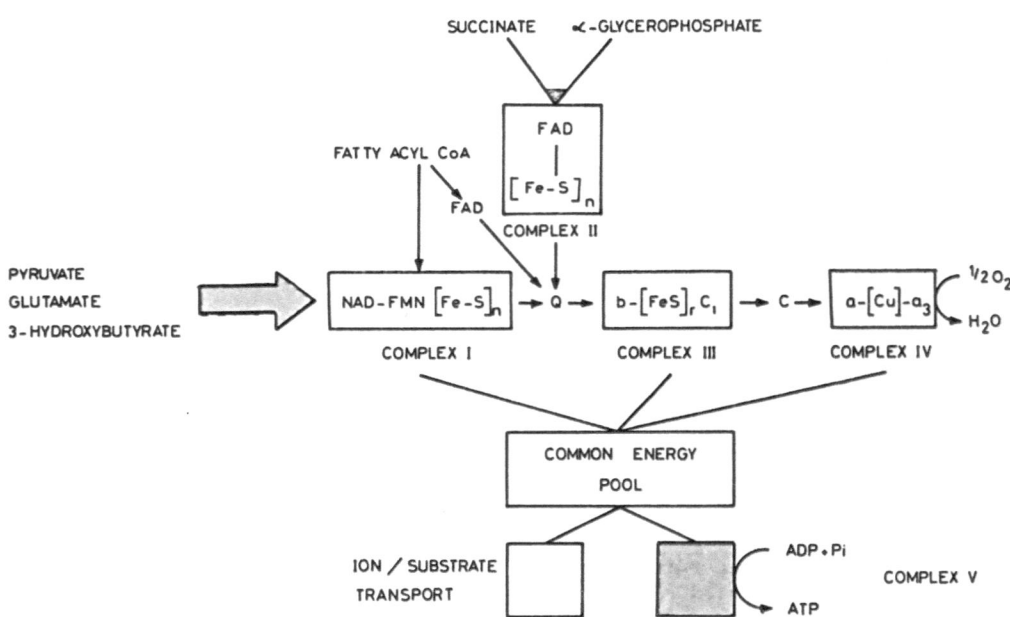

Figure 3 A diagramatic view of the mammalian respiratory chain. The oxidative route for major substrates is also illustrated. [Fe–S] = iron–sulphur protein

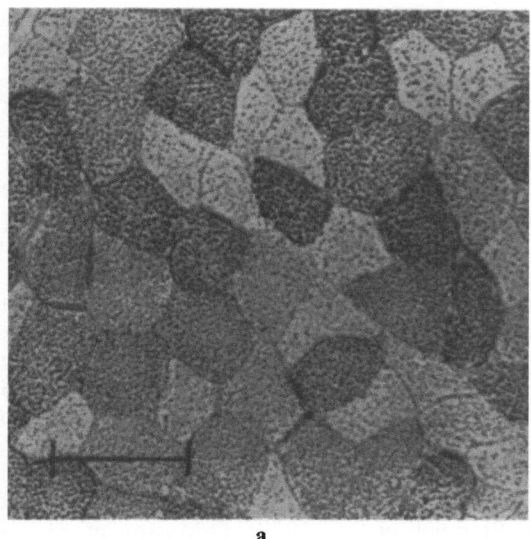
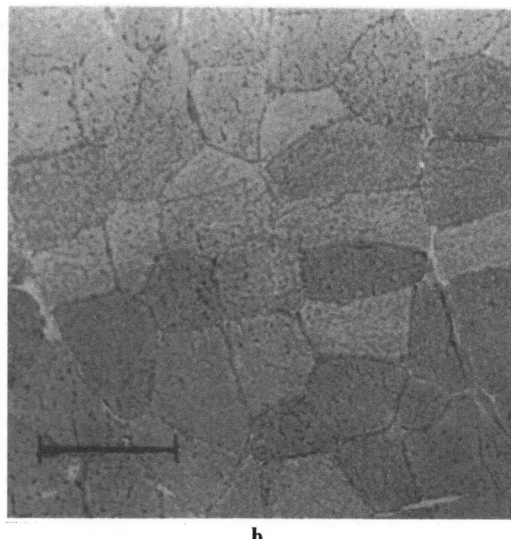

a   b

Figure 4 Muscle biopsies – histological appearance before and after oral carnitine treatment (6 g/day) in one patient. The patient (family 1) presented as a typical lipid storage myopathy; (a) shows abnormal lipid accumulations with the sudan back stain; (b), after 14 months on oral carnitine therapy, the patient was rebiopsied and there was no evidence to suggest any lipid accumulation. Scale bar = 100 μm

(2 ± 0.7 [SD, $n = 28$] μmol/g wet weight). Oxygen uptake studies on isolated muscle mitochondria revealed that NAD-linked substrates were poorly utilized, whilst that of succinate, and ascorbate + tetramethylphenylenediamine (TMPD) were within the normal range (Table 3). However, with the TMPD shunt (Lee et al., 1967) the rates of oxygen uptake with NAD-linked substrates were stimulated. These data suggested that the defect was localized within the NADH-CoQ portion of the respiratory chain. The activity of NADH-ferricyanide reductase (823 nmol/min per mitochondrial protein) was such that it would not be expected to limit respiration and the cytochrome levels and citric acid cycle enzyme activities were within the normal range. The defect thus might be located at one of

the iron–sulphur centres (for reviews see Beinert, 1977; Fleischer and Packer, 1978) within complex I.

The patient's mother gave a long history of muscle pain weakness and fatigue. A muscle biopsy showed lipid accumulation in type 1 fibres and a muscle carnitine level which was 52% of the mean control value. In vitro mitochondrial studies revealed an almost identical pattern of abnormality to that of her daughter (Table 3). These findings suggest that both mother and daugher have a defect located within complex I associated with a lipid storage myopathy.

Two sisters in a second family presented with lifelong muscle weakness and severe exercise intolerance (Morgan-Hughes et al., 1979). A standard exercise test was performed and lactate levels were grossly abnormal. Muscle biopsies revealed 'ragged red' fibres, but there was no evidence to suggest a lipid storage myopathy and the muscle carnitine level in one sister was within the normal range. In vitro mitochondrial studies showed low but coupled respiration rates with NAD-linked substrates (Morgan-Hughes et al., 1979, and Table 4) but normal activities with succinate. These data suggested that the defect was localized within the NADH-CoQ portion of the respiratory chain. The reasons why some defects located in complex I are associated with a carnitine deficient lipid storage myopathy whereas others are not is as yet unclear (Morgan-Hughes et al., 1984).

The mitochondrial myopathies (and multisystem disease states) highlight a unique genetic problem since the mitochondrion contains its own functional DNA (mt DNA; for review, see Schatz and Mason, 1974; Tzagoloff et al., 1979; Grivell, 1983). Mammalian mt DNA has a circular structure approximately 16 000 nucleotides in length and its sequence in man has recently been published (Anderson et al., 1981). Mt DNA is thought to be maternally inherited (Giles et al., 1980; Brown et al., 1981; Lansman et al., 1983) and has

Table 3 Respiratory activities at 25 °C of isolated human skeletal muscle mitochondria from a patient with mitochondrial myopathy, lipid storage myopathy and carnitine deficiency and her mother (family 1) (expressed as natmsO/min per mg mitochondrial protein)

Substrate	Patient		Mother	
	State 3	+TMPD[a]	State 3	+TMDP[a]
Pyruvate + malate	24	141	18	62
Glutamate + malate	0	277	30	142
Succinate + rotenone	97	ND	89	67
Palmitoylcarnitine + malate	0	258	ND	ND
Ascorbate	—	427	—	235

See Table 2 for details
[a] Respiration in the presence of TMPD, i.e. the TMPD shunt (see Lee et al., 1967)

Table 4 **Respiratory activities at 25 °C of isolated human skeletal muscle mitochondria (from a patient with mitochondrial myopathy and NADH-CoQ reductase deficiency (family 2) (expressed as natmsO/min per mg mitochondrial protein)**

Substrate	Patient State 3	RCR	Control: range State 3	RCR
Pyruvate + malate	17	4.3	90–149	2.6–4.1
Glutamate + malate	17	4.3	141–147	2.7–5.5
Succinate + rotenone	50	2.1	55–185	1.7–4.1
Ascorbate + TMPD	68	—	177–493	—

See Tables 2 and 3 for details
Control range taken from Makinen and Lee, 1968, Max *et al.*, 1972, Scholte *et al.*, 1981 and Schotland *et al.*, 1976

13 reading frames, some proteins of which have been identified, namely subunits I, II and III of the cytochrome oxidase complex, cytochrome b and subunit VI of the ATPase. The remaining proteins of the respiratory chain and the vast majority of other mitochondrial proteins are coded for by the nuclear DNA synthesizing systems (see Schatz and Mason, 1974; Tzagoloff *et al.*, 1979). The importation of these proteins from the cytosol into the mitochondrion is a highly complex process and many problems remain to be solved (Schatz, 1979). However, considerable information has been derived from the studies of Schatz and his colleagues on yeast mutants (Daum *et al.*, 1982a, b; Gasser *et al.*, 1982; Maccecchini *et al.*, 1979; Ohashi *et al.*, 1982; Reid and Schatz, 1982a, b; Reid *et al.*, 1982; Solioz and Schatz, 1979; Suissa and Schatz, 1982). A synopsis of their work is that (1) mitochondrial proteins are usually synthesized as larger precursors, (2) the importation of these into the mitochondrion may be energy dependent, (3) the transfer of the precursor proteins across the inner mitochondrial membrane may be coincident with a proteolytic cleavage step(s) and (4) in the case of cytochromes, the attachment of the haem group is important to membrane transferral. Mutations of mt DNA whether by nucleotide substitution, insertion, deletion, etc. are rapidly fixed or lost within the germ cell lineage (Birky *et al.*, 1983; Chapman *et al.*, 1982). There also appears to be a heterogeneous population of mt DNA within the germ cell lineage (see Hanswirth and Laipis, 1982) and the distribution of these at cell division determines the phenotype (Birky *et al.*, 1983). Indeed studies on Chinese hamster cell lines resistant to chloramphenicol suggests that there must be a greater than threshold level of mutant mt DNA in any one cell before the phenotype is expressed (Howell, 1983).

The application of the techniques used in the above studies would give valuable insight into the genetic character of the mitochondrial myopathies. Some of the reported mitochondrial lesions allow one to speculate upon the mode of inheritance and/or site of mutation. The mother and daughter presented in this paper may imply maternal inheritance, although two other sisters, whilst showing slight muscle weakness, have muscle carnitine levels within the normal range. However, the phenotypic expression of the defect may be dependent upon the number of mutant DNA molecules in any one cell/tissue (see Howell, 1983) or the defect may give rise to an activity which, although impaired, is still sufficient to provide for the 'critical flux' of the pathway in question (Kark and Becte, 1981). Another consideration raised by the mother/daughter study presented in this paper is that if their defect is maternally inherited then some translation product essential for the functional integrity of complex I (Ragan, 1976) and/or the fatty acyl-carnitine system must be coded for by mt DNA. Such lesions, i.e. defects of particular proteins in a respiratory complex where the protein in question is coded for by mitochondrial DNA, have been reported, e.g. combined deficiencies of cytochrome b and cytochrome oxidase (Van Biervliet *et al.*, 1977; DiMauro *et al.*, 1980; Stansbie *et al.*, 1982). Furthermore this particular combination of deficiencies has also been shown to be present in numerous yeast strains (Solioz and Schatz, 1979; Nobrega and Tzagoloff, 1980a,b). These yeast cells contained abnormal cytochrome b polypeptides and lacked subunit I of the cytochrome oxidase complex. The combined defect was shown to be due to the split nature of the cytochrome b gene and the faulty processing of the precursor RNA for the cytochrome b and cytochrome oxidase subunit I (Solioz and Schatz, 1979). However, the human mt DNA does not contain any split genes (Anderson *et al.*, 1981) but this does not preclude the sharing of RNA processing enzymes.

In conclusion, these mitochondrial myopathies not only provide an interesting clinical situation but also pose some very fundamental biochemical problems, e.g. what role does oxidative phosphorylation as opposed to glycolytic ATP production play in the contractile process? In the case of one of the families (two sisters), we have been able to study their biochemistry using ^{31}P-NMR. In this study (Radda *et al.*, 1982) both sisters exercised their forearm in the NMR magnet. Spectral studies demonstrated that the creatine phosphate level fell rapidly and after exercise ceased, took seven times longer to return to normal resting concentrations than normal control subjects. Interestingly the intramuscular pH returned to the resting level within the normal time course despite the obvious production of lactate during exercise (see Morgan-Hughes *et al.*, 1979). This may imply that these sisters have evolved more efficient mechanism(s) for exporting muscle lactate. We have also studied an animal model using this ^{31}P-NMR technique (see Clark *et al.*, 1983; Hayes *et al.*, unpublished observations) in which skeletal muscle showed an impairment in oxidative capacity. This model displayed an eightfold longer time course in creatine phosphate recovery after 1 cycle/second stimulation (for 10 min) than controls (Hayes *et al.*, unpublished observations). However, the intramuscular pH remained below baseline throughout the experiment, indicating a slow clearance of lactate or a continued acceleration of glycolysis. Using the animal model it is hoped to increase our understanding of the roles played by aerobic and anaerobic ATP production in muscle function and also to provide some means of therapy for individuals suffering from this situation.

This work was supported by the Brain Research Trust (D.J.H.) and the Muscular Dystrophy Group of Great Britain (J.M.H.) We also thank Dr G. K. Radda and his colleagues of Oxford University for the use of their NMR facilities. The electron micrograph was kindly provided by Dr D. N. Landon (Institute of Neurlogy, London).

References

Anderson, S., Bankier, A. T., Barrell, B. G., de Bruijn, M. M. L., Coulson, A. R., Drouin, J., Eperon, I. C., Mierlich, P., Roe, B. A. Sanger, F., Schreier, P. H., Smith, A. J. M., Staden, P. and Young, I. G. S. Sequences and organisation of the human mitochondrial genome. *Nature (London)* 290 (1981) 457–465

Beinert, H. Iron sulphur centres of the mitochondrial electron transfer system — recent developments. In Lovenberg, W. (ed.) *Iron-Sulfur Proteins*, Vol. III, Academic Press, New York, 1977

Birky, C. W., Acton, A. R., Dietrich, R. and Carver, M. Mitochondrial transmission genetics: replication, recombination and segregation of mitochondrial DNA and its inheritance crosses. In Slonimski, P., Borst, P. and Attardi, G. (eds.) *Mitochondrial Genes*, Cold Spring Harbor Laboratory, N.Y. (Symp. Quant. Biol), 1982, pp. 333–348

Birky, C. W., Maruyama, T. and Fuerst, P. Population and evolutionary genetic theory for genes in mitochondria and chloroplasts. *Genetics* 103 (1983) 513–527

Blass, J. P., Avigon, J. and Uhlendorf, B. W. A defect in pyruvate decarboxylase in a child with an intermittent movement disorder. *J. Clin. Invest.* 49 (1970) 423–432

Brown, G. G., Castora, F. J., Frantz, S. C. and Simpson, M. V. Mitochondrial DNA polymorphism: evolutionary studies on the genus Rattus. *Ann. N Y Acad. Sci.* 361 (1981) 135–153

Cerri, C. G., Meola, G. and Scarlato, G. Biochemical and morphological studies on a case of systemic carnitine deficiency. *Acta Neuropathol.* 7 (1981) 219–220

Chapman, R. W., Stephens, J. C., Lansman, R. A. and Avise, J. C. Models of mitochondrial DNA transmission genetics and evolution in higher eucaryotes. *Genet. Res.* 40 (1982) 41–57

Clark, J. B., Hayes, D. J., Byrne, E. and Morgan-Hughes, J. A. Mitochondrial myopathies – defects in mitochondrial metabolism in human skeletal muscle. *Biochem. Soc. Trans.* 11 (1983) 626–627

Daum, G., Bohni, P. C. and Schatz, G. Import of proteins into mitochondria. Cytochrome b_2 and cytochrome c peroxides are located in the intermembrane space of yeast mito-chondria. *J. Biol. Chem.* 257 (1982a) 13028–13033

Daum, G., Gasser, S. M. and Schatz, G. Import of proteins into mitochondria. Energy dependent, two step processing of the intermembrane space enzyme cytochrome b_2 by isolated yeast mitochondria. *J. Biol. Chem.* 257 (1982b) 13075–13080

DiDonato, S., Castiglione, A., Rinold, M., Cornelio, F., Vendemia, F., Cardace, G. and Bertagnolio, B. Heterogeneity of carnitine palmitoyl transferase deficiency. *J. Neurol. Sci.* 50 (1981) 207–215

DiDonato, S., Cornelio, F., Pacini, L., Peluchetti, D. and Rimoldi, M. Muscle carnitine palmitoyl transferase deficiency. A case with enzyme deficiency in cultured fibroblasts. *Ann. Neurol.* 4 (1978) 465–467

DiMauro, S. Metabolic myopathies. In Vinken, P. J. *et al.* (eds.) *Handbook of Clinical Neurology*, North Holland, Amsterdam, 1979, pp. 175–234

DiMauro, S., Bonilla, E., Lee, C. P., Schotland, D. L., Scarpa, A., Conn, H. and Chance, B. Lufts disease: further biochemical and ultrastructural studies of skeletal muscle in the 2nd case. *J. Neurol. Sci.* 27 (1972) 217–232

DiMauro, S., Schotland, D. L., Bonilla, E., Lee, C. P., Gambetti, P. L. and Rowland, L. P. Progressive ophthalmo-plegia, glycogen storage and abnormal mitochondria. *Arch. Neurol.* 29, (1973) 170–179

DiMauro, S., Mendell, J. R., Sahenk, Z., Bachman, D., Scarpa, A., Scofield, R. M. and Reiner, C. Fatal infantile mitochondrial myopathy and renal dysfunction due to cytochrome C oxidase deficiency. *Neurology* 30 (1980) 795–804

Engel, A. G. and Angelini, C. Carnitine deficiency of human skeletal muscle with associated lipid storage myopathy. A new syndrome. *Science* 179 (1973) 889–902

Fleischer, S. and Packer, L. (eds.) Biological oxidations. Mitochondrial and microbial systems. *Meth. Enzymol.* (1978) LIII

Gasser, S. M., Daum, G. and Schatz, G. Import of proteins into mitochondria. Energy-dependent uptake of precursors by isolated mitochondria. *J. Biol. Chem.* 257 (1982) 13034–13041

Giles, C., Blanc, H., Cann, H. M. and Wallace, D. C. Maternal inheritance of human mitochondrial DNA. *Proc. Natl. Acad. Sci. USA* 77 (1980) 6715–6719

Grivell, L. A. Mitochondrial DNA. *Sci. Am.* 248 (1983) 60–73

Hanswirth, W. W. and Paipis, P. J. Rapid variation in mammalian mitochondrial genotypes: Implications for the mechanism of a maternal inheritance. In Slonimski, P., Borst, P. and Attardi, G. (eds.), *Mitochondrial Genes*, Cold Spring Harbor Laboratory, NY (Symp. Quant. Biol.), 1982, pp. 137–142

Hayes, D. J., Summers, B. A., Morgan-Hughes, J. A. and Clark, J. B. A combined deficiency of muscle carnitine and mitochondrial ATPase activity in a patient with multisystem disease partially responsive to oral carnitine. In *Proceedings of the 5th International Congress on Neuromuscular Diseases*, Marseilles, 1982, Abstr. 16.4

Heiman-Patterson, T. D., Bonilla, E., DiMauro, S., Foreman, J. and Schotland, D. L. Cytochrome c oxidase deficiency in a floppy infant. *Neurology* 32 (1982) 898–900

Hosking, G. P., Cavanagh, N. P. C., Smyth, D. P. L. and Wilson, J. Oral treatment of carnitine myopathy. *Lancet* 1 (1977) 853

Howell, N. Origin, cellular expression and hybrid transmission of mitochondrial CAP-R, Pyr-INDr OLI-r mutant pheno-types. *Somatic Cell Genet.* 9 (1983) 1–24

Kark, R. A. P. and Becte, D. M. Multiple genotypes, multiple phenotypes and partial defects. *Muscle Nerve* 4 (1981) 31–40

Kark, R. A. P., Rodriguez-Budelli, M. and Blass, J. P. Evidence for a primary defect of lipoamide dehydrogenase in Friedreich's ataxia. *Adv. Neurol.* 21 (1978) 163–180

Karpati, G., Carpenter, S., Engel, A., Watters, G., Allen, J., Rothman, S., Klassen, G. and Mamer, O. A. The syndrome of systemic carnitine deficiency. *Neurology* 25 (1975) 16–24

Land, J. M. and Clark, J. B. Mitochondrial myopathies. *Biochem. Soc. Trans.* 7 (1979) 231–245

Land, J. M., Morgan-Hughes, J. A. and Clark, J. B. Mitochondrial myopathy – biochemical studies revealing a deficiency of NADH–cytochrome b reduction activity. *J. Neurol. Sci.* 50 (1981) 1–13

Lansman, R. A., Avise, J. C. and Huettel, M. D. Critical experimental test of the possibility of 'paternal leakage' of mitochondrial DNA. *Proc. Natl. Acad. Sci. USA* 80 (1983) 1969–1971

Layzer, R. B., Havel, R. J. and McIlroy, M. B. Partial deficiency of carnitine palmitoyl transferase: physiological and biochemical consequences. *Neurology* 30 (1980) 627–633

Lee, C. P., Sottocasa, E. L. and Ernster, L. Use of artificial electron acception for abbreviated phosphorylating electron transport: flavin cytochrome c. *Meth. Enzymol.* X (1967) 33–37

Luft, R., Ikkos, D., Palmieri, G., Ernster, L. and Afzelius, B. A case of severe hypermetabolism of non-thyroid origin with a defect in the maintenance of respiratory control: a correlated clinical, biochemical and morphological study. *J. Clin. Invest.* 41 (1962) 1776–1804

Maccecchini, M. L., Ruhin, Y., Blobel, G. and Schatz, G. Import of proteins into mitochondria: precursor forms of the extra-mitochondrially made F_1-ATPase subunits in yeast. *Proc. Natl. Acad. Sci. USA* 76 (1979) 343–347

Makinen, M. W. and Lee, C. P. Biochemical studies of skeletal muscle mitochondria I. Microanalysis of cytochrome content, oxidative phosphorylative activities of mammalian skeletal muscle mitochondria. *Arch. Biochem. Biophys.* 126 (1968) 75–82

Max, S. R., Garbus, J. and Wehman, H. J. Simple procedure for the rapid isolation of functionally intact mitochondria from human and rat skeletal muscle. *Anal. Biochem. Sci.* 46 (1972) 576–584

Morgan-Hughes, J. A. Defects of the energy pathways of skeletal muscle. In Matthews, W. B. and Glaser, G. H. (eds.) *Recent Advances in Clinical Neurology*, Churchill Livingstone, Edinburgh, 1982, pp. 1–46

Morgan-Hughes, J. A. Disorders of mitochondrial metabolism; some clinical biochemical mechanisms. In Saunders, K. B. (ed.) *Advanced Medicine 19*, Pitman, London, 1983, pp. 243–260

Morgan-Hughes, J. A., Darveniza, P., Kahn, S. M., Landon, D. N., Sherratt, R. M., Land, J. M. and Clark, J. B. A mitochondrial myopathy characterised by a deficiency in reducible cytochrome b. *Brain* 100 (1977) 617–640

Morgan-Hughes, J. A., Darveniza, P., London, D. N., Land, J. M. and Clark, J. B. A mitochondrial myopathy with a deficiency of respiratory chain NADH-CoQ reductase activity. *J. Neurol. Sci.* 43 (1979) 27–46

Morgan-Hughes, J. A., Hayes, D. J. and Clark, J. B. Mitochondrial myopathies. In Serratrice, G. *et al.* (eds.) *Neuromuscular Diseases*, 1984, Raven Press, New York, pp. 79–87

Morgan-Hughes, J. A., Hayes, D. J., Clark, J. B., Landon, D. N., Swash, M., Stark, R. J. and Rudge, P. Mitochondrial encephalomyopathies. Biochemical studies in two cases revealing defects in the respiratory chain. *Brain* 105 (1982) 553–582

Nobrega, F. G. and Tzagoloff, A. Assembly of mitochondrial membrane system complete restriction map of the cytochrome b region of mitochondrial DNA in *S. cerevisiae*. *J. Biol. Chem.* 255 (1980a) 9821–9827

Nobrega, F. G. and Tzagoloff, A. Assembly of mitochondrial membrane system: DNA sequence and organisation of the cytochrome b gene in *S. cervisiae*. *J. Biol. Chem.* 255 (1980b) 9828–9837

Ohashi, A., Gibson, J., Gregor, I. and Schatz, G. Import of proteins into mitochondria. The precursor of cytochrome c_1 is processed in two steps, one of them home dependent. *J. Biol. Chem.* 257 (1982) 13042–13047

Olson, W., Engel, W. K., Walsh, G. O. and Einaugler, R. Oculo cranio somatic neuromuscular disease with 'ragged red' fibres. *Arch. Neurol.* 26 (1972) 193–211

Prick, M., Gabreëls, F., Renier, W., Trijbels, F., Jasper, H., Lamen, H. and Kok, J. Pyruvate dehydrogenase deficiency restricted to brain. *Neurology* 31 (1981) 227–230

Radda, G. K., Bore, P. J., Gadian, G. D., Ross, B. D., Styles, P., Taylor, D. J. and Morgan-Hughes, J. A. ^{31}P NMR

examination of 2 patients with NADH-CoQ reductase deficiency. *Nature (London)* 295 (1982) 608–609

Ragan, C. I. NADH-ubiquinone oxido reductase. *Biochim. Biophys. Acta* 456 (1976) 249–290

Reid, G. A. and Schatz, G. Import of proteins into mitochondria. Yeast cells grown in the presence of carbonyl cyanide m-chlorophenyl-hydrazone accumulate massive amounts of some mitochondrial precursor polypeptides. *J. Biol. Chem.* 257 (1982a) 13056–13061

Reid, G. A. and Schatz, G. Import of proteins into mitochondria. Extramitochondrial pools and post translational import of mitochondrial protein precursors *in vivo*. *J. Biol. Chem.* 257 (1982b) 13062–13067

Reid, G. A., Yonetani, T. and Schatz, G. Import of proteins into mitochondria. Import and maturation of the mitochondrial intermembrane space enzymes cytochrome b_2 and cytochrome c peroxidase in intact yeast cells. *J. Biol. Chem.* 257 (1982) 13068–13074

Robinson, B. H. and Sherwood, W. G. Pyruvate dehydrogenase phosphatase deficiency: a cause of congenital chronic lactic acidosis in infancy. *Pediatr. Res.* 9 (1975) 935–939

Robinson, B. H., Taylor, J. and Sherwood, W. G. Deficiency of dihydrolipoyl dehydrogenase (a component of pyruvate and α ketoglutarate dehydrogenase complexes). A cause of congenital chronic lactic acidosis in infancy. *Pediatr. Res.* 11 (1977) 1198–1202

Schatz, G. How mitochondria import proteins from the cytoplasm. *FEBS Lett.* 103 (1979) 201–211

Schatz, G. and Mason, T. C. The biosynthesis of mitochondrial proteins. *Annu. Rev. Biochem.* 43 (1974) 51–87

Scholte, H. R., Busch, H. F. M. and Luft-Houwen, I. E. M. Functional disorders of mitochondria in muscle diseases – respiratory chain phosphorylation – the carnitine system. In Busch, H. F. M., Jennekens, G. G. J. and Scholte, H. R. (eds.) *Mitochondria and Muscular Diseases*, Mefar b.v., The Netherlands, 1981, pp. 133–145

Schotland, D. L., DiMauro, S., Bonilla, F., Scarpa, A. and Lee, C. P. Neuromuscular disorder associated with a defect in mitochondrial energy supply. *Arch. Neurol.* 33 (1976) 475–479

Smyth, D. P. L., Lake, B. D., MacDermot, J. and Wilson, J. Inborn error of carnitine metabolism (carnitine deficiency) in man. *Lancet* 1 (1975) 1198–1199

Solioz, M. and Schatz, G. Mutations in putative intervening sequences of the mitochondrial cytochrome b gene of yeast produce abnormal cytochrome b polypeptides. *J. Biol. Chem.* 254 (1979) 9331–9334

Spiro, A. J., Moore, C. L., Prineas, J. W., Strasberg, P. M. and Rapin, I. A cytochrome related inherited disorder of the nervous system and muscle. *Arch. Neurol.* 23 (1970) 103–112

Stansbie, D., Dormer, R. L. and Hughes, I. A. Mitochondrial myopathy with skeletal muscle cytochrome-c-oxidase deficiency. *J. Inher. Metab. Dis.* 5 (1982) 27

Suissa, M. and Schatz, G. Import of proteins into mitochondria. Translatable mRNAs for imported mitochondrial proteins are present in free as well as mitochondria-bound cytoplasmic polysomes. *J. Biol. Chem.* 257 (1982) 13048–13055

Tzagoloff, A., Macino, G. and Sebalb, W. Mitochondrial genes and translation products. *Annu. Rev. Biochem.* 48 (1979) 419–441

Van Biervliet, J. P. G. M., Bruinis, L., Ketting, D., de Bree, P. K., Van der Heiden, C., Wadman, S. K., Willems, J. L., Bookelman, H., Van Haelst, V. and Monnens, A. H. Hereditary mitochondrial myopathy with lactic acidaemia – a de Toni–Fanconi–Debré Syndrome and a defective respiratory chain in voluntary striated muscle. *Pediatr. Res.* 11 (1977) 1088–1090

J. Inher. Metab. Dis. 7 Suppl. 1 (1984) 69–73

Lactic Acidaemia

B. H. ROBINSON and W. G. SHERWOOD

Research Institute, The Hospital for Sick Children, 555 University Avenue, Toronto, Ontario, Canada, M5G 1X8 and the Departments of Pediatrics and Biochemistry, University of Toronto, Ontario, Canada

Congenital childhood lactic acidaemia is a poorly understood group of genetic diseases. The most common underlying inherited defect encountered in this group is deficiency of the pyruvate dehydrogenase complex. Of 23 cases we have diagnosed, 18 have a deficiency in the first component of the complex, the E_1 decarboxylase, while the other five have multiple α-keto acid dehydrogenase deficiency due to a defect in lipoamide dehydrogenase. In addition to the lactic acidosis associated with pyruvate decarboxylase deficiency, ten of the cases showed evidence of facial dysmorphism consisting of a narrow head, wide nasal bridge and flared nostrils or gross microcephaly. Two further patients had agenesis of the corpus callosum. Isolated pyruvate carboxylase deficiency was found to present in two different forms, one with lactic acidaemia and mental retardation, the other with lactic acidaemia, hyperammonaemia citrullinaemia and hyperlysinaemia. The former presentation we have shown to be associated with the presence of a biotinylated pyruvate carboxylase protein of the correct subunit molecular weight (125 kd) which has no catalytic activity (CRM + ve). The latter we have shown to be associated with the absence of any recognizable pyruvate carboxylase protein (CRM − ve).

INTRODUCTION

Congenital childhood lactic acidaemia is a poorly understood group of genetic diseases. Because lactic acid accumulation in this syndrome is in general (but not always) a function of pyruvate accumulation, anything that interferes with the metabolism of pyruvate has the potential to cause lactic acidaemia. Thus lactic acidaemia is known to be present in the acute stages of many of the organic acidurias such as propionic, methylmalonic and 3-hydroxy-3-methylglutaric aciduria probably because of the interference with coenzyme A metabolism in relation to its role in the pyruvate dehydrogenase complex. Lactic acidaemia may also arise because of the failure of an organ system which plays an important role in lactic acid removal, this being a common feature of hereditary diseases where liver function is compromised. In recent years we have been concerned with identifying inborn errors of pyruvate metabolism that result in primary lactic acidaemia and we have found that there is considerable heterogeneity among this group.

PYRUVATE DEHYDROGENASE DEFICIENCY

By far the most common inherited defect encountered is deficiency of the pyruvate dehydrogenase complex (EC 1.2.4.1) (Blass *et al.*, 1970, 1971a, b; Farmer *et al.*, 1973; Farrel *et al.*, 1975; Strömme *et al.*, 1976). In cultured skin fibroblasts we have been able to identify a total of 23 cases and these resolve into two distinct types. Eighteen cases (Table 1) have a deficiency in the first component of the complex, the E_1 pyruvate decarboxylase (EC 4.1.1.1; McKusick 20880) (Robinson *et al.*, 1980; Robinson, 1982). A smaller group of five show not only a deficiency of the pyruvate dehydrogenase complex but also of the α-ketoglutarate dehydrogenase and the branched chain keto acid dehydrogenase complexes (Munnich *et al.*, 1982; Robinson *et al.*, 1981; Taylor *et*

al., 1978). Isolated deficiency of the other α-keto acid dehydrogenase complexes are known, deficiency of the E_1 component of the branched chain α-keto acid dehydrogenase (EC 1.2.4.3) complex resulting in maple syrup urine disease (McKusick 24680) (Chuang *et al.*, 1982) and deficiency of the E_1 component of the 2-oxoglutarate dehydrogenase complex (EC 1.2.4.2) resulting in 2-oxoglutaric aciduria (Kohlschütter *et al.*, 1982). Combined deficiency of the α-keto acid dehydrogenase complexes in some cases can definitively be ascribed to a deficiency of lipoamide dehydrogenase (EC 1.6.4.3), the third component of the three complexes (Robinson *et al.*, 1978, 1981). In other cases the situation is unclear, there being a partial deficiency of lipoamide dehydrogenase which on its own could not account for the observed deficiencies in the three α-keto acid dehydrogenase complexes (Munnich *et al.*, 1982). We hypothesized that in such cases the catalytic activity of the lipoamide dehydrogenase was not greatly compromised by the mutation but the ability to interact with the transacetylases in the reaction sequence of each complex was curtailed.

A number of important points arise about the clinical and biochemical presentation of pyruvate dehydrogenase E_1 deficiency (Table 1). Firstly, the defect in enzyme activity is nearly always partial, the activities ranging from 11 to 38% of the mean of control values except for one patient who had 2% of normal activity (cell line 1373). Secondly, in the patients where blood lactate/pyruvate ratios have been measured, the ratios are either the same as or only slightly above those measured in normal children (Robinson *et al.*, 1983b). The prognosis for pyruvate dehydrogenase deficiency patients in general is very poor. There is a gradation of the severity and course of the disease process which to a certain extent appears to be a function of the blood lactate concentration. In six cases there was death in the neonatal period accompanied by severe acidosis.

Journal of Inherited Metabolic Disease. ISSN 0141-8955. Copyright © SSIEM and MTP Press Limited, Queen Square, Lancaster, UK.

Table 1 Presentation of deficiency of the pyruvate dehydrogenase complex (E_1 component)

Strain No.	PDH complex activity native	Ca^{2+} activated	Typical blood lactate (mmol/l)	Dysmorphism	Age	Proven structural brain damage
811	0.172 ± 0.035(8)	0.180 ± 0.045(9)	5	Facial	†4y	PM dysmyelination of cortex
936	0.118 ± 0.15(3)	0.118 ± 0.015(3)	9	—	†Neonate	—
1118	0.142 ± 0.032(5)	0.134 ± 0.020(7)	4	Facial	3y	—
1108	0.097 ± 0.028(7)	0.061 ± 0.020(7)	10	Facial	†Neonate	CT hydrocephalic partial agenesis of corpus callosum
1122	0.139 ± 0.051(5)	0.075 ± 0.027(7)	13	—	†Neonate	CT cysts in cerebral cortex
984	0.105 ± 0.025(5)	0.162 ± 0.057(5)	5–10	—	†4y	—
1083	0.236 ± 0.042(6)	0.231 ± 0.033(7)	2–5	—	†Neonate	—
1159	0.255 ± 0.045(6)	0.208 ± 0.036(5)	4–7	Facial	1y	CT cystic lesions in cerebral cortex and brainstem
1288	0.090 ± 0.029(10)	0.101 ± 0.031(10)	8–17	—	†Neonate	PM Poor differentiation of grey and white matter
1368	0.100 ± 0.017(11)	0.073 ± 0.037(3)	7	—	†2y	—
1290	0.177 ± 0.045(12)	0.207 ± 0.052(12)	5–7	Microcephalic	10y	—
1360	0.089 ± 0.022(4)	0.073 ± 0.024(4)	8–11	Facial	8 months	—
1343	0.211 ± 0.027(9)	0.188 ± 0.053(9)	4–7	Microcephalic	1y	CT hydrocephalus optic atrophy
825	0.112 ± 0.022(4)	0.096 ± 0.037(4)	2–3	Facial	5y	—
828	0.106 ± 0.033(4)	0.087 ± 0.021(5)	2–3	Facial	6y	—
911	0.065 ± 0.016(5)	0.060 ± 0.010(5)	2–3	—	8y	CT cortical cyst
1216	0.061 ± 0.032(9)	0.048 ± 0.030(9)	3–4	Facial	†2y	CT cortical atrophy
1373	0.010 ± 0.008(7)	0.012 ± 0.008(7)	18	—	†Neonate	CT hydrocephalus PM cystic basal ganglia. Agenesis of corpus callosum ectopic olivary nuclei
Controls	0.344 ± 0.017(47)	0.532 ± 0.017(50)	—	—	—	

Values for PDH activity are given as the mean ± SEM expressed in nmol/min per mg protein in the native and Ca^{2+} activated state (Robinson et al., 1980). The number of determinations is given in parenthesis. † = deceased

Another four died at 2, 4, 4, and 6 years of age, respectively, after a course of unremitting lactic acidaemia and neurological dysfunction. The remaining surviving cases have chronic lactic acidaemia accompanied by varying degrees of physical and mental retardation. In ten of the cases there was some facial dysmorphism which consisted of a narrowed head, wide nasal bridge and flared nostrils or gross microcephaly. Two patients with neonatal death showed malformation of the brain at autopsy. In one patient there was partial agenesis of the corpus callosum and in another there was agenesis of the corpus callosum with ectopic olivary nuclei. A patient with pyruvate dehydrogenase E_1 deficiency was also described by Wick *et al.* (1978) to have agenesis of the corpus callosum. Ten of the patients showed structural brain damage either determined at autopsy or by CT scanning. Most commonly observed were cystic lesions in the cerebral cortex and in the brainstem, as had been described previously by others (Reynolds and Blass, 1976). The reason why such extensive damage occurs in the brain relates to the fact that the rate of glucose utilization by the brain in most species generates pyruvate at a rate which is close to the capacity of pyruvate dehydrogenase to oxidize it (Cremer and Teal, 1974; Robinson *et al.*, 1977). This situation, coupled with the fact that the brain cannot use fatty acids as an alternative fuel, dictates not only that the brain will be the primary pathological target in pyruvate dehydrogenase deficiency but also that partial defects in this enzyme complex may cause considerable morbidity. The combination of being in the main energy generating pathway and being rate limiting (or close to rate limiting) is a unique situation. The only other fuel which can possibly supply the brain in this condition is ketone bodies and for this reason low carbohydrate, high fat diets have been tried on children with pyruvate dehydrogenase deficiency (Cederbaum *et al.*, 1976). Three of the patients diagnosed by us responded to a high fat diet by lowering the levels of blood lactate, one of them with signs of clinical improvement. Three patients were tried on the high fat diet with no response either in the blood lactate or the clinical signs.

When all three α-keto acid dehydrogenase complexes are deficient as in lipoamide dehydrogenase deficiency, the prognosis is again poor, death occurring early in life (Munnich *et al.*, 1982; Robinson *et al.*, 1978, 1981). Postmortem examination shows the brain in these cases to have necrotization and vacuolation in the basal ganglia.

Pyruvate dehydrogenase phosphatase (EC 3.1.3.43) deficiency has been described in one patient with severe lactic acidaemia and carbohydrate intolerance (Robinson *et al.*, 1975) and also in a number of cases of Leigh's disease (De Vivo *et al.*, 1979; Sorbi and Blass, 1982). In this deficiency the phosphatase that converts pyruvate dehydrogenase from its phosphorylated inactive form to its non-phosphorylated active form (Linn *et al.*, 1969; Wieland and Jagow-Westermann, 1972; Pettit *et al.*, 1975) is found to be lacking in activity. This has had the effect of keeping the activity of the complex lower than it otherwise would be. The diagnosis of Leigh's disease has also been made in conjunction with a case of pyruvate dehydrogenase E_1 deficiency (Toshima *et al.*, 1982) and also in a case of muscle cytochrome oxidase (EC 1.9.3.1) deficiency (Willems *et al.*, 1977). The similarity of the pathologic lesions in the brain stem in Leigh's disease, chronic thiamine deficiency and pyruvate dehydrogenase deficiency of various kinds suggests that the mechanisms underlying this pathology have some common feature.

PYRUVATE CARBOXYLASE DEFICIENCY

It has been intimated for some time that there are two rather different presentations for classical pyruvate carboxylase (EC 6.4.1.1) deficiency which are quite different again from the biotin responsive multiple carboxylase deficiency (Saunders *et al.*, 1979; Bartlett and Gompertz, 1978) which will be described in detail by Bartlett in this symposium (Bartlett *et al.*, 1984). In classical pyruvate carboxylase deficiency the measurable activity of enzyme is less than 5% of that found in control fibroblasts (Robinson *et al.*, 1980; De Vivo *et al.*, 1977; Atkin *et al.*, 1979). The patients originally described from North America were described as presenting with moderate to severe lactic acidaemia accompanied by psychomotor retardation, sometimes with neonatal death as the outcome (Robinson *et al.*, 1980; De Vivo *et al.*, 1977; Atkin *et al.*, 1979; Haworth *et al.*, 1981). Those described from France had the lactic acidaemia and neurological problems but accompanied by hyperammonaemia, citrullinaemia, hyperlysinaemia and altered redox state (Saudubray *et al.*, 1976; Coudé *et al.*, 1981). Two individuals with this form of presentation were diagnosed recently by our group as having pyruvate carboxylase deficiency. When cultured skin fibroblasts from these patients were examined for their ability to synthesize [^{3}H]-biotin containing proteins it was found that they did not produce an [^{3}H]-biotin containing protein of the correct subunit molecular weight ($M_r = 125$ kd) corresponding to pyruvate carboxylase (Robinson *et al.*, 1983a, 1984). The patients with the simple presentation all showed a [^{3}H]-biotin containing protein of 125 kd. They also showed a protein of 125 ku immunoprecipitable by antipyruvate carboxylase antiserum when the cells were labelled with ^{35}S-methionine. On the other hand the two atypical patients showed no immunoprecipitable protein corresponding to pyruvate carboxylase (Robinson *et al.*, 1984). Thus we have been able to show that the presentation of pyruvate carboxylase deficiency with associated hyperammonaemia, hyperlysinaemia and citrullinaemia is associated with the absence of a biotinylated, cross-reacting pyruvate carboxylase protein (CRM − ve).

The uncomplicated presentation of pyruvate carboxylase is associated with a demonstrable biotinylated cross-reacting pyruvate carboxylase protein (CRM + ve). The difference in the biochemical presentation of these patients must emanate from the lack of ability to generate oxaloacetate and aspartate in CRM − ve patients, thus compromising the urea cycle and the homeostatic mechanisms involved in regulating cytosolic and mitochondrial redox states (Coudé *et al.*, 1981; Robinson *et al.*, 1984).

COMPROMISED PYRUVATE OXIDATION WITH NORMAL PYRUVATE DEHYDROGENASE AND PYRUVATE CARBOXYLASE

A number of patients have come to our attention with the presentation of lactic acidaemia in whom we are unable to demonstrate any defect in either pyruvate dehydrogenase, pyruvate carboxylase or phosphoenol-pyruvate carboxykinase (EC 4.1.1.32). In our patients there was a defect in the ability of the cultured skin fibroblasts to oxidize pyruvate and lactate which could be relieved by the addition of methylene blue (Goodyer and Lancaster, 1981). This together with the very high lactate to pyruvate ratios measured in the blood of these children was indicative of a redox disequilibrium which could be altered by adding an electron acceptor. One of the patients (Goodyer and Lancaster, 1981) responded to administration of methylene blue with a fall in the blood lactate level. However, all three patients eventually died, two of them in the neonatal period. Our further investigations showed that the isolated mito-chondria from the fibroblasts of our two patients were able to oxidize pyruvate at normal rates. For this reason, we proposed that a disequilibrium of reducing power must be present in the cytosol of these cells, which we confirmed by measuring a lower NAD/NADH ratio in fibroblast cell extracts (Robinson et al., 1983b). The exact site where the defective gene product exerts its influence in this redox type of lactic acidaemia remains to be determined. It may be that other individuals with a similar presentation may have defects in oxidative phosphorylation or the respiratory chain.

We thank the Canadian Medical Research Council (MR 6573) and The Beta Sigma Phi Society for their support of this work.

References

Atkin, B. M., Utter, M. F. and Weinberg, M. B. Pyruvate carboxylase and phosphoenol-pyruvate carboxykinase activity in leucocytes and fibroblasts from a patient with pyruvate carboxylase deficiency. *Pediatr. Res.* 13 (1979) 38–43

Bartlett, K. and Gompertz, D. Biotin activation of carboxylase activity in cultured fibroblasts from a child with combined carboxylase defect. *Clin. Chim. Acta* 84 (1978) 399–401

Bartlett, K., Ghneim, H. K., Stirk, J.-H., Dale, G. and Alberti, K. G. M. M. Pyruvate carboxylase deficiency. *J. Inher. Metab. Dis.* 7, Suppl. 1 (1984) 74–78

Blass, J. P., Avigan, J. and Uhlendorf, B. W. A defect in pyruvate decarboxylase in a child with an intermittent movement disorder. *J. Clin. Invest.* 49 (1970) 423

Blass, J. P., Kark, R. A. P. and Engel, W. K. Clinical studies of a patient with pyruvate decarboxylase deficiency. *Arch. Neurol.* 25 (1971a) 449–460

Blass, J. P., Lonsdale, D., Uhlendorf, B. W. and Ham, E. Intermittent ataxia with pyruvate decarboxylase activity. *Lancet* 1 (1971b) 1302

Cederbaum, S. D., Blass, J. P., Minkoff, N., JannBrown, W., Cotton, M. E. and Harris, S. H. Sensitivity to carbohydrate in a patient with familial intermittent lactic acidosis and pyruvate dehydrogenase deficiency. *Pediatr. Res.* 10 (1976) 713–720

Chuang, D. T., Ku, L. S. and Cox, R. P. Thiamine-responsive maple syrup urine disease: Decreased affinity of the mutant branched chain α-keto acid dehydrogenase for α-ketoisovalarate and thiamine pyraphosphate. *Proc. Nat. Acad. Sci. USA* 79 (1982) 3300–3304

Coudé, F. X., Ogier, H., Marsac, C., Munnich, A., Charpentier, C. and Saudubray, J. M. Secondary citrullinemia with hyperammonemia in four neonatal cases of pyruvate carboxylase deficiency. *Pediatrics* 68 (1981) 914

Cremer, J. E. and Teal, H. M. Development of pyruvate dehydrogenase in rat brain. *FEBS Lett.* 39 (1974) 17–20

De Vivo, D., Haymond, M. W., Leckie, M. P., Bursmann, Y. L., McDougal, D. B. and Pagliara, A. S. Clinical and biochemical implications of pyruvate carboxylase deficiency. *J. Clin. Endocr. Metab.* 45 (1977) 1281–1296

De Vivo, D. C., Haymond, M. W., Obert, K. A., Nelson, J. S. and Pagliara, A. S. Defective activation of the pyruvate dehydrogenase complex in subacute necrotising encephalo-myelopathy (Leigh's disease). *Ann. Neurol.* 6 (1979) 483–494

Farmer, T. W., Veath, L., Miller, A. L., O'Brien, J. S. and Rosenberg, R. M. Pyruvate decarboxylase deficiency in a patient with subacute necrotising encephalomyelopathy. *Neurology* 23 (1973) 423

Farrel, D. F., Clark, A. F., Scott, R. C. and Wennberg, R. P. Absent pyruvate decarboxylase in man. A cause of congenital lacticacidosis. *Science* 187 (1975) 1082–1084

Goodyer, P. R. and Lancaster, G. Effect of methylene blue on fibroblasts in lactic acidosis. *Pediatr. Res.* 15 (1981) 562

Haworth, J. C., Robinson, B. H. and Perry, T. L. Lactic acidosis due to pyruvate carboxylase deficiency. *J. Inher. Metab. Dis.* 4 (1981) 57–58

Kohlschütter, A., Behbehani, A., Langenbeck, U., Albani, M., Heidemain, P., Hoffmann, G., Klemike, J., Lehnert, W. and Wendel, U. A familial progressive neurodegenerative disease with 2-oxoglutaric aciduria. *Eur. J. Pediatr.* 138 (1982) 32–37

Linn, T. E., Pettit, F. H., Hucho, F. and Reed, L. J. Keto acid dehydrogenase complexes XI. Comparative studies of regulatory properties of the pyruvate dehydrogenase complexes from kidney heart and liver mitochondria. *Proc. Nat. Acad. Sci. USA* 64 (1969) 227–234

Munnich, A., Saudubray, J. M., Taylor, J., Charpentier, C., Marsac, C., Roccichioli, F., Amédée-Menesme, O., Frézal, J. and Robinson, B. H. Congenital lactic acidosis α-ketoglutaric aciduria and variant form of maple syrup urine disease due to a single enzyme defect. Dihydrolipoyl dehydrogenase deficiency. *Acta Paediatr. Scand.* 71 (1982) 167–171

Pettit, F. H., Pelley, J. W. and Reed, L. J. Regulation of pyruvate dehydrogenase kinase and phosphatase by acetyl-CoA/CoA and NADH/NAD ratios. *Biochem. Biophys. Res. Commun.* 65 (1975) 575–582

Reynolds, S. F. and Blass, J. P. A possible mechanism for selective cerebellar damage in partial pyruvate dehy-drogenase deficiency. *Neurology* 26 (1976) 625–628

Robinson, B. H. Inborn errors of metabolism leading to lactic-acidemia. *Trends Biochem. Sci.* 7 (1982) 151–153

Robinson, B. H. Inborn errors of pyruvate metabolism. *Trans. Biochem. Soc.* 11 (1983) 623–626

Robinson, B. H., Oei, J., Saunders, M. and Gravel, R. ³H-Biotin labelled proteins in cultured human skin fibroblasts from patients with pyruvate carboxylase deficiency. *J. Biol. Chem.* 258 (1983a) 6660–6664

Robinson, B. H., Oei, J., Sherwood, W. G., Applegarth, D., Wong, L., Haworth, J., Goodyer, P., Casey, R. and Zaleski, L. A. The molecular basis for the two different clinical presentations of classical pyruvate carboxylase deficiency. *Am. J. Hum. Genet.* Accepted for publication (1984)

Robinson, B. H. and Sherwood, W. G. Pyruvate dehy-drogenase phosphatase deficiency. A cause of chronic congenital lacticacidosis in infancy. *Pediatr. Res.* 9 (1975) 935–939

Robinson, B. H., Sherwood, W. G. and Oei, J. The development of pyruvate dehydrogenase in the subhuman primate *Macacca mulatta. Biol. Neonate* 32 (1977) 154–157

Robinson, B. H., Taylor, J., Francois, B., Baudet, A. and Peterson, D. F. Lacticacidosis, neurological deterioration and compromised cellular pyruvate oxidation due to a defect in the reoxidation of cytoplasmically generated NADH. *Eur. J. Pediatr.* 140 (1983b) 98–101

Robinson, B. H., Taylor, J., Kahler, S. G. and Kirkman, H. N. Lactic acidemia neurologic deterioration and carbohydrate dependance in a girl with dihydrolipoyl dehydrogenase deficiency. *Eur. J. Pediatr.* 136 (1981) 35–39

Robinson, B. H., Taylor, J. and Sherwood, W. G. Deficiency of dihydrolipoyl dehydrogenase: A cause of congenital lactic acidosis in infancy. *Pediatr. Res.* 11 (1978) 1198–1202

Robinson, B. H., Taylor, J. and Sherwood, W. G. The genetic heterogeneity of lactic acidosis: occurrence of recognizable inborn errors of metabolism in a pediatric population with lactic-acidosis. *Pediatr. Res.* 14 (1980) 956–982

Saudubray, J. M., Marsac, C., Charpentier, C., Cathelineau, L., Besson, L. M. and Leroux, J. P. Neonatal congenital lactic acidosis with pyruvate carboxylase deficiency in two siblings. *Acta Pediatr. Scand.* 65 (1976) 717–724

Saunders, M., Sweetman, L., Robinson, B., Roth, K., Conn, R. and Gravel, R. A. Biotin responsive organic aciduria. Multiple carboxylase defect and complementation studies with propionic aciduria in cultured fibroblasts. *J. Clin. Invest.* 64 (1979) 1695–1702

Sorbi, S. and Blass, J. P. Abnormal activation of pyruvate dehydrogenase in Leigh disease fibroblasts. *Neurology* 32 (1982) 555–558

Strömme, J. H., Borud, O. and Moe, P. J. Fatal lactic acidosis in a newborn attributable to a congenital defect of pyruvate dehydrogenase. *Pediatr. Res.* 10 (1976) 60–66

Taylor, J., Robinson, B. H. and Sherwood, W. G. A defect in branched-chain amino acid metabolism in a patient with congenital lacticacidosis due to dihydrolipoyl dehydrogenase deficiency. *Pediatr. Res.* 12 (1978) 60

Toshima, K., Kuroda, Y., Hashimoto, T., Ho, M., Watanabi, T., Migano, M. and Li, K. Enzymologic studies and therapy of Leigh's disease associated with pyruvate decarboxylase deficiency. *Pediatr. Res.* 16 (1982) 430–435

Wick, H., Schweizer, K. and Baumgartner, R. Thiamine dependency in a patient with congenital lacticacidemia due to pyruvate dehydrogenase deficiency. *Agents Actions* 7 (1978) 405–408

Wieland, O. H. and Jagow-Westermann, B. ATP-dependent inactivation of heart muscle pyruvate dehydrogenase and reactivation of Mg^{++}. *FEBS Lett.* 3 (1972) 271–274

Willems, J. L., Monnens, A. H., Trijbels, J. M. T., Veerkamp, J. H., Meyer, A. E. T. H., Van Dam, K. and Van Haelst, U. Leigh's encephalomyopathy in a patient with cytochrome C oxidase deficiency of muscle tissue. *Pediatrics* 60 (1977) 850–855

J. Inher. Metab. Dis. 7 Suppl. 1 (1984) 74–78

Pyruvate Carboxylase Deficiency

K. BARTLETT, H. K. GHNEIM, J.-H. STIRK, G. DALE and K. G. M. M. ALBERTI
Department of Clinical Biochemistry and Metabolic Medicine, University of Newcastle upon Tyne, Newcastle upon Tyne NE1 7RU, UK

The causes of congenital lactic acidaemia are outlined. Isolated pyruvate carboxylase deficiency is reviewed in detail with a report of a recent case and a discussion of the biochemical consequences. Other causes of defective pyruvate carboxylation are described, particularly the combined carboxylase defects.

INTRODUCTION

Lactic acidaemia is a common finding and it is important to establish that it is not the consequence of either muscular exercise or stress. A screaming but perfectly normal infant can generate extremely high blood lactate concentrations (Kollee *et al.*, 1977). Similarly we have observed that a fitting child produced a marked lactic acidaemia of 16 mmol/l. Thus it is not surprising that lactic acidaemia is found in some children with neurological damage in whom there is no other evidence of biochemical disorder. Lactic acidaemia may be a perfectly normal response to a number of situations and does not necessarily indicate either a primary defect of pyruvate metabolism or a secondary effect of some other organic acidaemia. However, deficiencies of pyruvate carboxylase, pyruvate dehydrogenase, phosphoenolpyruvate carboxykinase, glucose-6-phosphatase and terminal electron transport are known to result in a lactic acidaemia. The remainder of this discussion will be limited to pyruvate carboxylase (PC; Pyruvate:CO_2 ligase (ADP) EC 6.4.1.1) and its disorders. The known disorders of PC are summarized in Table 1.

PYRUVATE CARBOXYLASE STRUCTURE AND FUNCTION

The place of PC in intermediary metabolism is well known. PC has a dual role; it is essential for gluconeogenesis from lactate and pyruvate in which it is probably rate-determining, but it also has an anaplerotic function. PC is a biotin-dependent carboxylase. Biotin is attached to the apocarboxylase via the ε-amino group of a lysine residue in a two step process with the

Table 1 Causes of defective pyruvate carboxylase

---

(1) Isolated pyruvate carboxylase deficiency
(2) Combined carboxylase deficiency
    (a) Holocarboxylase synthetase deficiency
    (b) Biotinidase deficiency
    (c) Defective gut absorption
    (d) Defective renal reabsorption
    (e) Dietary biotin deficiency
(3) Secondary to other organic acidaemias

---

intermediate formation of biotinyl adenylate. The reaction is catalysed by holocarboxylase synthetase, thought to be a single enzyme although it has not been purified to homogeneity. The reaction catalysed by PC can be expressed as two partial reactions: firstly the MgATP-dependent carboxylation of the enzyme-bound biotin, and secondly the binding of pyruvate with transfer of CO_2 to yield oxaloacetate. The native enzyme is a tetramer of identical subunits, each with a molecular weight of 12.5 kd. There is one biotin and one acetyl CoA binding site per monomer. The enzyme is activated by K^+, Mg^{2+} and acetyl CoA and inhibited by MgADP and some acyl-CoA esters. These and other properties of PC have been reviewed in detail elsewhere (Utter *et al.*, 1975). Liver and kidney show the highest activities of PC, although the enzyme can be detected in most tissues.

Available evidence suggests that the gut uptake of biotin required for PC and the other biotin-dependent carboxylases is facilitated (Berger *et al.*, 1972). The biotin is carried in the circulation to tissues where it enters cells by a carrier mediated process (Ghneim and Bartlett, unpublished findings). Biotinylation of apoPC, apopropionyl CoA carboxylase and apo-3-methylcrotonyl CoA carboxylase occurs in the mitochondrion. The turnover of the biotin-dependent enzymes yields biocytin, the lysyl derivative of biotin, rather than free biotin. There exists a specific hydrolase, biotinidase (EC 3.5.1.12), to regenerate free biotin. Biotinidase is present in plasma at about the same specific activity as in liver on a gram wet weight basis, although its function in plasma is unknown. The functional relationship of endogenous recycled biotin and biotin derived from the diet also remains uncertain.

ISOLATED PC DEFICIENCY—A CASE REPORT

The patient (M.K.) was born full term to unrelated parents after an uneventful pregnancy and was the first child. At 36 h he was found to be hypothermic, hypotonic and refused to feed. He was transferred to the special care baby unit where he was found to be acidaemic (pH 6.92, pCO_2 3.0 kPa), his urine contained ketones and there was an anion gap of 31 mmol/l. Urinary organic acid screening showed a raised lactate (10.4 mmol/mmol creatinine) and 3-hydroxybutyrate (0.56 mmol/mmol creatinine). The urinary amino acids were also abnormal. Citrulline, arginine and lysine were

Journal of Inherited Metabolic Disease. ISSN 0141-8955. Copyright © SSIEM and MTP Press Limited, Queen Square, Lancaster, UK.

elevated (107, 26 and 460 μmol/μmol creatinine respectively), the other amino acids, alanine in particular, were normal. The plasma amino acids showed gross disturbances and are given in Table 2. There was normoglycaemia (8.3 mmol/l), hyperketonaemia (3-hydroxybutyrate = 1.22 mmol/l) and a marked lactic acidaemia (10.8 mmol/l) with an abnormally high lactate/pyruvate ratio (25.6). Measurement of leukocyte carboxylases showed a complete absence of pyruvate carboxylase, a result which was subsequently confirmed in cultured fibroblasts. The acidaemia was partially controlled with bicarbonate and therapy with biotin and aspartate attempted, neither of which altered his lactic acidaemia or clinical state. He remained hypotonic and unresponsive with increasing dyspnoea until his death at about 3 months of age. Autopsy was refused by the parents. The mother subsequently became pregnant, refused antenatal diagnosis and a second child was born who has proved not to have the disease.

ISOLATED PC DEFICIENCY

There have been about 20 cases of isolated PC deficiency described (De Vivo *et al.*, 1977; Robinson *et al.*, 1980; Wolf and Feldman, 1982). In most the presentation is in early life with hypotonia, metabolic acidosis, developmental delay, and death within the first few years of life. Surviving patients are severely retarded. There have been suggestions that PC deficiency is the underlying defect in the subacute necrotizing encephalomyelopathy of Leigh (SNE) (Tada *et al.*, 1973). Indeed the first

patient with hepatic PC deficiency reported by Hommes *et al.* (1968) was described as a case of SNE. In several recent studies of autopsy-proven SNE, however, PC has been shown to be entirely normal (Hansen *et al.*, 1982; Atkin *et al.*, 1979). Previous reports of the association of PC with SNE were ascribed to poor technique – the estimation of PC in liver biopsy being notoriously unreliable (Murphy *et al.*, 1981). It seems therefore that SNE and PC deficiency are separate entities, and that if a deficiency in cultured cells or leukocytes cannot be shown then a diagnosis of PC deficiency is excluded. Isolated PC deficiency is inherited as an autosomal recessive condition (Atkin, 1979) and prenatal diagnosis has been reported (Marsac *et al.*, 1981, 1982).

Even if the reports of hepatic PC deficiency are discounted there still remains heterogeneity with respect to age at presentation, severity and metabolic consequences of PC deficiency. Somatic cell hybridization has, however, failed to demonstrate complementation (Feldman and Wolf, 1980) although biochemical heterogeneity has been shown (Hansen *et al.*, 1983; Robinson *et al.*, 1983; Robinson and Sherwood, 1984).

BIOCHEMICAL CONSEQUENCES OF ISOLATED PC DEFICIENCY

The citrullinaemia was the most striking of the amino acid changes observed in our patient. This has been observed previously in four patients reported by Coude *et al.* (1981), and is probably a result of aspartate shortage due to oxaloacetate depletion. This interpretation is consistent with the low level of TCA intermediates in liver (De Vivo *et al.*, 1977). Attenuation of the urea cycle due to substrate depletion is probably the mechanism of the hyperammonaemia sometimes seen. Although PC is essential for gluconeogenesis from lactate and pyruvate, hypoglycaemia was never observed in our patient and seems to be an inconsistent finding. Hyperketonaemia is however usually observed. It has been suggested that this is due simply to overflow of acetyl CoA from pyruvate due to oxaloacetate depletion. However, this is unlikely since pyruvate dehydrogenase is inactivated by high acetyl CoA/CoA ratios (Randle *et al.*, 1979). Since the insulin/glucagon ratio is low in PC deficiency (De Vivo *et al.*, 1977), there will be increased lipolysis with increased delivery of fatty acids to the liver. Furthermore since liver citrate is low, cytosolic acetyl CoA and hence malonyl CoA will be low, allowing unrestricted entry of fatty acids into the mitochondrial compartment and hence increased β-oxidation and ketogenesis (McGarry *et al.*, 1977).

A feature of some patients with PC deficiency is a raised lactate/pyruvate ratio indicating that the cytosol is more reduced than normal. The reverse is true of the 3-hydroxybutyrate/acetoacetate couple probably because of impaired activity of redox shuttles due to oxaloacetate shortage.

TREATMENT OF ISOLATED PC DEFICIENCY

There appears to be no effective treatment for isolated PC deficiency. High fat diets exacerbate the hyperketonaemia, whereas high carbohydrate diets cause

Table 2 Plasma amino acids in Patient M.K. with pyruvate carboxylase deficiency

Amino acid	μmol/l	
	Patient M.K.	Normal range
Aspartate	40	20–70
Threonine	307	100–400
Serine	112	50–350
Asparagine	79	0–175
Glutamate	58	0–250
Glutamine	534	400–1600
Proline	0	50–450
Glycine	1637	200–600
Citrulline	392	0–40
Alanine	1477	100–800
1/2 Cystine	103	0–100
Valine	475	50–400
Methionine	67	0–80
Isoleucine	200	0–150
Leucine	382	20–180
Tyrosine	342	30–135
Phenylalanine	156	40–110
Histidine	224	45–150
Tryptophan	18	0–50
Ornithine	117	25–225
Lysine	1292	105–315
Arginine	229	10–70

Amino acids in **bold** type indicate concentrations >5 SD from the mean increased lactic acidaemia (De Vivo *et al.*, 1977). Aspartate treatment has been reported in a child with mild lactic acidaemia (1.9 mmol/l), low hepatic PC activity but normal leukocyte and fibroblast enzyme (Baal *et al.*, 1981). Thiamine has also been reported to produce an amelioration of the lactic acidaemia (Brunette *et al.*, 1972). Thiamine as its pyrophosphate is an inhibitor of PDH kinase and thus high thiamine may result in increased activity of PDH and therefore diversion of pyruvate to acetyl CoA (Randle, 1982). Biotin, when it has been tried, has never produced any clinical or biochemical response.

PC DEFICIENCY IN COMBINED CARBOXYLASE DEFICIENCY

Combined or multiple carboxylase deficiency (CCD) is a heterogenous group of disorders which have in common the excretion of a constellation of abnormal metabolites characteristic of defective activity of all three mitochondrial carboxylases, defective activity of these enzymes in leukocytes and a marked and dramatic clinical and biochemical biotin-responsiveness (Leonard *et al.*, 1981; Wolf and Feldman, 1982). Two variants have been distinguished on the basis of age at presentation–i.e. early- and late-onset CCD (Sweetman, 1981). In most instances the late-onset form is also characterized by the stigmata of dietary biotin deficiency, i.e. alopecia and skin rash (Sweetman *et al.*, 1981), in addition to the metabolic changes seen in the early-onset form of the disease. In early-onset CCD we have shown that there is defective activity of all three mitochondrial carboxylases in cultured cells, which can be reversed by the addition of large amounts of biotin to the culture medium (Bartlett *et al.*, 1980). In these individuals there is defective activity of the enzyme which attaches biotin to the apocarboxylases, holocarboxylase synthetase (Burri *et al.*, 1981; Ghneim and Bartlett, 1982). However, in late-onset CCD no carboxylase defects can be demonstrated in cultured fibroblasts no matter what the concentration of biotin in the medium (Figure 1) although there is a marked

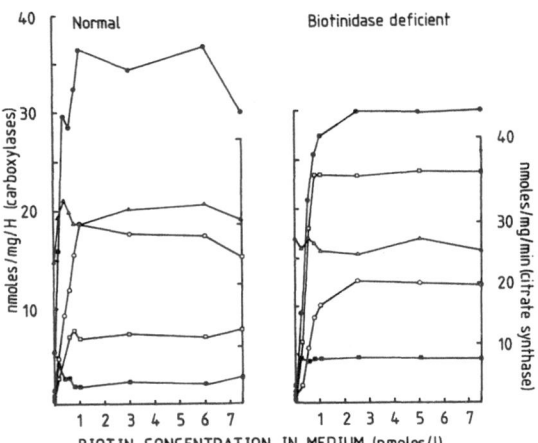

Figure 1 The specific activities of propionyl CoA carboxylase (●——●), 3-methylcrotonyl CoA carboxylase (○——○), pyruvate carboxylase (□——□), acetyl CoA carboxylase (■——■) and citrate synthase (△——△) in biotin-deficient fibroblasts from control and biotinidase-deficient subjects cultured in the presence of increasing concentrations of biotin

deficiency of all four enzymes in leucokytes which is reversed by biotin treatment (Table 3). This paradox has been recently resolved by the elegant studies of Wolf and his co-workers (Wolf *et al.*, 1983a, b), who demonstrated that some patients with late-onset CCD have defective activity of biotinidase. These individuals become functionally biotin-deficient because they are unable either to recycle endogenous biotin derived from the turnover of the biotin-dependent enzymes, or to liberate dietary protein-bound biotin. There have been reports of defective gut transport and renal reabsorption (Munnich *et al.*, 1981; Baumgartner *et al.*, 1982), although the interpretation of the former has been questioned (Thoene and Wolf, 1983). We have confirmed biotinidase deficiency in a total of six cases, including the patient shown in Table 3 and Figure 1, of late-onset CCD using both the original colorimetric

Table 3 Leukocyte carboxylase activity in a patient with biotinidase deficiency before and after biotin treatment

Enzyme	nmol mg^{-1} h^{-1}			
	Pre-biotin	*2 months post-biotin*	*12 months post-biotin*	*Normal range*
Propionyl CoA carboxylase	0.04	1.7	6.2	1.6–3.7
3-Methylcrotonyl CoA carboxylase	0.004	0.9	4.5	0.2–1.3
Pyruvate carboxylase	0	0.2	0.6	0.1–0.5
Acetyl CoA carboxylase	0	0.04	0.33	0.06–0.2
Citrate synthase*	7.3	5.9	10.4	5.5–17.3

* Units: nmol mg^{-1} min^{-1}

assay of Knappe *et al.* (1963) and a new sensitive fluorimetric assay we have developed (Wastell, Dale and Bartlett, 1984).

We have recently drawn attention to the auditory and visual defects in these children, a previously unrecognized problem of biotinidase deficiency treated with high doses of biotin (Taitz *et al.*, 1983). At present it is not clear if this is a consequence of early metabolic insult, biotin treatment or the accumulation of biocytin. The early reports of low to normal biotin in these children must now be discounted because existing biotin assays do not distinguish biotin and biocytin.

PC DEFICIENCY SECONDARY TO OTHER ORGANIC ACIDAEMIAS

Lactic acidaemia is frequently observed in patients in whom there is clearly no primary defect in pyruvate metabolism and is secondary to some other organic acidaemia. It is possible that this is due to inhibition of PC by the accumulation of abnormally high concentrations of acyl-CoA esters within the mitochondrial matrix. Evidence for this mechanism has been recently reported (Stirk *et al.*, 1983). Pyruvate carboxylation was measured in intact rat liver mitochondria and was inhibited by some acids. This inhibition could be partially relieved by glycine, presumably because formation of the corresponding acylglycine lowered the matrix concentration of abnormal acyl-CoA. Similar effects on PDH have been reported (Gregersen, 1981), which would of course also contribute to impaired pyruvate disposal.

References

Atkin, B. M. Carrier detection of pyruvate carboxylase in fibroblasts and lymphocytes. *Pediatr. Res.* 13 (1979) 1101–1104

Atkin, B. M., Buist, N. M. R., Utter, M. F., Leiter, A. B. and Banker, B. Q. Pyruvate carboxylase deficiency and lactic acidosis in a retarded child without Leigh's disease. *Pediatr. Res.* 13 (1979) 109–116

Baal, M. G., Gabreels, F. J. M., Renier, W. O., Hommes, F. A., Gijshers, Th. H. J., Lamers, K. J. B. and Kok, J. C. N. A patient with pyruvate carboxylase deficiency in the liver: treatment with aspartatic acid and thiamine. *Dev. Med. Child. Neurol.* 23 (1981) 521–530

Bartlett, K., Ng, H. and Leonard, J. V. A combined defect of three mitochondrial carboxylases presenting as biotin-responsive 3-methylcrotonylglycinuria and 3-hydroxy-isovaleric aciduria. *Clin. Chim. Acta* 100 (1980) 183–185

Baumgartner, R., Suormala, T., Wick, H., Geisert, J. and Lehnert, W. Infantile multiple carboxylase deficiency: Evidence for normal absorption but renal loss of biotin. *Helv. Paediatr. Acta* 37 (1982) 499–502

Berger, E., Long, E. and Semenza, G. The sodium activiation of biotin absorption in hamster small intestine *in vitro*. *Biochem. Biophys. Acta* 255 (1972) 873–887

Brunette, M. G., Delvin, E., Hazel, B. and Scriver, C. R. Thiamine-responsive lactic acidosis in a patient with deficient low-K_m pyruvate carboxylase in liver. *Paediatrics* 50 (1972) 702–711

Burri, B. J., Sweetman, L. and Nyhan, W. L. Mutant holocarboxylase synthetase: evidence for the enzyme defect in early infantile biotin-responsive multiple carboxylase deficiency. *J. Clin. Invest.* 68 (1981) 1491–1495

Coude, F. X., Ogier, H., Marsac, C., Munnich, A., Charpentier, C. and Saudubray, J.-M. Secondary citrullinaemia with hyperammonaemia in four neonatal cases of pyruvate carboxylase deficiency. *Paediatrics* 68 (1981) 914

De Vivo, D. C., Haymond, M. W., Leckie, M. P., Bussman, Y. L., McDougal, D. B. and Pagliara, A. S. The clinical and biochemical implications of pyruvate carboxylase deficiency. *J. Clin. Endocrinol. Metab.* 45 (1977) 1281–1296

Feldman, G. L. and Wolf, B. Evidence for two complementation groups in pyruvate carboxylase-deficient human fibroblast cell lines. *Biochem. Genet.* 18 (1980) 617–624

Ghneim, H. K. and Bartlett, K. Mechanism of biotin-responsive combined carboxylase deficiency. *Lancet* 1 (1982) 1187–1188

Gregersen, N. The specific inhibition of the pyruvate dehydrogenase complex from pig kidney by propionyl-CoA and isovaleryl-CoA. *Biochem. Med.* 26 (1981) 20–27

Hansen, T. L., Christensen, E. and Brandt, N. J. Studies of pyruvate carboxylase, pyruvate decarboxylase and lipo-amide dehydrogenase in subacute necrotizing encephalomyelopathy. *Acta Paediatr. Scand.* 71 (1982) 263–267

Hansen, T. L., Christensen, E., Willems, J. L. and Trijbels, J. M. F. A mutation of pyruvate carboxylase in fibroblasts from a patient with severe, chronic lactic acidaemia. *Clin. Chim. Acta* 131 (1983) 39–44

Hommes, F. A., Polman, H. A. and Reerink, J. D. Leigh's encephalopathy: an inborn error of gluconeogenesis. *Arch. Dis. Child.* 43 (1968) 423–426

Knappe, J., Brummer, W. and Biederbick, K. Reinung und Eigenschaften der biotinidase aus schweinenieren und Lactobacillus Casei. *Biochem. Z.* 338 (1963) 599–613

Kollee, L. A. A., Willems, J. L., De Kort, A. F. M., Monnens, L. A. H. and Trijbels, J. M. F. Blood sampling technique for lactate and pyruvate estimation in children. *Ann. Clin. Biochem.* 14 (1977) 285–287

Leonard, J. V., Seakins, J. W. T., Bartlett, K., Hyde, J., Wilson, J. and Clayton, B. Inherited defects of 3-methylcrotonyl-CoA carboxylation. *Arch. Dis. Child.* 56 (1981) 53–59

McGarry, J. D., Mannaerts, G. P. and Foster, D. W. A possible rôle for malonyl-CoA in the regulation of hepatic fatty acid oxidation and ketogenesis. *J. Clin. Invest.* 60 (1977) 265–270

Marsac, C., Augereau, Ch., Boue, J. and Vidailhet, M. Antenatal diagnosis of pyruvate carboxylase deficiency. *Lancet* 1 (1981) 675

Marsac, C., Augereau, Ch., Feldman, G., Wolf, B., Hansen, T. L. and Berger, R. Prenatal diagnosis of pyruvate carboxylase deficiency. *Clin. Chim. Acta* 119 (1982) 121–127

Munnich, A., Saudubray, J.-M., Carre, G., Coude, F. X., Ogier, H., Charpentier, C. and Frezal, J. Defective biotin absorption in multiple carboxylase deficiency. *Lancet* 2 (1981) 263

Murphy, J. V., Isohashi, F., Weinberg, M. B. and Utter, M. F. Pyruvate carboxylase deficiency: An alleged biochemical cause of Leigh's disease. *Pediatrics* 68 (1981) 401–404

Randle, P. J. Congential lactic acidoses. In *Metabolic Acidoses* (Ciba Foundation Symposium No 87), Pitman Press, Bath, 1982, p. 354

Randle, P. J., Sugden, P. H., Kerbey, A. L., Radcliffe, P. M. and Hutson, N. J. Regulation of pyruvate oxidation and the conservation of glucose. *Biochem. Soc. Symp.* 43 (1979) 47–67

Robinson, B. H., Taylor, J. and Sherwood, W. G. The genetic heterogeneity of lactic acidosis: occurrence of recognisable inborn errors of metabolism in a paediatric population with lactic acidosis. *Paediatr. Res.* 14 (1980) 956–962

Robinson, B. H., Oei, J., Saunders, M. and Gravel. R. [^{3}H]Biotin-labelled proteins in cultured human skin fibroblasts from patients with pyruvate carboxylase deficiency. *J. Biol. Chem.* 258 (1983) 6660–6664

Robinson, B. H. and Sherwood, W. G. Lactic acidaemia. *J. Inher. Metab. Dis.* 7, Suppl. 1 (1984) 69–73

Stirk, J.-H., Bartlett, K. and Sherratt, H. S. A. The effects of some short-chain fatty acids on pyruvate carboxylase activity in intact isolated rat liver mitochondria. *Biochem. Soc. Trans.* 11 (1983) 286–287

Sweetman, L. Two forms of biotin-responsive multiple carboxylase deficiencies. *J. Inher. Metab. Dis.* 4 (1981) 53–54

Sweetman, L., Suhr, L., Baker, H., Petersen, R. M. and Nyhan, W. L. Clinical and metabolic disorders in a boy with dietary deficiency of biotin. *Pediatrics* 68 (1981) 553–558

Tada, K., Sugita, K., Fujikawi, K., Kesai, T., Takada, G. and Omura, K. Hyperalaninaemia with pyruvicaemia in a patient suggestive of Leigh's encephalomyelopathy. *J. Pediatr.* 109 (1973) 13–18

Taitz, L. S., Green, A., Strachan, I., Bartlett, K. and Bennet, M. Biotinidase deficiency and the eye and ear. *Lancet* 2 (1983) 918

Thoene, J. and Wolf, B. Biotinidase deficiency in juvenile multiple carboxylase deficiency. *Lancet* 2 (1983) 398

Utter, M. F., Barden, R. E. and Taylor, B. L. Pyruvate carboxylase: an evaluation of the relationships between structure and mechanisms and between structure and catalytic activity. *Adv. Enzymol.* 42 (1975) 1–72

Wastell, H., Dale, G. and Bartlett, K. A sensitive fluorometric rate assay for biotinidase using a new derivative of biotin, biotinyl-6-aminoquinoline. *Anal. Biochem.* (1984) in press

Wolf, B. and Feldman, G. L. The biotin-dependent carboxylase deficiencies. *Am. J. Hum. Genet.* 34 (1982) 699–716

Wolf, B., Grier, R. E., Parker, W. D., Goodman, S. I. and Allen, R. J. Deficient biotinidase activity in late-onset multiple carboxylase deficiency. *N. Engl. J. Med.* 308 (1983a) 161

Wolf, B., Grier, R. E., Allen, R. J., Goodman, S. I. and Kien, C. L. Biotinidase deficiency: the enzymatic defect in late-onset multiple carboxylase deficiency. *Clin. Chim. Acta* 131 (1983b) 273–281

J. Inher. Metab. Dis. 7 Suppl. 1 (1984) 79–89

Organic Acids in Urine of Patients with Congenital Lactic Acidoses: An Aid to Differential Diagnosis

R. A. CHALMERS

Paediatric Research Group, MRC Clinical Research Centre, Watford Road, Harrow HA1 3UJ, UK

The differential diagnosis of patients with apparent congenital lactic acidoses poses one of the most intractable problems in the study of patients with disorders of organic acid metabolism. An outline of the factors leading to a lactic acidosis, particularly in infants and young children, together with a brief review of the known causes of congenital lactic acidosis, are presented. Quantitative examination of the organic acids excreted by patients with proven enzyme deficiencies causing congenital lactic acidosis has demonstrated the characteristic patterns that are associated with specific disorders of this kind. After exclusion of uninherited, acquired and secondary metabolic causes of lactic acidosis, these quantitative patterns of organic acid excretion, together with other clinical and biochemical observations, provide valuable indicators of the area of the underlying primary metabolic disorder for subsequent selected, confirmatory, enzymology. The study of organic acids has a key and central role in the approach to the clinical and biochemical investigation and diagnosis of patients with congenital lactic acidoses.

The differential diagnosis of patients with apparent congenital lactic acidoses poses one of the most intractable problems in the study of patients with disorders of organic acid metabolism. Studies on patients with this group of disorders are characterized by the disconcertingly large number of patients with lactic acidosis in whom no enzyme deficiency can be demonstrated (Robinson *et al.*, 1980). This may be caused by incomplete initial biochemical investigations of the patients concerned before enzymology is undertaken. The present work and review examines the quantitative patterns of organic acid excretion into urine of patients with congenital lactic acidoses caused by clearly identified and proven enzyme deficiencies in order to define those features that are characteristic of a particular disorder, or group of disorders affecting one specific area (for example, the pyruvate dehydrogenase complex). These features can then be used as an aid, together with other clinical and biochemical characteristics, towards the differential diagnosis of other patients with suspected congenital lactic acidoses.

LACTIC ACIDOSIS

Lactate concentrations in urine and other body fluids depend upon the pyruvate concentration and upon the relative amounts of reduced and oxidized cytosolic NAD, these parameters being interrelated by the expression:

$$\frac{[\text{lactate}] \cdot [\text{NAD}^+]}{[\text{pyruvate}] \, [\text{NADH}] \, [\text{H}^+]} = K$$

where K is a constant. When NAD/NADH ratios are constant, changes in [lactate] depend upon the rate of pyruvate formation and the final pyruvate concentration. Thus, [lactate] may increase when NAD/NADH ratios fall and when [pyruvate] or [H$^+$] increase and a variety of causes may lead to a lactic acidosis (Chalmers and Lawson, 1982).

Lactic acidosis has been defined as a metabolic acidosis (i.e. a reduced base excess) associated with a blood lactate concentration of more than 2 mmol/l (18 mg per 100 ml), with a blood pH below 7.37. It is with this initial definition that diagnostic problems arise immediately, since if inadequate control is exercised over sampling methods and time of sampling, many patients without any primary metabolic disorder may show increased blood lactate concentrations. Patients with *congenital* lactic acidoses generally have blood lactate concentrations that are much greater (commonly 3–8 mmol/l or above) and that therefore exceed the renal reabsorptive thresholds, especially in infants and young children, with the appearance of lactate in the urine. Thus in the diagnosis of such patients, urine is the preferred body fluid, with the ratio of urine concentrations of lactate to creatinine being a useful parameter for initial assessment.

UNINHERITED AND OTHER CAUSES OF LACTIC ACIDOSIS AND LACTIC ACIDURIA

In addition to the initial problem of definition, several clinical conditions and situations unrelated to inherited disease may result in raised concentrations of lactic acid in blood and urine, particularly in the sick infant and young child. These include muscular exercise (for example, caused by convulsion and fitting), hyperventilation, hypoxia, septicaemia, circulatory shock, severe anaemia, and general liver failure. Some therapeutic measures being undertaken for other reasons may also produce the same effect. These include intravenous (i.v.) administration of glucose, fructose, bicarbonate and pyruvate and the use of certain drugs

Journal of Inherited Metabolic Disease. ISSN 0141–8955. Copyright © SSIEM and MTP Press Limited, Queen Square, Lancaster, UK. Printed in the Netherlands.

given to the newborn and even to the mother during the latter stages of pregnancy, causing a neonatal lactic acidosis. The use of i.v. glucose in special care and intensive care baby units is probably a major cause of lactic acidosis and lactic aciduria because of the inability of the newborn to utilize the administered glucose in the amounts given, resulting in a gluconic and lactic aciduria (Chalmers and Lawson, 1982). In such circumstances, the concomitant administration of insulin may be advised.

Lactic acidosis may also occur as a secondary phenomenon in other disorders of organic acid metabolism (Chalmers and Lawson, 1982), including isovaleric acidaemia, propionic acidaemia, methylmalonic aciduria, 3-hydroxy-3-methylglutaric aciduria and pyroglutamic aciduria. It may also arise more directly in multicarboxylase deficiency caused by deficiencies of holocarboxylase synthetase, biotinidase and other factors, where one of the secondarily-affected mitochondrial enzymes is pyruvate carboxylase (EC 6.4.1.1). Thus, in the study by Robinson et al. (1980), two of the 28 patients with 'unidentified disorders' in fact had the latter condition. All of these disorders are, however, readily excluded on the basis of their associated characteristic organic aciduria and such errors should not arise if adequate organic acid analyses are undertaken prior to expensive and time-consuming investigative enzymology.

THE CONGENITAL LACTIC ACIDOSES

The identified causes of congenital lactic acidosis include disorders of pyruvate metabolism, of gluconeogenesis and of the respiratory chain. Some disorders of the tricarboxylic acid (TCA) cycle may also be included, particularly where these are in closely related enzyme systems, for example the 2-oxoglutarate dehydrogenase complex (α kg DH) (EC 1.2.4.2).

Disorders affecting the pyruvate dehydrogenase (PDH) complex (EC 1.2.4.1) have been discussed by Robinson (1983) and Robinson and Sherwood (1984) and in reviews elsewhere (see e.g. Chalmers and Lawson, 1982): identified enzyme deficiencies include those of pyruvate decarboxylase (E1) (EC 4.1.1.1) (Farrell et al., 1975; Strömme et al., 1976; Robinson et al., 1980; Robinson and Sherwood, 1984) and lipoamide dehydrogenase (E3) (EC 1.6.4.3), the latter being associated with disordered metabolism of pyruvate, 2-oxoglutarate and branched-chain keto acids (Robinson et al., 1977, 1981; Taylor et al., 1978; Munnich et al., 1982; Kuhara et al., 1983), since all three dehydrogenase complexes share the same E3 enzyme. Few reports have appeared consistent with a deficiency of dihydrolipoyl transacetylase (E2) (EC 2.3.1.12), for which no direct enzyme assay exists at present, but the occurrence of patients with congenital lactic acidoses caused by deficiencies in this enzyme or its subunits appears most probable (Cederbaum et al., 1976). A patient with apparent deficiencies of the E1 enzymes of both the PDH and α kg DH complexes, with altered binding of thiamine pyrophosphate (TPP) has also been described (Kuroda et al., 1979). The common identity of some of the

subunits of all three enzymes involved in these complexes seems probable to explain some of the patients in whom such combined deficiencies have been reported. Patients with apparent deficiencies in the activating enzyme of the PDH complex, PDH phosphate phosphatase, have also been observed but only one report has appeared in detail (Robinson and Sherwood, 1975). The possibility of substrate transport, regulatory and structural defects affecting the activity of these enzyme complexes *in vivo* that are difficult to demonstrate *in vitro*, particularly in cultured skin fibroblasts, indicates the need for better diagnostic approaches, possibly using substrates labelled with stable isotopes for investigations *in vivo*.

The close association of the PDH and α kg DH complexes and their combined deficiencies indicates the close links between the TCA cycle and pyruvate and lactate metabolism. Many patients with congenital lactic acidoses caused by known enzyme deficiencies have increased concentrations of TCA cycle intermediates in their urine, indicating possible inhibition of the cycle caused by imbalance of the NAD/NADH ratio, lack of availability of NADH and possible inhibition of common transport systems. Several patients have been observed with moderate lactic acidoses but with more marked excretion of TCA cycle intermediates suggesting reduction of activity of specific TCA cycle enzymes themselves, with the lactic acidosis being a secondary phenomenon. The patients are generally characterized by severe progressive ataxia, neurological features and early death, indicating the severity of even partial deficiencies in the cycle.

Patients with disorders affecting pyruvate carboxylase (excluding multicarboxylase deficiencies) (Saudubray et al., 1976; De Vivo et al., 1977; Van Biervliet et al., 1977b; Atkin et al., 1979; Baal et al., 1981; Coudé et al., 1981) have been shown to include those who have enzyme protein present, albeit inactive or with reduced catalytic activity (cross-reacting material positive (CRM + ve)) and those who are totally deficient (CRM − ve) (Robinson, 1983; Robinson and Sherwood, 1984). The combination of clinical and biochemical symptoms including the hyperammonaemia, ketosis and citrullinaemia generally without hypoglycaemia (Saudubray et al., 1976; Coudé et al., 1981) associated with the CRM−ve variants, together with organic acid analysis (Van Biervliet et al., 1977b), should allow differentiation of these patients and indication of the appropriate enzymology to perform.

Disorders of gluconeogenesis, which may also cause congenital lactic acidosis, are not a primary subject under consideration in the present context, having recently been reviewed in detail elsewhere (Burman et al., 1980). These include fructose-1,6-bisphosphatase deficiency, glucose-6-phosphatase deficiency (types I and IB glycogen storage diseases) and phosphoenolpyruvate carboxykinase (PEPCK) (EC 4.1.1.32) deficiency (Fiser et al., 1974; Hommes et al., 1976; Vidnes et al., 1976). The first two disorders are characterized by fasting hypoglycaemia without ketosis and hepatomegaly and may be more easily distinguished from other causes of congenital lactic acidosis. They also have distinctive organic aciduria, however, and are included here for completeness. PEPCK deficiency is also characterized by non-ketotic hypoglycaemia but also by hypotonia and only moderate lactic acidosis, together with fatty deposits in liver and other tissues. The abnormal triglyceride metabolism associated with this and the other disorders of gluconeogenesis has not been satisfactorily explained but in PEPCK deficiency the combination of symptoms has been likened to those of systemic carnitine deficiency, which may give some clue to the underlying aetiology.

Disorders of the respiratory chain have been covered in elegant detail by Clark *et al.* (1983, 1984) and include deficiencies of single cytochromes, for example b, of cytochrome c oxidase, of more than one cytochrome, for example aa_3/b and ATPase. All of these patients are characterized by a mitochondrial myopathy and most patients have presented in older age groups including adults. However, some patients with generalized cytochrome c oxidase deficiency present acutely in early infancy with a rapidly lethal combination of mitochondrial myopathy, Fanconi syndrome and massive lactic acidosis (Van Biervliet *et al.*, 1977a) and such disorders should also be considered in the differential diagnosis of congenital lactic acidoses in infants.

THE ORGANIC ACIDURIA OF CONGENITAL LACTIC ACIDOSES

This brief summary of the known causes of the congenital lactic acidoses puts into perspective the complexity of their differential diagnosis, the major problem being the differentiation of the various disorders of pyruvate metabolism and of the TCA cycle. Chalmers *et al.* (1977) suggested from studies on a patient with pyruvate decarboxylase (E1) deficiency that the quantitative pattern of organic acids in such patients, together with the clinical and biochemical profiles of the patients, would allow indication of the area of the underlying primary enzyme deficiency, thereby reducing and refining the otherwise considerable amount of investigative and often frustrating enzymology required to achieve a diagnosis (Robinson *et al.*, 1980).

There have been few adequate reports on organic acids in patients with congenital lactic acidoses other than those of Van Biervliet and his co-workers (Van Biervliet *et al.*, 1977a,b; Willems, 1978) and of the author and his co-workers (Chalmers *et al.*, 1977, 1978), organic acid patterns in urine frequently being described as 'normal' (Baal *et al.*, 1981). In the present study, quantitative extraction methods have been used, based upon the use of DEAE Sephadex (see Chalmers and Lawson, 1982), combined with quantitative capillary gas chromatography on fused silica columns (Tracey *et al.*, 1983), and capillary gas chromatography–mass spectrometry. The latter included the use of extracted ion profiles of ions characteristic of the representative metabolites in these disorders and selected to give 'fingerprints' of the individual lactic acidoses (Chalmers, Whelan and Roe, unpublished). Urine specimens from 23 patients were examined (Table 1). While the numbers of patients included are relatively small, all had clearly

Table 1 Patients with proven causes of congenital lactic acidoses and included in the study

Deficiency	No. of patients
PDH complex	
E1	3
E3	1
PDH phosphate phosphatase	1
Pyruvate carboxylase, isolated	4
Gluconeogenesis	
GSD I	6
GSD IB	2
Fructose-1,6-bisphosphatase	2
Cytochromes	
cyt b	2
cyt aa_3/b	1
cyt c oxidase	1

demonstrated and unambiguous enzyme or cytochrome deficiencies (except those with GSDI B), clinical history was known and generally a number of specimens, taken at different times during the course of their illness, were available for analysis. Several have been published as individual case reports by the referring centres (for example, Strömme *et al.*, 1976; Van Biervliet *et al.*, 1977a,b; Chalmers *et al.*, 1977, 1978; Morgan-Hughes *et al.*, 1977). Specimens from several other patients not included here, with as yet unproven enzyme deficiencies, were also examined for comparative purposes, and included some with apparent TCA cycle defects.

The patterns and concentrations of organic acids observed are dependent upon the time of the sample in relation to the clinical condition of the patient and the treatment, including diet, employed. Specimens were examined wherever possible from before and during treatment periods. Insufficient space is available, however, to list in detail the observations made on individual patients and this report represents a summarized presentation of the available data. The quantitative patterns reported here as characteristic for a particular condition have been consistent for the untreated sick patients on presentation, at which time the initial samples are taken for diagnostic purposes. Wherever possible, reference has also been made to the literature reports where these are well documented, to confirm the present findings and to summarize the biochemical and clinical characteristics associated with a particular enzyme deficiency.

Cytochrome deficiencies

The most simple pattern is observed in patients with cytochrome deficiencies (Figure 1). Here a gross lactic aciduria is observed with a relatively normal pattern of other organic acids including those of the tricarboxylic acid cycle and such patients are generally easily distinguished from other patients with congenital lactic acidoses. Infantile patients with generalized cytochrome c oxidase deficiency show a Fanconi syndrome in addition to their mitochondrial myopathy and evidence

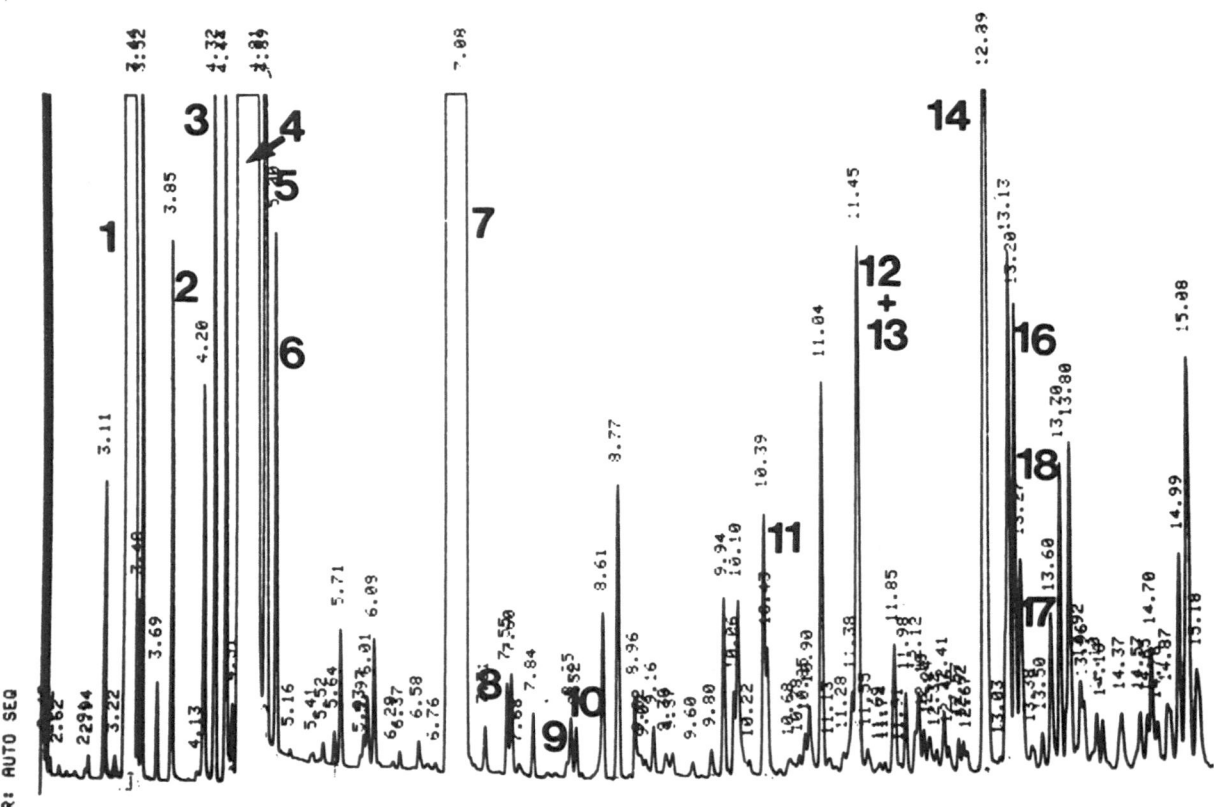

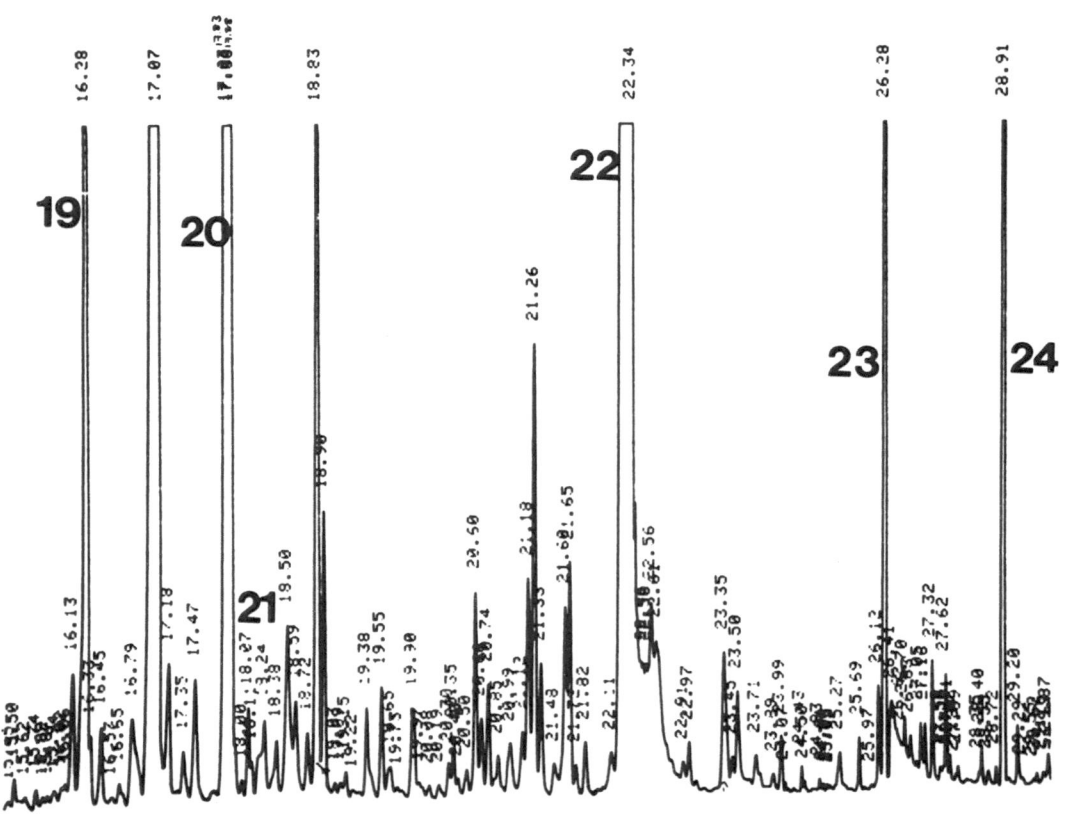

of greatly reduced energy availability and may thus be distinguished by their characteristic amino aciduria.

Disorders of gluconeogenesis

The gluconeogenic disorders tend to be distinguished clinically by their fasting hypoglycaemia and hepatomegaly but here again distinctive organic acid patterns are observed in urine (Figure 2). Patients show a gross lactic aciduria and only a very moderate pyruvic aciduria, increased [lactate]/[pyruvate] (L/P) ratio and a greatly increased 2-oxoglutaric aciduria with associated 2-hydroxyglutaric aciduria in the absence of increases in other TCA cycle intermediates. There may also be a moderate dicarboxylic aciduria in some patients indicating a disturbance of fatty acid β-oxidation. The patients show distinctive responses to glucose tolerance, glucagon and alanine loading tests that help with their differential diagnosis. The absolute diagnosis is made by enzymology on liver biopsy material, this being essential to finally distinguish GSD I, GSD IB and fructose-1,6-bisphosphatase deficiency. On treatment with, for example, nocturnal nasogastric and frequent daytime glucose feeding, the lactic aciduria may be almost abolished but the 2-oxoglutaric aciduria persists. The reason for the latter is still unclear, although it is probably caused by an excessive input of substrate into the TCA cycle combined with a retardation of the flux at the rate limiting step of the α kg DH complex (Kodama *et al.*, 1980). No specimens were available in the present study from a patient with PEPCK deficiency but these rare patients should be distinguished by their non-ketotic fasting hypoglycaemia, hypotonia and moderate lactic acidosis.

Disorders of pyruvate dehydrogenase and of the TCA cycle

Analysis of organic acids in urine may be of greatest value, however, in the differential diagnosis of disorders of pyruvate metabolism and of the TCA cycle. Pyruvate decarboxylase or E1 deficiency is characterized by greatly increased lactate and, particularly, pyruvate concentrations with the L/P ratio remaining normal. This may be ascribed to lack of pyruvate oxidation at the initial stage of the PDH complex with a disproportionate increase in pyruvate associated with increased alanine concentrations in blood. There is some increase in TCA cycle intermediates with 2-oxoglutarate being particularly increased with, of interest, much less increase in 2-hydroxyglutarate. Citrate excretion tends

to be reduced, probably because of the decreased flux of pyruvate to acetyl CoA combined with decreased activity of the TCA cycle itself but isocitrate may be increased (Figure 3). A similar pattern with normal citrate excretion was seen in the patient with an E3 deficiency, here accompanied by moderate increases in branched chain oxo acids and their hydroxy acid derivatives (but not to the concentrations observed in patients with classical branched chain ketoaciduria). Patients with E3 deficiency also show moderate increases in plasma branched chain amino acids and these features should provide good indicators of a probable E3 deficiency for final confirmation by enzymology. Other patients with PDH deficiencies that cannot be ascribed to E1 or E3 deficiencies (putative E2 deficiencies or other causes) show similarly greatly increased lactate, pyruvate and 2-oxoglutarate concentrations with relatively normal branched chain oxo acids. Patients with E3 deficiency probably have only a slowing of pyruvate oxidation *in vivo* since the deficient enzyme is responsible for the recycling of the lipoic acid cofactor for the E2 enzyme and not directly for pyruvate conversion to acetyl moeities. Patients with an E2 deficiency may also show only a slowing of pyruvate oxidation *in vivo* but should show a decreased acetyl CoA production comparable to that in patients with an E1 deficiency. The latter, with the initial oxidation of pyruvate itself greatly reduced, tend as a result to show the greatest increase in pyruvate concentrations and the most severe clinical symptoms. Patients with PDH phosphate phosphatase deficiency show only minimal increases in blood lactate concentrations and a normal quantitative organic acid pattern in urine, consistent with the primarily regulatory deficiency present *in vivo*.

Pyruvate carboxylase deficiency

Finally, the patterns and concentrations of organic acids in urine of patients with isolated pyruvate carboxylase deficiency are quite distinctive from those of patients with disorders of the PDH complex. In these patients lactate is again greatly increased but with only a moderate increase in pyruvate and thus a greatly increased L/P ratio (Figure 4). Blood alanine concentrations are normal. Citrate excretion is normal although there are increases in the TCA cycle intermediates that are precursors to oxaloacetate, particularly fumarate, malate, succinate and 2-oxoglutarate. The accumulation of these precursors indicates the close association, through pyruvate carboxylase, of

---

Figure 1 Organic acids in urine of a patient with congenital lactic acidosis, mitochondrial myopathy and a cytochrome (*b*) deficiency. Extracted using DEAE Sephadex and separated as their trimethylsilyl (TMS) and TMS-ethoxime derivatives using capillary gas–liquid chromatography on 25 m fused silica CP-SIL-5 columns with a split injection (70:1) of 2 μl sample at 200 °C. Temperature programming from 70 °C to 250 °C at 6 °C min^{-1} was used with helium carrier gas (1.4 ml min^{-1}).

Relevant peak identifications, confirmed using GC–MS, are: (1) lactate, (2) pyruvate, (3) 2-hydroxy-*n*-butyrate, (4) sulphate, (5) 3-hydroxy-*n*-butyrate, (6) acetoacetate, (7) phosphate, (8) succinate, (9) glycerate, (10) fumarate, (11) 2-deoxytetronate, (12) malate, (13) pyroglutamate, (14) erythronate, [(15) 2-hydroxyglutarate (not seen)], (16) threonate, (17) 3-hydroxy-3-methylglutarate, (18) 2-oxoglutarate, (19) aconitate (presumed *cis*), (20) citrate, (21) isocitrate, (22) urate, (23) *n*-tetracosane internal standard and (24) *n*-hexacosane internal standard.

(The small numbers where seen are retention times in minutes)

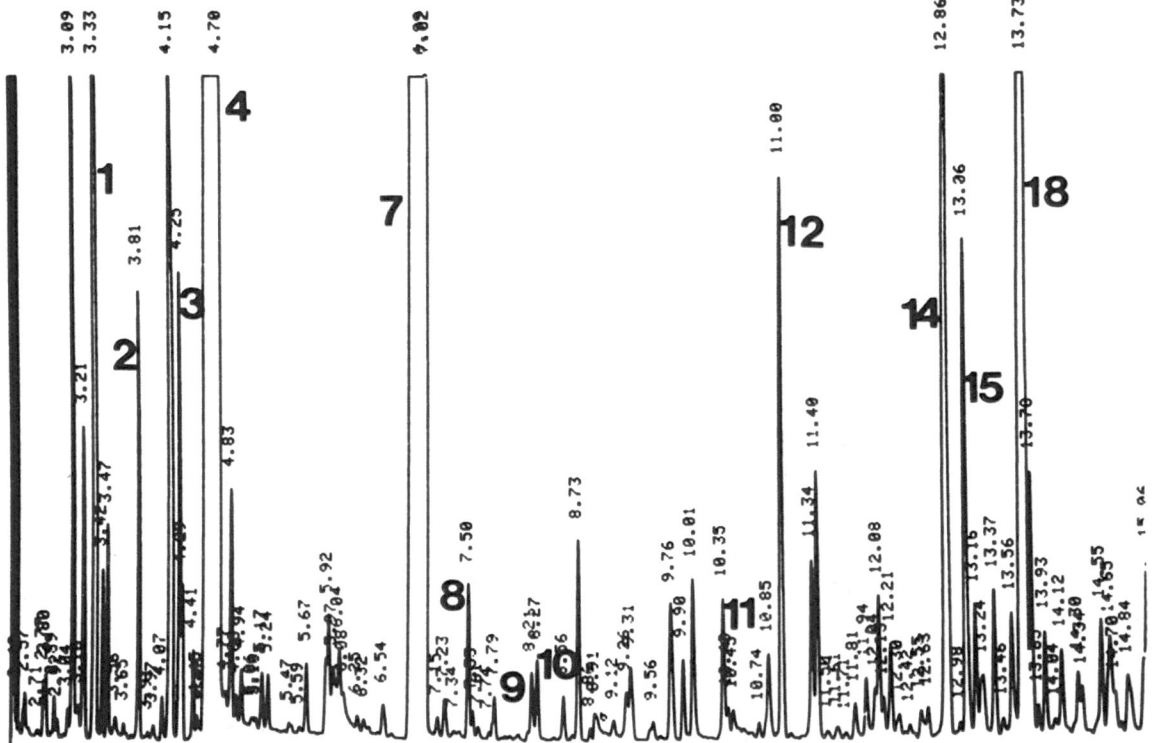

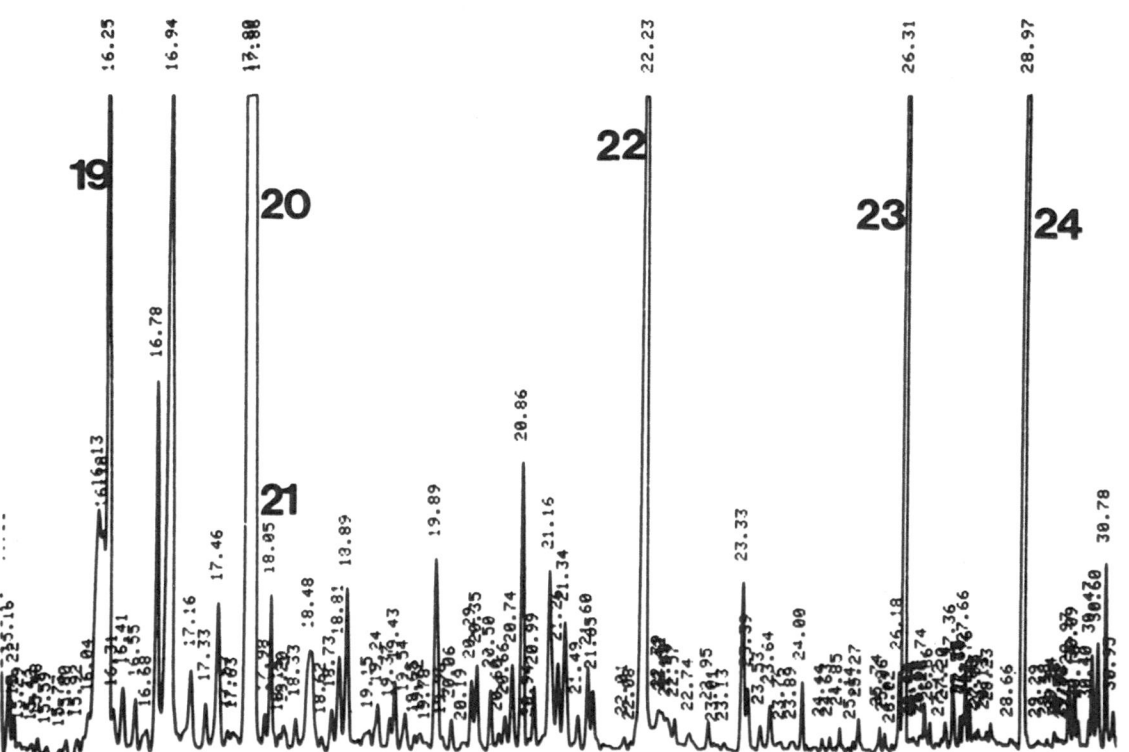

Figure 2 Organic acids in urine of a patient with congenital lactic acidosis and glucose-6-phosphatase deficiency (glycogen storage disease, GSD, type I). Chromatographic conditions and peak identifications are as given in the legend to Figure 1

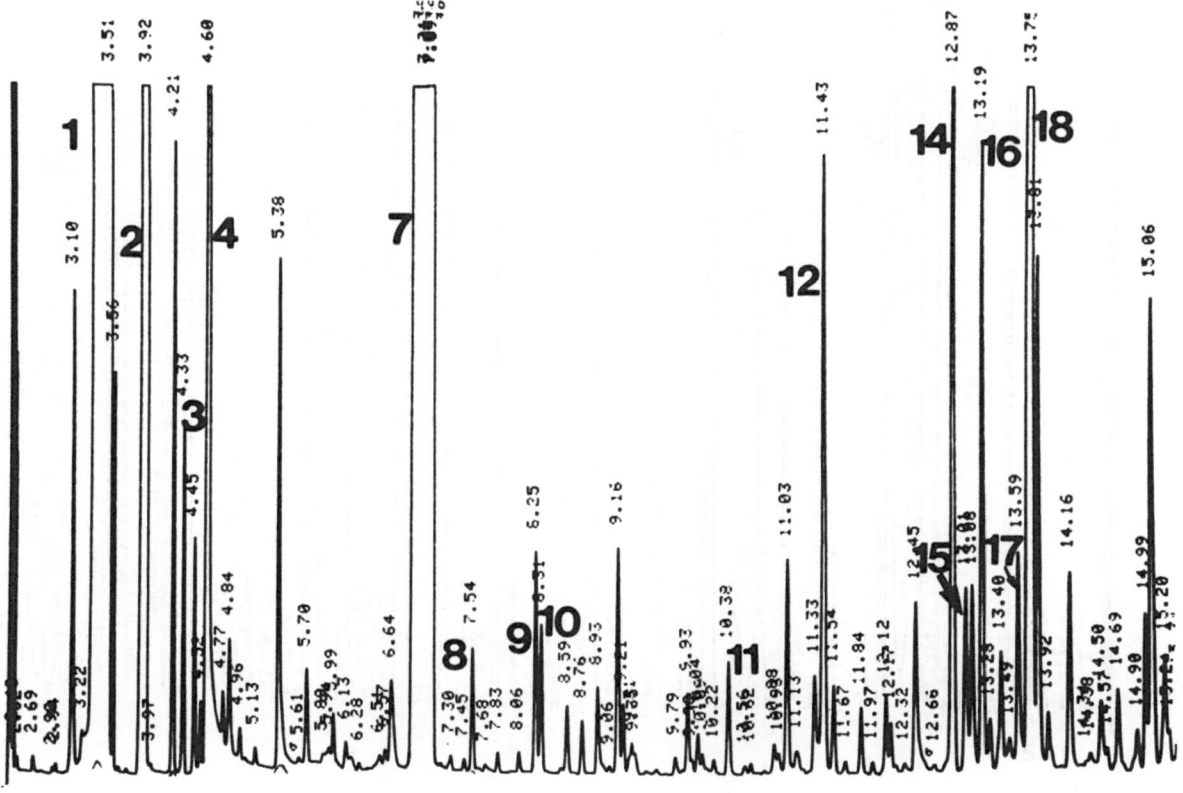

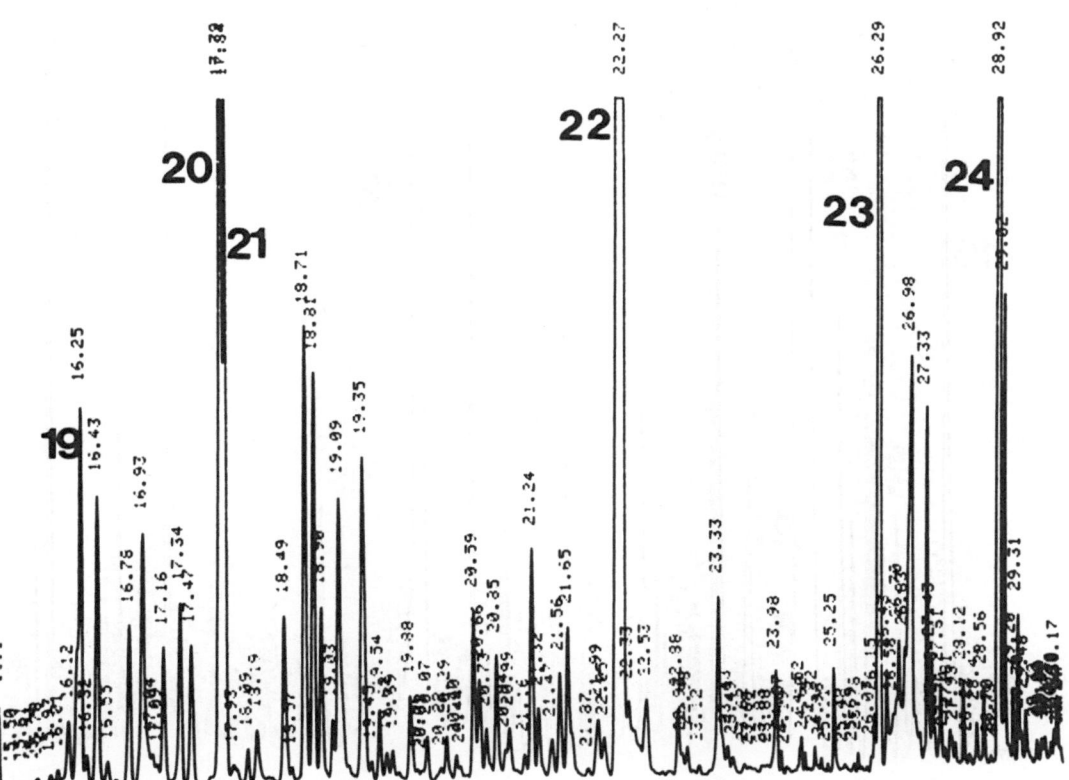

Figure 3 Organic acids in urine of a patient with congenital lactic acidosis and pyruvate decarboxylase (E1) deficiency. Chromatographic conditions and peak identifications are as given in the legend to Figure 1

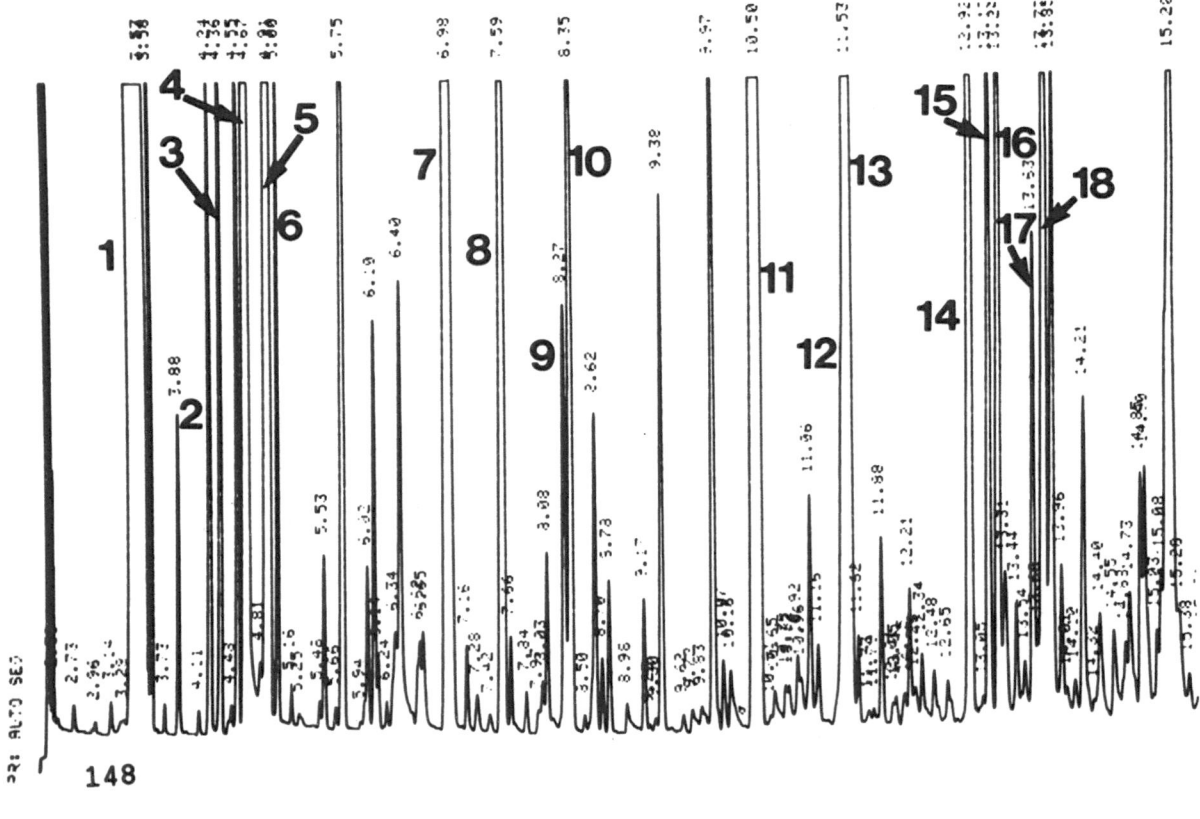

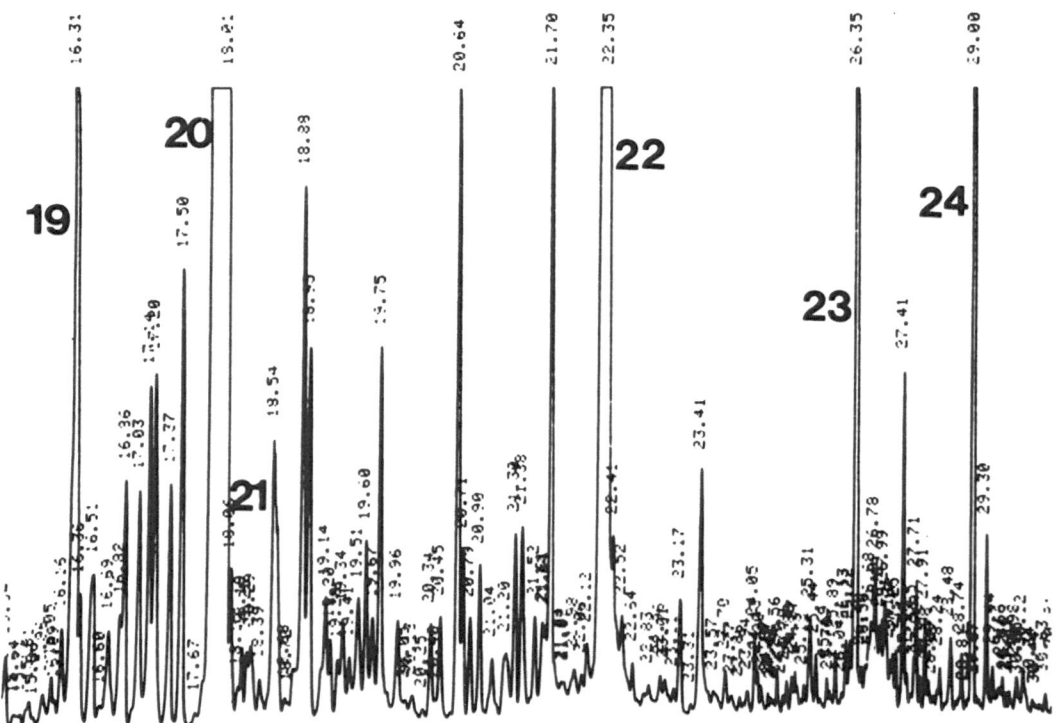

Figure 4 Organic acids in urine of a patient with congenital lactic acidosis and pyruvate carboxylase deficiency. Chromatographic conditions and peak identifications are as given in the legend to Figure 1

pyruvate with the TCA cycle and the imbalance of $NAD^+/NADH$ ratios in this condition. They may also explain the general absence of hypoglycaemia in patients with pyruvate carboxylase deficiency. These patients also generally show increased concentrations of 3-hydroxybutyrate and acetoacetate in contrast to the non-ketotic hypoglycaemia in disorders of gluconeogenesis and the CRM–ve patients also show hyperammonaemia with associated glutaminuria, glutamic aciduria and pyroglutamic aciduria. Thus the organic acid pattern and concentrations in urine may be particularly useful to distinguish patients with pyruvate carboxylase deficiency prior to confirmatory enzymology.

CONCLUSIONS: THE DIFFERENTIAL DIAGNOSIS OF CONGENITAL LACTIC ACIDOSES

These observations form the basis of a scheme for the differential diagnosis of patients with congenital lactic acidoses. After exclusion of uninherited, acquired and other secondary causes of lactic acidosis, the quantitative pattern of organic acids in urine, summarized in Table 2, together with other clinical and biochemical observations, provides valuable indicators of the area of the underlying primary metabolic disorder. The approach to the investigation of the patient with a lactic acidosis (Figure 5) must include an initial careful clinical and biochemical investigation followed by quantitative analysis of organic acids in urine and blood plasma. The results of these observations should exclude the uninherited and acquired causes of the lactic acidosis and other disorders of organic acid metabolism, giving at the same time indication of the possible cause of the congenital lactic acidosis present. These observations, supported by loading tests (for example, glucose and alanine) and other investigations (for example, exercise tests) where appropriate, are followed by *selected* enzymology on cultured skin fibroblasts, liver biopsy or

muscle biopsy material to give a final definitive diagnosis. The use *in vivo* of metabolic precursors labelled with stable isotopes may be expected to have a place in the differential diagnosis of the congenital lactic acidoses in the future. Further detailed observations of individual new patients with proven enzyme deficiencies are required to establish further the quantitative organic acid patterns indicated in this paper. The data summarized here indicate clearly that the study of organic acids has a key and central role in the clinical and biochemical investigation and diagnosis of patients with congenital lactic acidoses.

The rarity of individual patients with these disorders makes a study of this kind of necessity a collaborative exercise. I am indebted to the many paediatricians and biochemists who have shared specimens from their patients, particularly Drs O. Borud, N. J. Brandt, E. Christensen, M. Duran, N. Gregersen and S. K. Wadman, and who were closely involved in the earlier part of this study on the congenital lactic acidoses. I am most grateful to Mrs B. M. Tracey and Mr D. Watson for their invaluable technical collaboration in this work.

References

Atkin, B. M., Buist, N. R. M., Utter, M. F., Leiter, A. B. and Banker, B. Q. Pyruvate carboxylase deficiency and lactic acidosis in a retarded child without Leigh's disease. *Pediatr. Res.* 13 (1979) 109–116

Baal, M. G., Gabreëls, F. J. M., Renier, W. O., Hommes, F. A., Gijsbers, Th. H. J., Lamars, K. J. B. and Kok, J. C. N. A patient with pyruvate carboxylase deficiency in the liver: Treatment with aspartic acid and thiamine. *Dev. Med. Child Neurol.* 23 (1981) 521–530

Burman, D., Holton, J. B. and Pennock, C. A. *Inherited Disorders of Carbohydrate Metabolism*, MTP Press, Lancaster, 1980

Cederbaum, S. D., Blass, J. P., Minkoff, N., Brown, W. J., Cotton, M. E. and Harris, S. H. Sensitivity to carbohydrate in a patient with familial intermittant lactic acidosis and pyruvate dehydrogenase deficiency. *Pediatr. Res.* 10 (1976) 713–720

Chalmers, R. A. and Lawson, A. M. *Organic Acids in Man. The Analytical Chemistry, Biochemistry and Diagnosis of the Organic Acidurias*, Chapman & Hall, London, 1982

Chalmers, R. A., Lawson, A. M. and Borud, O. Gas chromatographic and mass spectrometric studies on urinary organic acids in a patient with congenital lactic acidosis due to pyruvate decarboxylase deficiency. *Clin. Chim. Acta* 77 (1977) 117–124

Chalmers, R. A., Ryman, B. E. and Watts, R. W. E. Studies on a patient with *in vivo* evidence of type I glycogenosis and normal enzyme activities *in vitro*. *Acta Paediatr. Scand.* 67 (1978) 201–207

Clark, J. B., Hayes, D. J., Byrne, E. and Morgan-Hughes, J. A. Mitochondrial myopathies: defects in mitochondrial metabolism in human skeletal muscle. *Biochem. Soc. Trans.* 11 (1983) 626–627

Clark, J. B., Hayes, D. J., Morgan-Hughes, J. A. and Byrne, E. Mitochondrial myopathies: disorders of the respiratory chain and oxidative phosphorylation. *J. Inher. Metab. Dis.* 7 Suppl. 1 (1984) 62–68

Coudé, F. X., Ogier, H., Marsac, C., Munnich, A., Charpentier, C. and Saudubray, J. M. Secondary citrullinemia with hyperammonemia in four neonatal cases of pyruvate carboxylase deficiency. *Pediatrics* 68 (1981) 914 (C)

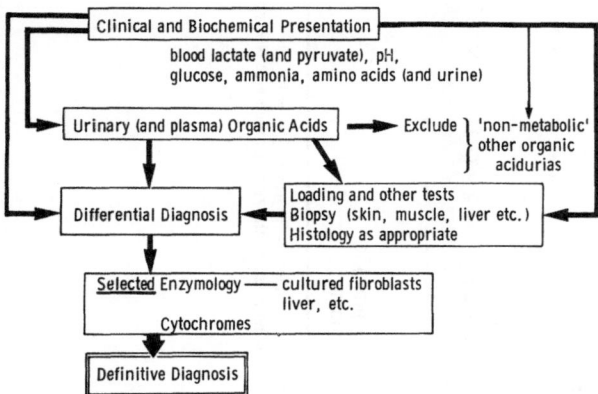

Figure 5 Scheme for the approach to the clinical and biochemical investigation of the patient with suspected congenital lactic acidosis

Table 2 Organic acid patterns in urine of patients with congenital lactic acidoses: an aid to their differential diagnosis

Disorder (Enzyme deficiency)	Organic acids								L/P ratio	Other observations
	Lactic	Pyruvic	2-Oxoglutaric	Citric	Isocitric	Fumaric	Malic	Succinic		
Pyruvate dehydrogenase										
E1	++++	+++	++	−	+	+	++	N	N	−
E3	++++	+	++	+	+	N	++	++	++	Branched-chain keto and hydroxy aciduria; branched-chain amino acidaemia
Other	+++	++	++	−	+	+	+	+	N	−
Pyruvate carboxylase	+++	(+)	++	+	+	++(+)	++(+)	++(+)	++(+)	Ketosis; CRM − ve with hyperammonaemia and citrullinaemia
Gluconeogenic:										
Fructose-1,6-bisphosphatase	+	N	+(+)	N	N	N	N	N	(+)	Hypoglycaemia, no ketosis, hypertriglyceridaemia, fatty liver, hepatomegaly
Glucose-6-phosphatase (GSD I/IB)	++	N	++(+)	N	N	N	+	+	+	
Cytochromes b, aa_3/b, cytochrome c oxidase	+++(+)	N	N	N	N	N	+	+	++	Mitochondrial myopathy; Fanconi in cyt aa_3/b and generalized cytochrome c oxidase
Normal ranges (approx.) in mmol/mol creatinine	5–40	<1–20	10–30	200–1500	20–150	<1–10	10–30	10–30	10–20	

L/P ratio is the ratio of [lactate]/[pyruvate]; N = 10–20
Quantitative levels indicated by the symbols used are: N = normal; − = 0.5 × N; + = (3–5) × N; + + = (10–50) × N; + + + = (100–500) × N; + + + + = (1000–5000) × N

De Vivo, D. C., Haymond, M. W., Leckie, M. P., Bursmann, Y. L., McDougal, D. B. and Pagliara, A. S. The clinical and biochemical implications of pyruvate carboxylase deficiency. *J. Clin. Exp. Med.* 45 (1977) 1281–1296

Farrell, D. F., Clark, A. F., Scott, R. C. and Wennberg, R. P. Absence of pyruvate decarboxylase activity in man: A cause of congenital lactic acidosis. *Science* 187 (1975) 1082–1084

Fiser, R. H., Melsher, H. L. and Fisher, D. A. Hepatic phosphoenolpyruvate carboxykinase (PEPCK) deficiency. A new cause of hypoglycemia in childhood. *Pediatr. Res.* 8 (1974) 432 (Abstr.)

Hommes, F. A., Bendien, K., Elema, J. D., Bremer, H. J. and Lombeck, I. Two cases of phosphoenolpyruvate carboxy-kinase deficiency. *Acta Paediatr. Scand.* 65 (1976) 233–240

Kodama, H., Okada, S., Inui, K., Yutaka, T. and Yabuchi, H. Studies on α-ketoglutaric aciduria in type I glycogenosis. *Tohoku J. Exp. Med.* 131 (1980) 347–353

Kuhara, T., Shinka, T., Inoue, Y., Matsumoto, M., Yoshvio, M., Sakaguchi, Y. and Matsumoto, I. Studies of urinary organic acid profiles of a patient with dihydrolipoyl dehydrogenase deficiency. *Clin. Chim. Acta* 133 (1983) 133–140

Kuroda, Y., Kline, J. J., Sweetman, L., Nyhan, W. L. and Groshong, T. D. Abnormal pyruvate and α-ketoglutarate dehydrogenase complexes in a patient with lactic acidemia. *Pediatr. Res.* 13 (1979) 928–931

Morgan-Hughes, J. A., Darveniza, P., Kahn, S. N., Landon, D. N., Sherratt, R. M., Land, J. M. and Clark, J. B. A mitochondrial myopathy characterised by a deficiency in reducible cytochrome b. *Brain* 100 (1977) 617–640

Munnich, A., Saudubray, J. M., Taylor, J., Charpentier, C., Marsac, C., Rocchiccioli, F., Amédée-Manesme, O., Coudé, F. X. Frézal, J. and Robinson, B. H. Congenital lactic acidosis, α-ketoglutaric aciduria and variant form of maple syrup urine disease due to a single enzyme defect: Dihydrolipoyl dehydrogenase deficiency. *Acta Paediatr. Scand.* 71 (1982) 167–171

Robinson, B. H. Inborn errors of pyruvate metabolism. *Biochem. Soc. Trans.* 11 (1983) 623–626

Robinson, B. H. and Sherwood, W. G. Pyruvate dehydrogenase phosphatase deficiency: A cause of congenital chronic lactic acidosis in infancy. *Pediatr. Res.* 9 (1975) 935–939

Robinson, B. H. and Sherwood, W. G. Lactic acidaemia. *J. Inher. Metab. Dis.* 7 Suppl. 1 (1984) 69–73

Robinson, B. H., Taylor, J., Kahler, S. G. and Kirkman, H. N. Lactic acidemia, neurologic deterioration and carbohydrate dependence in a girl with dihydrolipoyl dehydrogenase deficiency. *Eur. J. Paediatr.* 136 (1981) 35–39

Robinson, B. H., Taylor, J. and Sherwood, W. G. Deficiency of dihydrolipoyl dehydrogenase (a component of the pyruvate and α-ketoglutarate dehydrogenase complexes): a cause of congenital chronic lactic acidosis in infancy. *Pediatr. Res.* 11 (1977) 1198–1202

Robinson, B. H., Taylor, J. and Sherwood, W. G. The genetic heterogeneity of lactic acidosis: Occurrence of recognisable inborn errors of metabolism in a paediatric population with lactic acidosis. *Pediatr. Res.* 14 (1980) 956–982

Saudubray, J. M., Marsac, C., Charpentier, C., Cathelineau, L., Besson Leaud, M. and Leroux, J. P. Neonatal congenital lactic acidosis with pyruvate carboxylase deficiency in two siblings. *Acta Paediatr. Scand.* 65 (1976) 717–724

Strömme, J. H., Borud, O. and Moe, P. J. Fatal lactic acidosis in a newborn attributable to a congenital defect of pyruvate dehydrogenase. *Pediatr. Res.* 10 (1976) 62–66

Taylor, J., Robinson, B. H. and Sherwood, W. G. A defect in branched-chain amino acid metabolism in a patient with congenital lactic acidosis due to dihydrolipoyl dehydrogenase deficiency. *Pediatr. Res.* 12 (1978) 60–62

Tracey, B. M., Stacey, T. E. and Chalmers, R. A. Urinary and plasma organic acids in dizygotic twin siblings with 3-hydroxy-3-methylglutaric aciduria, studied by gas chromatography and mass spectrometry using fused silica capillary columns. *J. Inher. Metab. Dis.* 6 Suppl 2 (1983) 125–126

Van Biervliet, J. P. G. M., Bruinvis, L., Ketting, D., de Bree, P. K., Van der Heiden, C., Wadman, S. K., Willems, J. L., Bookelman, H., Van Haelst, V. and Monnens, L. A. H. Hereditary mitochondrial myopathy with lactic acidaemia, a deToni–Fanconi–Debré Syndrome, and a defective respiratory chain in voluntary striated muscles. *Pediatr. Res.* 11 (1977a) 1088–1093

Van Biervliet, J. P. G. M., Bruinvis, L., Van der Heiden, C., Ketting, D., Wadman, S. K., Willems, J. L. and Monnens, L. A. H. Report of a patient with severe, chronic lactic acidaemia and pyruvate carboxylase deficiency. *Dev. Med. Child Neurol.* 19 (1977b) 392–401

Vidnes, J. and Søvik, O. Gluconeogenesis in infancy and childhood. III. Deficiency of extramitochondrial form of hepatic phosphoenolpyruvate carboxykinase in a case of persistent neonatal hypoglycaemia. *Acta Paediatr. Scand.* 65 (1976) 307–312

Willems, J. L. Disturbances in pyruvate metabolism. A biochemical and clinical investigation. Thesis, Catholic University of Nijmegen, 1978

J. Inher. Metab. Dis. 7 Suppl. 1 (1984) 90–92

4-Hydroxybutyric Aciduria: A New Inborn Error of Metabolism

The three papers below describe the clinical and laboratory evidence for a new inborn error of metabolism, 4-hydroxybutyric aciduria, together with evidence for the cause being a deficiency of succinic semialdehyde dehydrogenase. The disorder is apparently inherited in an autosomal recessive mode.

The clinical and biochemical findings in four patients with 4-hydroxybutyric aciduria are reviewed. The prominent clinical features are marked hypotonia, non-progressive ataxia of the trunk and limbs, ocular dyspraxia and mental retardation. GC–MS examination of urinary organic acids and short chain fatty acids resulted in the identification of 4-hydroxybutyric acid (GHB) and succinic semialdehyde (SSA). GHB was also elevated in blood and c.s.f. In the older patients a continuous improvement in the atactic symptoms was observed over several years coincident with a significant fall in the plasma GHB. GHB and SSA are metabolites of 4-aminobutyric acid (GABA) and an increased concentration of GABA was observed in the c.s.f. of one patient so studied. Studies of lysates of lymphocytes isolated from whole blood of two of the patients showed the molecular defect to be a deficiency of succinic semialdehyde dehydrogenase. Additional studies of enzyme activities in family members gave results consistent with an autosomal recessive mode of inheritance.

4-Hydroxybutyric Aciduria: A New Inborn Error of Metabolism. I. Clinical Review

D. Rating, F. Hanefeld, H. Siemes and J. Kneer
Department of Pediatrics, Free University of Berlin, Kaiserin Auguste Victoria Haus, Heubnerweg 6, D-1000 Berlin 19, G.F.R.

C. Jakobs
Present address: Department of Pediatrics, Academic Hospital of the Free University of Amsterdam, De Boelelaan 1117, 1007 MB Amsterdam, The Netherlands

M. Hermier and P. Divry
Laboratoire de Biochimie, Hôpital Debrousse, 29 rue Soeur Biovier, 69332, Lyon, Cedex 5, France

Atactic syndromes in childhood are difficult to classify and only few conditions are well defined and characterized by specific biochemical abnormalities e.g. IgA deficiency in Louis Bar syndrome (McKusick 20890), elevated serum levels of phytanic acid in Refsum's disease (McKusick 26650) or a β-lipoproteinaemia in Bassen–Kornzweig syndrome (McKusick 20010). In 1981 we observed a Turkish boy who suffered from a non-progressive ataxia with muscular hypotonia. He excreted large amounts of 4-hydroxybutyric acid (GHB) in his urine. The biochemical findings in this boy led us to postulate a deficiency of succinic semialdehyde (SSA) dehydrogenase, as the first recognized inborn error of GABA metabolism (Jakobs et al., 1981).

This paper summarizes the relevant clinical findings in our index patient as well as in two other siblings with similar biochemical abnormalities seen by us in Berlin and of a further case observed by Dr Divry in Lyon (Divry et al., 1983).

Case 1: B.S. (born in 1977) is the first child of related Turkish parents. He has a younger healthy sister. Pregnancy and delivery were normal. His psychomotor development was retarded from the beginning: he started to sit at about 8–10 months only. Until the age of 17 months no attempts were made to stand or walk. Though he was said to understand he was unable to speak any syllables or simple words.

On the first examination at our hospital in 1979 (Table 1) we saw a 1½-year-old attentive and mildly mentally retarded boy with a marked truncal and a moderate limb ataxia with very unstable sitting and crawling. He was unable to stand without support. He had a marked muscular hypotonia but no weakness. The plantar responses were flexor. There was no sensory loss and no pathological tonic reflex pattern. His ocular mobility resembled mild ocular apraxia, with normal vision. Both fundi were normal. The physical examination was otherwise normal, especially there were no skin changes or enlargement of internal organs.

Cases 2 and 3 come from an unrelated Lebanese family with five more healthy children of both sexes. F.R. was

Table 1 4-Hydroxybutyric aciduria: clinical signs in three patients at diagnosis

	B.S. (2 years)	M.R. (9 years)	F.R. (11 years)
Mental retardation	Mild	Mild	Mild
Ataxia			
Gait	+ + +	+	+ +
Intention tremor	+ + +	+ +	+ +
'Ocular dyspraxia'	+ + +	+	+ + +
Dysarthria		+ + +	+
Muscular hypotonia	+ + +	0	+
Pyramidal signs	0	0	0
Sensory deficit	0	0	0
Telangiectasia	0	+	+
Tendon reflexes	((+))	(+)	(+)
Epilepsy	???	0	0
Nerve conduction velocity	Normal	Normal	Normal

+ + + = marked,   + + = moderate,   + = slight,   (+) = discrete, ((+)) = minimal; 0 = absent

born in 1970. Pregnancy and delivery were normal. Her psychomotor development was retarded and she could not walk unsupported until the age of 4 years. On the first examination in 1980 (Table 1) at the age of 11 years she had a mild mental retardation, and a moderate ataxia of the trunk and limbs, with a moderate intention tremor. There was a mild muscular hypotonia but no weakness. The deep tendon reflexes were difficult to elicit. There were no pyramidal signs and no sensory disturbances. Her eyes showed bilateral telangiectatic vascular changes of the conjunctivae resembling Louis Bar syndrome. Voluntary conjugate gaze movements were reduced horizontally in both directions without nystagmus. Her speech was slightly dysarthric. The physical examination was otherwise normal.

M.R., her younger brother, was born in 1972. Pregnancy and delivery were normal. In contrast to his elder sister his early motor milestones were normal. He started walking at about 1 year. Though he was said to understand, his active language development was grossly retarded. On the first examination in 1980 (Table 1), aged 9 years, he had a mild mental retardation, with a slight ataxia of the trunk and moderate ataxia of the limbs. There was an only slight ocular dyspraxia. Though he showed no unusual hypotonia or weakness his deep tendon reflexes were difficult to elicit. As with his sister the physical examination otherwise was normal with the exception of striking conjunctival telangiectasias.

Case 4: B.R. was born in 1977 to related Algerian parents. An older sister is said to have been very floppy and died at the age of 4 months without a diagnosis. There is a healthy younger sister. Pregnancy was normal but after birth an intracranial haemorrhage was suspected. However, neither pneumencephalography nor CT scans revealed any lesion. The further development of this boy was characterized by marked ataxia of the trunk and limbs, and marked muscular hypotonia. At the end of the first year of life seizures occurred which were controlled partially by valproate

and phenobarbitone. At the age of 6 years the boy is mentally retarded. He can hardly stand and can not walk.

In all four cases increased amounts of GHB in the urine were found (see Jakobs *et al.*, 1984) while other laboratory investigations were normal including screening for aminoaciduria, determination of phytanic acids and immunoglobulins, nerve conduction velocity, c.s.f. agarose gel electrophoresis.

Increased concentrations of GHB were also found in the c.s.f. in cases 1 and 4. Our index case showed in addition increased levels of GABA in his c.s.f. (GABA-c.s.f.: 654 pmol/ml, controls: mean 148 (range 90–243) pmol/ml). In all four cases there was a continuous fall in the GHB concentration in plasma. Treatment with isoniazid and valproate was tried only in our index case. However, this did not produce any changes of his clinical signs nor of GHB concentration in plasma or urine. Ethosuccimide seemed to worsen the muscular hypotonia and ataxia, the boy became more apathic and showed a change in his mood.

At follow-up, cases 1 and 4 were found to be stable. No progression of the atactic symptoms or of neurological signs could be observed. However, both siblings showed a dramatic improvement of the cerebellar symptoms over the years. Two years later both children showed only very discrete ataxia of the trunk and the limbs, and in the girl only a slight ocular dyspraxia was left (Table 2).

DISCUSSION

The changed pattern of GABA metabolism shown in the urine and plasma of our patients (Jakobs *et al.*, 1984) and the enzyme studies done (Gibson *et al.*, 1983, 1984) demonstrate that the four patients suffer from a non-progressive ataxia due to an SSA dehydrogenase deficiency. GHB is a natural occurring metabolite in human brain (Roth and Giarman, 1969), though it can be found only in very small amounts of about 10^{-5} to 10^{-6} mol/g (Doherty *et al.*, 1978; Santaniello *et al.*, 1978; Roth and Giarman, 1969). GHB derives from glutamic acid and GABA via SSA. The significance of brain GHB is indicated by a highly specific SSA reductase as demonstrated in the brain of rats (Rumigny *et al.*, 1981). It is very likely that the increased c.s.f. concentrations of GHB found in two cases and that of GABA in one case, reflect alterations of GHB and GABA

Table 2 4-Hydroxybutyric aciduria: follow-up in three patients

	B.S. (5 years)	M.R. (11 years)	F.R. (13 years)
Mental state	Stable	Stable	Stable
Speaking	0	Improved	Normal
Ataxia	Unchanged	Improved	Improved
Gait	+ + +	+ + → (+)	+ + → (+)
Intention tremor	+ + +	+ + → (+)	+ + → (+)
'Ocular dyspraxia'	+ + +	+ → (+)	+ + + → +
Muscular hypotonia	+ + +	0	+ → 0

Symbols as in Table 1

metabolism in the cerebrum. There is no clearcut relationship between GHB plasma levels and the severity of cerebellar symptoms in our patients. However, plasma GHB concentrations might not reflect levels of GHB in the c.s.f. or the brain.

With the current state of knowledge we can only speculate whether GHB or GABA concentrations are responsible for the cerebellar symptoms in the patients. Ando *et al.* (1979) highlighted the possibility of a particular effect of GHB on the clinical state when they described increased concentrations of GHB in the striatum, pallidum and the substantia nigra despite decreased GABA levels in patients with Huntington's chorea. Nahorski *et al.* (1972) found no effect of ethosuccimide on GABA levels, whereas it produced

most profound GHB changes. In rats the acute intake of ethosuccimide is followed by an increase of GHB and chronic intake by a decrease of GHB concentration in the cerebellar cortex (Snead *et al.*, 1980). Therefore, we can not assume that the adverse effects seen in our case after ethosuccimide might be primarily related to changes of GHB concentrations. From the clinical point of view the improvement of cerebellar symptoms, particularly of the ataxia in the two siblings and the non-progressive course in the other two patients, is a most remarkable observation, because most atactic syndromes in childhood tend to be stable or slowly progressive.

For References see p. 96.

J. Inher. Metab. Dis. 7 Suppl. 1 (1984) 92–94

4-Hydroxybutyric Aciduria: A New Inborn Error of Metabolism. II. Biochemical Findings

C. Jakobs*, J. Kneer, D. Rating and F. Hanefeld
Department of Pediatrics, Free University of Berlin, Kaiserin Auguste Victoria Haus, Heubnerweg 6, D-1000 Berlin 19, G.F.R.

P. Divry and M. Hermier
Laboratoire de Biochimie, Hôpital Debrousse, 29 rue Soeur Bouvier, 69322, Lyon, Cedex 5, France

The urinary excretion of 4- or γ-hydroxybutyric acid (GHB) was first reported by Jakobs *et al.* (1981) in a child with neurological abnormalities (B.S., male, born 1977 of related Turkish parents). In an addendum to their paper this West Berlin group reported the discovery of siblings (F.R., female, born 1970, and M.R., male, born 1972, from non-related Lebanese parents) with metabolic profiles identical to that of their first case. Another patient with γ-hydroxybutyric aciduria (B.R., male, born 1975 of related Algerian parents) was recently described by Divry *et al.* (1983) from Lyon. The purpose of this communication is to review the biochemical findings in these four patients.

In all four patients routine laboratory tests did not provide any clue to the diagnosis. There was no acidosis. Ion exchange column chromatography of the amino acids was normal. Gas chromatographic–mass spectrometric (GC–MS) examination of the organic acids and short chain fatty acids (SCFA), however, showed abnormal profiles. Ethylacetate solvent extraction of the urine after prior oxime formation of possibly present

keto- or aldo-acids, TMS-derivatization and GC-separation on a packed (3% OV-17) column revealed a number of abnormal compounds (Jakobs *et al.*, 1981). The most prominent one was identified as GHB by GC–MS, using authentic GHB for comparison. A small peak in the GC profile had the same retention time and mass spectrum as the second of two oxime-TMS derivatives (syn- and antigeometrical isomers) of authentic succinic semialdehyde (SSA). The first peak of SSA in the urine co-eluted with succinic acid (SA) on the packed column. In addition 3,4-dihydroxybutyric acid (normally not seen using solvent extraction) was found to be elevated.

Identification was performed by comparison of the mass spectrum of this urinary compound with that provided in the literature. Finally GC–MS evidence was obtained for the presence of 3-keto-4-hydroxybutyric acid. However, the authentic compound for unambiguous identification was not available. 3,4-Dihydroxybutyric acid and 3-keto-4-hydroxybutyric acid are believed to arise from β-oxidation of GHB. GC analysis of the SCFA-fraction revealed a further unknown peak. The mass spectrum of this peak differed strongly from those normally seen for SCFA, and was shown to be identical to that of authentic γ-butyrolactone (GBL). GBL can be formed by ring

---

* To whom requests for reprints should be addressed. Present address: Department of Pediatrics, Academic Hospital of the Free University of Amsterdam, De Boelelaan 1117, 1007 MB Amsterdam, The Netherlands.

closure of GHB and when an aqueous solution of GHB was subjected to the same procedure as for the SCFA the peak of GBL was observed. The importance of this finding is evident as the Lyon patient was mainly discovered by his 'unknown' peak in the SCFA profile which later proved to be GBL by GC–MS (Divry *et al.*, 1983). In this patient initial GC–MS analysis of urinary organic acids as methyl esters revealed no major abnormalities but the interpretation was difficult because the patient was on valproic acid therapy. However, after the valproate treatment was stopped, the presence of GHB was demonstrated in a new urine sample. The conversion of GHB to GBL offers an elegant method for a fast and sensitive determination of GHB in urine, blood and spinal fluid. The quantification of urinary SSA was performed only on a few occasions in the Berlin patient B.S., using the oxime-TMS derivative (both isomers), on a glass capillary (SE-30) column. In three investigated samples the urinary GHB/SSA ratio was consistently close to 35.

Table 1 shows some of the results on GHB in urine, plasma and spinal fluid found in the four patients. There was no correlation between urinary excretion and plasma concentration. Plasma GHB concentrations tended to decrease with time in all four patients.

GHB, previously only found in mammalian brain, is known to be a metabolite of γ--aminobutyric acid (GABA). Its biosynthesis from GABA via the trans-amination product SSA· has recently been reviewed (Davidson, 1980). The reduction of SSA to GHB involves two different NADPH-linked reductases (Cash *et al.*, 1979). However, this seems to be only a minor pathway for the degradation of GABA. The oxidation of SSA to succinic acid (SA) in a reaction which is catalysed by

SSA dehydrogenase (SSADH, EC 1.2.1.24) seems to be the major route because of the high affinity of this enzyme for SSA, permitting entry into the Krebs cycle. Certainly the metabolism of GABA is not limited to central nervous tissue. Lancaster *et al.* (1973) and White and co-workers (White and Sato, 1978; White, 1979) have shown that GABA is metabolized in liver, kidney and blood platelets. For the biochemical correlations within the GABA-metabolite pathway, see Figure 1.

It is interesting to note that GHB itself was introduced about 1960 as an analogue of GABA for use as an intravenous anesthetic, but neuropharmacological and neurophysiological side-effects precluded the clinical use of the drug in humans. Since that time, however, a large number of experimental studies on the pharmaco-kinetics and mechanism of action of the drug have been made (Snead, 1977). The half-life of the drug GHB is somewhat longer then 1 h in humans and GHB is nearly completely eliminated by biotransformation; only a small amount can be detected unmetabolized in the urine. The route of metabolism was until recently assumed to involve β-oxidation (Lee, 1977). Later experiments, however, favour the conversion via SSA to SA which subsequently enters into the Krebs cycle (Doherty and Roth, 1978). For these metabolic interconversions also see Figure 1.

Divry *et al.* (1983) showed that glutamic acid indeed is a precursor. Their patient was loaded with L-glutamic acid (100 mg/kg orally) and a late but significant increase in plasma GHB was found (149, 166, 171, 177, 249 and 170 μmol/l at respectively $T = 0$, $+1$ h, $+2$ h, $+3$ h, $+4$ h and $+48$ h).

The elevated concentration of GHB in blood and spinal fluid (not detected in normals) and the high

Table 1 GHB-concentrations in urine, plasma and spinal fluid

Patients	Sample	Urine (μmol/g creat.)	Plasma (μmol/l)	C.s.f. (μmol/l)
B. S. (W. Berlin), born 1977	08.01.79	2907		
	09.03.79		1010	
	28.09.79	1978	943	596
	08.10.80	3383	385	
	26.11.80	857	290	
	23.05.81	3390		
	23.02.83	435	40	
F. R. (W. Berlin), born 1970	29.08.80	1863		
	08.10.80		96	
	06.12.81	805	154	
	01.03.83	402	15	
M. R. (W. Berlin), born 1972	29.08.80	1706		
	08.10.80		202	
	06.12.81	1153	202	
	01.03.83	1154	35	
B. R. (Lyon), born 1975	13.12.79	1593	301	
	21.01.80	797	194	245
	12.06.81	2540	220	
	18.06.81	611	130	350
	10.02.83	310	51	

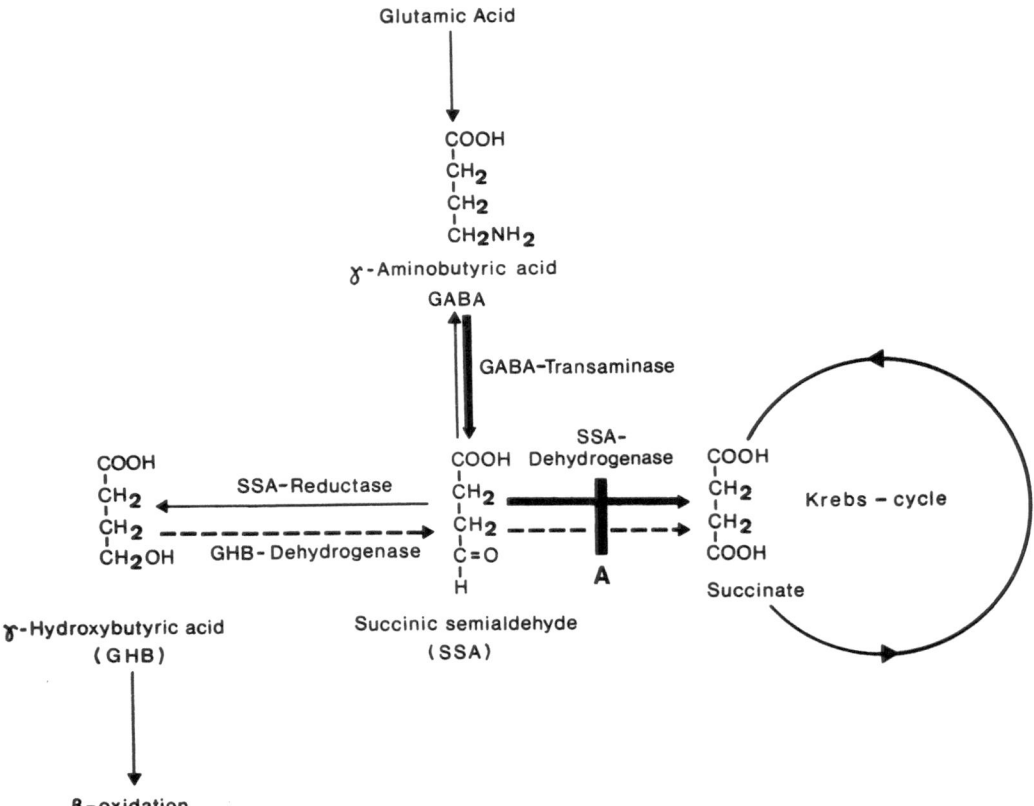

Figure 1 Biochemical correlations between GABA, SSA and GHB. Fat arrow, main degradation pathway for GABA; dotted arrow, main biotransformation pathway for the drug GHB. **A**, likely site of the enzyme defect in the patients presented in this paper. (Reprinted with permission of the authors and publisher of Jakobs *et al.*, 1981)

excretion of GHB in the urine of the patients described here indicate the possibility of an error of metabolism. The findings mentioned above can be explained by a lack, or abnormal kinetics, of the SSADH. In that case SSA degraded from GABA cannot enter into the Krebs cycle and will be reduced by the SSA-reductases. When this main pathway via the Krebs cycle is blocked, the β-oxidation of GHB probably becomes more important. This pathway has as intermediates 3,4-dihydroxybutyric acid and 3-keto-4-hydroxybutyric acid. In the West Berlin patient, B.S., both metabolites were believed to be elevated.

Recently we heard of two newly discovered cases of γ-hydroxybutyric aciduria from Dr Goodman, Denver, USA, and Dr Haan, Melbourne, Australia. From this and our findings in the four patients presented here (of whom two were siblings and each of the two other patients had related parents) we believe that γ-hydroxybutyric aciduria is a clinical entity, presumably of an autosomal inherited character. A deficiency in SSADH is postulated. The enzyme studies recently published by Gibson *et al.* (1983) strongly support our hypothesis.

For References see p. 96.

J. Inher. Metab. Dis. 7 Suppl. 1 (1984) 95–96

4-Hydroxybutyric Aciduria: A New Inborn Error of Metabolism. III. Enzymology and Inheritance

K. M. Gibson, I. Jansen, L. Sweetman and W. L. Nyhan

Departments of Chemistry, Medicine and Pediatrics, University of California, San Diego, La Jolla, CA 92093, USA

D. Rating

Department of Pediatrics, Free University of Berlin, Kaiserin Auguste Victoria Haus, Heubnerweg 6, D-1000 Berlin 19, G.F.R.

C. Jakobs

Department of Pediatrics, Academic Hospital of the Free University of Amsterdam, De Boelelaan 1117, 1007 MB Amsterdam, The Netherlands

P. Divry

Laboratoire de Biochimie, Hôpital Debrousse, 29 rue Soeur Bouvier, 69322 Lyon Cedex 5, France

4-Hydroxybutyric aciduria is an inborn error in the metabolism of 4-aminobutyrate (GABA) that is of particular interest because of the accumulation of a neuropharmacologically active compound (Jakobs *et al.*, 1981; Divry *et al.*, 1983). We have localized the defect in this condition to succinic semialdehyde dehydrogenase activity (SSDH, succinic semialdehyde: NAD^+ oxidoreductase, EC 1.2.1.24) using an indirect coupled assay in which the precursor was $U-^{14}C$-GABA. Heterozygosity could not be demonstrated with that assay. We have now developed a sensitive direct assay for SSDH using enzymatically prepared $U-^{14}C$-succinic semialdehyde. Lysates of lymphocytes have been employed and the enzymatic product, ^{14}C-succinic acid, has been quantified by liquid partition chromatography (LPC). It is the purpose of this report to present the activities of SSDH in lysates of lymphocytes isolated from whole blood of two patients with this disorder, their parents and siblings. The data establish the molecular defect as a deficiency of succinic semialdehyde dehydrogenase and are consistent with an autosomal recessive mode of inheritance.

METHODS

Whole venous blood was drawn from patients and relatives and the isolated lymphocytes sent from West Berlin to San Diego and kept at $-70\,°C$ in complete media containing 10% DMSO for a year prior to analysis. Lymphocytes were isolated by density centrifugation on Ficoll gradients (Gibson *et al.*, 1983). Assay of SSDH was performed in lysates of lymphocytes using a modification of the procedure of Cash *et al.* (1979). Control samples were assayed without freezing. Frozen lymphocyte suspensions were thawed at $37\,°C$, isolated by centrifugation, washed with PBS and resuspended in 0.3 ml of 100 mmol/l Tris–HCl buffer, pH 8.0, and lysed by sonication (Gibson *et al.*, 1983). The final assay mixture contained (in a volume of 100 µl): 0.3 mmol/l NAD^+, 100 mmol/l KCL, 0.25 mmol/l dithiothreitol, 100 mmol/l Tris–HCl, pH 8.0, 20 µl of cell extract (equivalent to approximately 15 µg of lymphoblast protein) and 0.15 mmol/l succinic semialdehyde (specific activity 3.2 mCi/mmol). Incubation was carried out for 30 minutes at $37\,°C$. The reaction was stopped by the addition of 10 µl of 4.2 mol/l $HClO_4$. After neutralization by addition of 6 mol/KOH, ^{14}C-succinic semialdehyde and ^{14}C-succinic acid were separated and identified by isocratic elution with 7% v/v 2-methyl-2-butanol in chloroform from silicic acid columns (Gibson *et al.*, 1983). SSDH activity was linear with time and protein content up to 45 minutes and 50 µg of protein. $U-^{14}C$-succinic semialdehyde was prepared by oxidation of purified $U-^{14}C$-GABA using bovine plasma monoamine oxidase and purified by cation-exchange chromatography. Propionyl CoA carboxylase (PCC) was assayed as a control on cell integrity and protein concentration determined (Gibson *et al.*, 1983). Individual assays were done in duplicate on each lymphocyte lysate. Lymphocytes from five control individuals were studied.

RESULTS

The activities of SSDH in patients, controls and family members are shown in Table 1. The activities of SSDH in the patients were 14 and 19% of the control mean. That of the mother was 28%, while that of the father was 64% of control. The mean activity for PCC in lymphocyte lysates of the family members was similar to the same mean activity in control lymphocyte lysates, indicating that conditions of storage did not adversely affect enzyme activity. The ratio of SSDH to PCC was employed in an attempt to correct for conditions of shipment, freezing and storage. The values in the patients were 8 and 11% of the mean control ratio of 1.13. The values in the parents were 25 and 46% of control, and 36 and 100% in the siblings.

Journal of Inherited Metabolic Disease. ISSN 0141–8955. Copyright © SSIEM and MTP Press Limited, Queen Square, Lancaster, UK.

Table 1 Activity of succinic semialdehyde dehydrogenase in lymphocytes

Specimen	SSDH	PCC	$\dfrac{SSDH}{PCC}$
	(pmol of product min^{-1} mg^{-1} protein)		
Patient (male)	64	547	0.12
Patient (female)	47	506	0.09
Mother	93	336	0.28
Father	210	404	0.52
Sibling (female)	424	374	1.13
Sibling (male)	143	345	0.41
Control mean ($\pm$ 1 SD)	330 $\pm$ 85 (range 259–470)	303 $\pm$ 109 (range 185–456)	1.13 $\pm$ 0.19 (range 0.91–1.43)

DISCUSSION

These data provide direct evidence for the localization of the molecular defect in 4-hydroxybutyric aciduria. The deficiency of SSDH leads to accumulation of succinic semialdehyde which is then reduced to form 4-hydroxybutyric acid, a compound known to have effects on the central nervous system. The results are consistent with those of our earlier indirect assay which depended on endogenous activity of GABA transaminase. The direct assay yields considerably higher activity for the enzyme, permitting an assessment of family members for the presence of heterozygosity. The parents and one sibling were interpreted to be heterozygotes. These data are consistent with an autosomal recessive mode of inheritance for SSDH deficiency. This is consistent with information from pedigrees. In this family there were affected male and female siblings and normal parents, and two of the known patients with this disorder are products of consanguineous matings.

REFERENCES TO PAGES 90–96

Ando, N., Gold, B. J., Bird, E. D. and Roth, R. H. Regional brain levels of γ-hydroxybutyrate in Huntington's disease. *J. Neurochem.* 32 (1979) 617–622

Cash, C. D., Maitre, M. and Mandel, P. Purification from human brain and some properties of two NADPH linked aldehyde reductases which reduce succinic semialdehyde to 4-hydroxybutyrate. *J. Neurochem.* 33 (1979) 1169–1175

Divry, P., Baltassat, P., Rolland, M. O., Cotte, J., Hermier, M., Duran, M. and Wadman, S. K. A new patient with 4-hydroxybutyric aciduria, a possible defect of 4-aminobutyrate metabolism. *Clin. Chim. Acta* 129 (1983) 303–309

Doherty, J. D. and Roth, R. H. Metabolism of γ-hydroxy-(1-^{14}C) butyrate by rat brain: relationship to the Krebs cycle and metabolic compartmentation of amino acids. *J. Neurochem.* 30 (1978) 1305–1309

Gibson, K. M., Jansen, I., Sweetman, L., Nyhan, W. L., Rating, D., Jakobs, C. and Divry, P. 4-Hydroxybutyric aciduria: a new inborn error of metabolism. III. Enzymology and inheritance. *J. Inher. Metab. Dis.* 7 Suppl. 1 (1984) 95–96

Gibson, K. M., Sweetman, L., Nyhan, W. L., Jakobs, C., Rating, D., Siemes, H. and Hanefield, F. Succinic semialdehyde dehydrogenase deficiency: an inborn error of gamma-aminobutyric acid metabolism. *Clin. Chim. Acta* 133 (1983) 33–42

Jakobs, C., Bojasch, M., Mónch, E., Rating, D., Siemes, H. and Hanefeld, F. Urinary excretion of gamma-hydroxybutyric acid in a patient with neurological abnormalities. The probability of a new inborn error of metabolism. *Clin. Chim. Acta* 111 (1981) 169–178

Jakobs, C., Divry, P., Kneer, J., Rating, D., Hanefeld, F. and Hermier, M. 4-Hydroxybutyric aciduria: a new inborn error of metabolism: II. Biochemical findings. *J. Inher. Metab. Dis.* 7 Suppl. 1 (1984) 92–94

Lancaster, G., Mohyuddin, F., Scriver, C. R. and Whelan, D. T. A gamma-amino butyrate pathway in mammalian kidney cortex. *Biochem. Biophys. Acta* 297 (1973) 229–240

Lee, C. R. Evidence for the β-oxidation of orally administered 4-hydroxybutyrate in humans. *Biochem. Med.* 17 (1977) 184–192

Nahorski, S. R. Biochemical effects of the anticonvulsants trimethadione, ethosuximide, and chlordiazepoxide in rat brain. *J. Neurochem.* 19 (1972) 1937–1946

Roth, R. H. and Giarman, N. J. Conversion in vivo of γ-aminobutyric to γ-hydroxybutyric acid in the rat. *Biochem. Pharmacol.* 18 (1969) 247–150

Rumigny, J. F., Maitre, M., Cash, C. and Mandel, P. Regional and subcellular localization in rat brain of the enzymes that can synthesize γ-hydroxybutyric acid. *J. Neurochem.* 36 (1981) 1433–1438

Santaniello, E., Manzocchi, and Tosi, L. Evaluation of gamma-hydroxybutyrate formed from L-glutamate by mouse brain homogenate. *J. Neurochem.* 31 (1978) 1117–1118

Snead, O. C. Gamma-hydroxybutyrate. *Life Sci.* 20 (1977) 1935–1943

Snead, O. C., Bearden, L. J. and Pegram, V. Effect of acute and chronic anticonvulsant administration on endogenous γ-hydroxybutyrate in rat brain. *Neuropharmacology* 19 (1980) 47–52

White, H. L. 4-Aminobutyrate: 2-oxoglutarate aminotransferase in blood platelets. *Science* 205 (1979) 696–698

White, H. L. and Sato, T. L. GABA-transaminases of human brain and peripheral tissues – kinetic and molecular properties. *J. Neurochem.* 31 (1978) 41–47

Preface to Short Communications

This issue is devoted to short communications based on oral and poster presentations at the free sessions of the Annual Meeting of the Society for the Study of Inborn Errors of Metabolism, held in Lyon, France, 6–9 September 1983. Due to the record number of free presentations at this meeting, we have been able to publish only a selection of the short communications offered. The free communications not reported elsewhere in this issue are listed below. Many of the short communications were submitted for the Noel Raine Award which commemorates the founding editor of the *Journal of Inherited Metabolic Disease*. Because of the quality and quantity of entrants two prizes were awarded, one to W. J. Rhead and B. A. Amendt for their paper 'Electron-transferring flavoprotein deficiency in the multiple acyl-CoA dehydrogenation disorders, glutaric aciduria type II and ethylmalonic-adipic aciduria', the other to S. L. C. Woo, J. H. Robson and F. Güttler for their paper 'The possibility for prenatal diagnosis of PKU by linkage analyses based on phenylalanine hydroxylase locus specific DNA-polymorphisms'.

With pressure on space in all scientific journals we hope that contributors and users will accept our suggestion that these papers be generated and used as short communications rather than as preliminary abstracts, at least in part. Since all must be subjected to critical scrutiny by an informed committee and by an international audience at the meeting some element of appraisal is inherent in their production. It is clear to the editors that some are preliminary communications which allow priority to be established. However, others are worthwhile additional records which are adequate in themselves as contributions to our accumulated experience and may not require additional recording.

We shall try to produce these short communications rapidly and we hope that they can continue to be an open channel of communication for members of the SSIEM and their colleagues.

R. A. Harkness
R. J. Pollitt

Free Communications

Cystic fibrosis: A disorder of the mitochondrial membrane possibly induces changes of Ca^{2+} and energy metabolism. *A. Von Ruecker, R. M. Bertele, H. K. Harms, Y. S. Shin and W. Endres*

Clinical heterogeneity in patients with cytochrome deficiency. *R. C. A. Sengers, J. C. Fischer, J. M. F. Trijbels, J. A. J. M. Bakkeren, W. Ruitbeek and A. M. Stadhouders*

A new patient with dicarboxylic aciduria presenting as Reye's syndrome. *J. A. del Valle, M. Martinez-Pardo, C. Ludena, C. Camarero, R. del Olmo, M. J. Garcia, B. Merinero, C. Perez-Cerda, F. Roman, A. Jimenez and L. Ugarte*

Mitochondrial myopathy and lactic acidosis associated with deficiency of several components of complex III of the respiratory chain. *N. G. Kennaway, V. Darley-Usmar, N. R. M. Buist, A. Papadimitriou, S. Di Mauro and R. Capaldi*

Estimation of pyruvate dehydrogenase complex, pyruvate carboxylase, and phosphoenolpyruvate carboxykinase activities in fibroblasts for the differential diagnosis of congenital lactic acidosis. *H. Wick and R. Baumgartner*

Maternal phenylketonuria. *D. P. Brenton, P. J. Garrod, S. Krywawych, M. Lilburn and A. Stewart*

Specificity of succinylacetone formation in tyrosinaemia type I. Application to prenatal diagnosis. *M. O. Rolland, E. Durif and P. Divry*

Glutaric aciduria type II: Clinical and biochemical observations and riboflavin treatment in four sisters. *R. B. H. Schutgens, H. R. Scholte, I. E. M. Luythouwen, H. A. Veder, M. De Visser and J. Bethlem*

In vivo metabolism of 1-[^{13}C]propionate in patients with propionic acidaemia, methylmalonic acidaemia and biotin responsive multiple carboxylase deficiency. *I. Yoshida, L. Sweetman, J. Wolff, W. L. Nyhan, M. Smith and A. Ajami*

Rapid differential diagnosis of carboxylase deficiencies and evaluation for biotin responsiveness in a single blood sample. *T. Suormala, R. Baumgarter, H. Wick and J. P. Bonjour*

A new sensitive fluorometric assay for biotinidase and its application to the elucidation of the primary defect in some patients with combined carboxylase deficiency. *K. Bartlett, H. J. Wastell, J. H. Stirk, M. J. Bennett, J. V. Leonard, L. S. Taitz and J. M. Saudubray*

Deficient liver biotinidase activity in multiple carboxylase deficiency. *A. Munnich, J. M. Saudubray, M. Gaudry, H. Ogier, G. Mitchell, C. Marsac, M. Causse, A. Marquet and J. Frezal*

Neonatal methylmalonic aciduria: treatment by forced diuresis. *H. Ogier, G. Mitchell, J. Rousselot, D. Devictor, C. Charpentier, J. M. Saudubray and A. Lemonnier*

Therapeutic trial in a patient with methylmalonic aciduria due to cob(I)alamin adenosyltransferase deficiency. *N. J. Brandt, B. Beck, E. Christensen and V. Faurholt Pedersen*

Neonatal and long term management of methylmalonic aciduria. *B. M. Tracey, C. de Sousa, T. E. Stacey, P. Timbrell and R. A. Chalmers*

Pyroglutamic aciduria in propionyl-CoA carboxylase deficiency. *H. Morishita, S. Nagaya, T. Nakazima, A. Kawase, Y. Hokazono, M. Kobayashi, Y. Ogawa and Y. Wada*

Report of a patient with acute neonatal isovaleric acidaemia. *J. Hyanek, S. K. Wadman, M. Duran, M. Zapadlo, J. Zeman and H. Houstkova*

Metabolism of isovaleryl-CoA in isovaleric acidaemia. *W. Lehnert*

Malonyl coenzyme A decarboxylase deficiency. *G. K. Brown, R. D. Scholem, A. Bankier and D. M. Danks*

Identification of the β-ketothiolase defect in α-methylacetoacetic-aciduria. *B. Middleton, R. B. H. Schutgens and K. Bartlett*

A new case of ketothiolase deficiency with favourable evolution. *G. Sabetta, C. Bachmann, O. Giardini, M. Castro, P. D'Eufemia, R. Lubrano and M. Gambarara*

Blood and urine carnitine values in different cases of oganic acidaemia and aminoacidopathies. *B. Cartier, P. Divry and M. Mathieu*

Labelled propionate uptake and methylmalonyl-CoA mutase activity in cultured skin fibroblasts and amniotic fluid cells. *B. Fowler, K. Mills and I. B. Sardharwalla*

Treatment of non-ketotic hyperglycinaemia with γ-aminobutyric acid, methionine, folic acid and pyridoxin. *M. Rodes, J. Sabater, L. Alvarez and M. Pineda*

Decreased glycine cleavage activity in liver of a patient with multiple α-ketoacidaemia and lactic acidaemia with lipoamide dehydrogenase deficiency. *M. Yoshino, Y. Koga, Y. Sakaguchi, F. Yamashita and T. Hayashi*

Renal clearance of branched chain α-keto acids in patients with maple syrup urine disease. *U. Langenbeck and U. Wendel*

Branched chain amino acid metabolism in cultured fibroblasts from patients with maple syrup urine disease and branched chain ketoacid dehydrogenase deficiency with lactic acidosis. *I. Yoshida, L. Sweetman and W. L. Nyhan*

L-Norvaline induced hyperammonaemia in the rat: Enhancement of hippurate production, after benzoate administration, by glyoxylate. *J. M. Tetau, C. Charpentier, M. P. Doussau and A. Lemonnier*

A microcomputer program to plan diets for infants with branched chain ketoaciduria. *P. B. Acosta, B. Kennedy and K. Anderson*

Leucinosis: Prenatal diagnosis and enzymatic study in several families. *P. Baltassat, R. Dumoulin, M. Mathieu and J. Cotte*

A method suitable for the diagnosis of cystinosis and the study of the *in vitro* action of cysteamine on cystinotic fibroblasts. *R. Dumoulin, P. Baltassat, M. Jaud, M. T. Zabot and J. Cotte*

Factor VII deficiency in homocystinuria. *M. D. Dautzenberg, J. M. Saudubray, R. Girot, A. Munnich, A. M. Fischer and S. Beguin*

Adult homocystinuria (cystathionine synthase deficiency) presenting with thromboembolism. *V. E. Shih, E. H. Picard and B. Fowler*

Two cases of neonatal argininosuccinic aciduria. *S. Krywawych, D. P. Brenton, E. Cady, M. Friedman, P. J. Garrod, D. K. Walker and D. V. Walters*

Diagnosis and treatment of argininaemia. Characteristics of arginase in human erythrocytes and tissues. *W. Endres, R. Schaller, Y. S. Shin and C. Bachmann*

Uracil and citrulline: the indexes for GC/MS screening of ornithine carbamyl transferase deficiency. *I. Matsumoto, Y. Inoue, T. Kuhara and T. Shinka*

Biochemical markers of treatment for ornithine carbamyl transferase deficiency during the first 48 hours of life. *J. Hammond, M. Potter and N. Howard*

Richner-Hanhart syndrome in two siblings of a consanguineous marriage. *E. Bonifazi, F. Carnevale, G. Di Bitonto and G. Krajewska*

Expression of *S*-adenosylmethionine synthetase isozymes in liver from patients with type I hereditary tyrosinaemia. *R. Berger, H. Van Faassen, G. P. A. Smit and J. Fernandes*

Paired comparisons between early treated PKU children and their matched sibling controls on intelligence test and school achievement test results at eight years of age. *R. Koch, C. Azen, E. G. Friedman and L. Williamson*

Consideration on the psychomotor development in a late treated phenylketonuric child with recurrent comatose condition, hyperammonemia and epilepsy. *G. Krajewska, F. Carnevale, G. Di Bitonto and L. Filannino*

Difficulties returning to diet therapy in patients with phenylketonuria: implications for child bearing. *K. Michals, H. Dominik, V. Schuett and E. Brown*

Betaine for treatment in 5,10-methylenetetrahydrofolate reductase deficiency. *U. Wendel and H. J. Bremer*

Computer simulation of phenylalanine metabolism in normal subjects and patients with phenylketonuria. *M. Hjelm, R. I. Kitney and J. W. Seakins*

Kinetic analysis of renal excretion of acidic metabolites of phenylalanine in six adult patients with phenylketonuria. *U. Langenbeck, F. Baum and A. Behbehani*

Age dependence of urinary levels of acidic phenylalanine metabolites in phenylketonuria (PKU). *A. E. Behbehani and U. Langenbeck*

Interaction between catecholic and phenolic monoamines in phenylketonuria. *S. B. Holiday, J. A. Hoskins and A. Tippett*

Heterogeneity of the biopterin synthesis defects. *R. Matalon, K. Michals, B. Rouse, G. Hoganson, S. Berlow, J. Israel, P. Supple and W. Seifert*

Dicarboxylic aciduria in patients with muscle disease. *S. Krywawych, D. P. Brenton, R. H. T. Edwards, K. Gohil and M. Hardy*

A case of ethylmalonic aciduria. *C. Boujet, A. Joannard and A. Favier*

Multiple acyl-CoA dehydrogenase deficiency responsive to riboflavin. *J. P. Harpey, C. Charpentier and S. I. Goodman*

Fatty acid β-oxidation defects: diagnosis in fibroblast culture. *G. Mitchell, J. M. Saudubray, Y. Benoit, J. C. Labarthe, H. Ogier, P. Divry and J. Frezal*

On the inheritance of glutaric aciduria type II. *W. J. Rhead, K. S. Fritchman, A. Moon and A. Grundmeyer*

Prenatal diagnosis of multiple acyl-CoA dehydrogenation deficiency. *B. Steinmann, A. Niederwieser, Th. Kuster, H. U. Bucher, A. Huch and U. Wendel*

Prenatal diagnosis and biochemical investigations of a child with multiple defects in fatty acid and lysine oxidation (glutaric aciduria type II). *R. G. F. Gray, M. J. Bennett, A. D. Patrick, D. A. Curnock, D. Hull and R. J. Pollitt*

Possible implications in glutaric aciduria of a novel peroxisomal enzyme. *J. Vamecq and F. Van Hoof*

Mitochondrial and peroxisomal fatty acid oxidation. *J. H. Veerkamp, H. T. B. Van Moerkerk and J. A. J. M. Bakkeren*

Evidence of peroxisomal β-oxidation of dicarboxylic acids. *S. Kølvraa, N. Gregersen and P. B. Mortensen*

Peroxisomal disturbances in the cerebro-hepato-renal syndrome of Zellweger. *F. Trijbels, L. Govaerts, L. Monnens, J. Bakkeren and A. Stadhouders*

Severe deficiency of plasmalogens in Zellweger syndrome. *R. B. H. Schutgens, H. V. D. Bosch, P. Borst, H. S. A. Heymans and W. H. H. Tegelaers*

A biochemical study of adrenoleukodystrophy. *C. J. Reinecke and P. J. Pretorius*

A mosaic of cytochrome oxidase positive and negative fibres in skeletal muscle. *H. S. A. Sherratt, M. A. Johnson and D. M. Turnbull*

Low skeletal muscle carnitine concentrations associated with deficiency of butyryl-CoA dehydrogenase activity. *K. Bartlett, M. Hardy, H. S. A. Sherratt, D. Stevens and D. M. Turnbull*

Mitochondrial myopathy with lactic acidosis and deficient activity of muscle succinate cytochrome-*c*-oxido-reductase. *A. W. Behbehani, H. Goebel, G. Osse, M. Gabriel, U. Langenbeck, J. Berden and R. B. H. Schutgens*

A familial progressive myopathy with core lesions: clinical and biochemical findings. *H. F. M. Busch, H. R. Scholte, W. F. M. Arts and I. E. M. Luyt-Houwen*

Pyruvate and acetate oxidation by CCCP-treated lymphocytes. *N. Venizelos and L. Hagenfeld*

Duchenne muscular dystrophy is a myopathy with abnormal mitochondria. *H. R. Scholte, H. F. M. Busch, F. G. I. Jennekens and I. E. M. Luyt-Houwen*

Method to reduce the spontaneous decarboxylation of $[^{14}C]$oxo-acids used in the study of the congenital lactic acidoses. *K. Hyland and J. V. Leonard*

Effects of short-chain fatty acids on pyruvate oxidation in cultured human fibroblasts and rat liver mitochondria. *Y. Koga, M. Yoshino and F. Yamashita*

A sensitive coupled fluorimetric rate assay for pyruvate dehydrogenase (EC.1.2.4.1) in cultured human fibroblasts. *M. Solomon and D. Stansbie*

Congenital lactic acidosis in two siblings. *U. Burger, T. Deufel, A. Otten, H. Wick, D. Peen, O. Klinge and H. Wolf*

Thiamine responsive lactic acidaemia. *N. Krawiecki, P. Hartlage, A. Roesel, L. Carter and F. A. Hommes*

Unusual organic acid and butanediol excretion in Wilson disease. *R. Libert, G. Cornu, E. de Hoffmann and F. Van Hoof*

Metabolic acidosis of the cerebrospinal fluid in a patient with primary lactic acidosis. *A. Superti-Furga, M. Di Rocco and P. Durand*

Rapid profiling of plasma organic acids by high performance liquid chromatography. *P. Daish and J. V. Leonard*

A novel method for the isolation of urinary organic acid prior to gas chromatography. *J. W. T. Seakins*

Organic aciduria in mental retardation. *C. J. Reinecke, L. J. Mienie and C. M. S. Rossouw*

Results of the selective screening for organic acid disorders. *M. Ugarte, M. J. Garcia, J. A. Del Valle, B. Merinero, C. Perez-Cerda, C. Hernandez, F. Roman and L. J. Kremer*

Urinary organic acid profile of normal newborn infants. *E. Lefebvre, M. Vidailhet and J. M. Rousselot*

The application of HPLC to a study of the urinary excretion of α-ketoacids in a patient with maple syrup urine disease during a metabolic crisis. *M. D. Boveda, J. M. Fraga, J. Pena and J. R. Alonso-Fernandez*

continued on p.152

J. Inher. Metab. Dis. 7 Suppl. 2 (1984) 99–100

Short Communication—Noel Raine Award

Electron-transferring Flavoprotein Deficiency in the Multiple Acyl-CoA Dehydrogenation Disorders, Glutaric Aciduria Type II and Ethylmalonic–adipic Aciduria

W. J. RHEAD and B. A. AMENDT

Department of Pediatrics, University of Iowa, Iowa City, IA 52242, USA

The multiple acyl-CoA dehydrogenation disorders (MADD), which include a severe variant, glutaric aciduria type II (MADD/S; GA-II; McKusick 30595; Przyrembel *et al.*, 1976) and a mild variant, ethyl-malonic–adipic aciduria (MADD/M; EMA; McKusick 23168; Mantagos *et al.*, 1979) are clinically and biochemically related inborn errors of organic acid metabolism. We and others have suggested that they are caused by deficient electron transfer from the acyl-CoA dehydrogenases (ADH; EC 1.3.99) to the electron-transport chain (Goodman *et al.*, 1982; Rhead *et al.*, 1980). Our preliminary data now demonstrate electron-transferring flavoprotein (ETF) deficiency in several cases of GA-II and EMA.

MATERIALS AND METHODS

Skin fibroblasts were obtained from two GA-II patients who presented in the neonatal period, one female (Goodman *et al.*, 1982) and one male (Drs P. Falace and L. Sweetman), two EMA patients, one female (Mantagos *et al.*, 1979), one male (Drs Walther, Niermeijer and Duran) and one adult female with mild GA-II (Dusheiko *et al.*, 1979), as well as five normal individuals. GA-II cells oxidized [1-^{14}C]butyrate and [2-^{14}C]leucine at less than 15% of control levels, and EMA/mild GA-II cells at 10–40% of control levels (Mantagos *et al.*, 1979; Dusheiko *et al.*, 1979; Rhead *et al.*, 1980; Rhead and Amendt, 1982; other data not shown); all cell lines oxidized [1,4-^{14}C]succinate normally. Fibroblasts were cultured in roller bottles and fibroblast mitochondria isolated as described earlier (Rhead *et al.*, 1980; Rhead and Tanaka, 1980), except that the digitonin step was omitted.

Mitochondrial medium chain ADH (MCADH; EC 1.3.99.3) and glutamate dehydrogenase (GDH; EC 1.4.1.4) were assayed as outlined previously (Rhead and Tanaka, 1980; Rhead *et al.*, 1983). Mitochondrial ETF activity was assayed by the dye reduction method described earlier (Rhead *et al.*, 1980), with the addition of 0.2 mmol/l *N*-ethylmaleimide (NEM; Rhead *et al.*, 1983). The reaction was initiated by 39 pmol of pure pig liver MCADH, as enzyme flavin.

RESULTS

Their organic acidurias suggest that the MADD result from generalized deficiencies of acyl-CoA dehydrogenation. In intact MADD fibroblasts, defective acyl-

CoA dehydrogenation blocks ^{14}C-labelled fatty acid, branched chain amino acid, and lysine catabolism. These oxidative defects are also demonstrable in intact fibroblast mitochondria, since GA-II mitochondria oxidize [1-^{14}C]octanoate, [1-^{14}C]palmityl CoA and [1,5-^{14}C]glutarate at less than 14% of control levels, while EMA/mild GA-II mitochondria oxidize these same substrates at 31–40% of control levels ($p < 0.05$; data not shown; Rhead and Amendt, 1982). [1,4-^{14}C]Succinate oxidation was normal in mitochondria from all cell lines, indicating that the tricarboxylic acid cycle functioned normally and that electron transport from succinate dehydrogenase to molecular oxygen was intact (Rhead and Amendt, 1982).

We have recently assayed dehydrogenases and ETF directly in 100 000 *g* mitochondrial sonic supernatants (MS) from GA-II and EMA fibroblasts (Table 1). Activity of GDH, a mitochondrial matrix marker enzyme, was identical in MS from all cell lines, confirming that all mitochondrial preparations were of comparable purity. As measured by a dye reduction assay, MCADH activity was 77% of control ($p > 0.1$) in EMA/mild GA-II MS and 55% of control ($p < 0.05$) in GA-II MS; isovaleryl CoA dehydrogenase (IVDH) activity was 91% of control in GA-II MS when measured with the same method (data not shown). Using a tritium release assay, IVDH and butyryl CoA dehydrogenase activities ranged from 70 to 113% of control in fibroblast MS derived from the first patient with GA-II (Przyrembel *et al.*, 1976; Rhead *et al.*, 1980). These data suggest that primary ADH deficiency is not the etiology of MADD, although variable, and possibly secondary, decreases in ADH activity are observed.

Since ETF catalyses the first step in electron transfer from the reduced ADH to coenzyme Q *in vivo*, we assayed ETF activity in MADD MS by modifying the dye reduction method for ADH. Addition of octanoyl CoA to purified pig liver MCADH yields reduced MCADH; ETF then catalyzes electron transfer from MCADH to the acceptor dye dichlorophenol indo-phenol (DCIP). In our assay, MADD MS represents the only source of ETF; thus the rate of DCIP reduction reflects MS ETF activity. The sulph-hydryl alkylating agent, NEM, inhibits artefactual DCIP reduction by CoASH derived from octanoyl CoA hydrolysis (Rhead *et al.*, 1983). Assayed with 39 pmol MCADH, ETF activity was 62% of control ($p < 0.05$) in EMA/mild GA-II MS and 29% of control in GA-II MS, lower than in EMA/mild GA-II MS ($p < 0.02$; Table 1). In more

Journal of Inherited Metabolic Disease. ISSN 0141–8955. Copyright © SSIEM and MTP Press Limited, Queen Square, Lancaster, UK.

Table 1   Activities (pmol production min^{-1} (mg protein)$^{-1}$ ± SEM) of dehydrogenases and electron-transferring flavoprotein in fibroblast mitochondria from patients with glutaric aciduria type II (GA-II), ethylmalonic–adipic aciduria (EMA) and from normal controls

Cell lines	Enzyme activity		
	Glutamate dehydrogenase (n = 19)	*Medium chain acyl-CoA dehydrogenase* (n = 10–15)	*Electron-transferring flavoprotein* (n = 8–12)
Normal controls	37 900 ± 3800	1577 ± 196	293 ± 46
EMA/mild GA-II	32 600 ± 4000	1214 ± 198	182 ± 26[1]
GA-II	36 600 ± 4800	874 ± 218[1]	86 ± 14[2]

[1] Different from normal control ($p < 0.05$)
[2] Different from EMA/mild GA-II ($p < 0.02$)

recent experiments, ETF activity in normal control MS increased three-fold when assayed with 165 pmol MCADH ($n = 6$) and was only 33% of control in EMA/mild GA-II MS ($n = 8$; $p < 0.05$). When compared to control values, ETF activity in GA-II MS fell dramatically to 11% of control ($n = 4$; $p < 0.01$; data not shown).

DISCUSSION

Clinically, the MADD are heterogenous and separate themselves into a neonatally fatal and severe variant (MADD/S, GA-II, GA-II-A) and a mild variant (MADD/M, EMA, GA-II-B). Our results confirm that the two MADD variants, while related biochemically, are distinct from one another at the enzymatic level, since mild and severe ETF deficiencies produce MADD/M and MADD/S, respectively. Our inability to demonstrate ETF deficiency in MS from the first patient with MADD/S (Przyrembel *et al.*, 1976) is probably related to artefactual DCIP reduction by CoASH in those experiments (Rhead *et al.*, 1980), since 'apparent' ETF activity in fibroblast MS falls 10-fold after NEM addition (Rhead *et al.*, 1983; unpublished data). However, ETF activity could be normal in patients with typical clinical, cellular and mitochondrial MADD phenotype(s), if ETF dehydrogenase (ETF DH) activity was deficient (Goodman *et al.*, 1982; Rhead *et al.*, 1980; Coude *et al.*, 1981). Deficiency of this iron–sulphur flavoprotein, which catalyses electron transfer from reduced ETF to coenzyme Q would secondarily inhibit all the ADH, producing the biochemical phenotype of MADD. Ultimately, ETF and ETF DH activities should be quantitated in all MADD patients before a specific enzymatic diagnosis is assigned. Such experiments are underway in our laboratory.

References

Coudé, F. X., Ogier, H., Charpentier, C., Thomassin, G., Checoury, A., Amedee-Manesme, O., Saudubray, J.-M. and Frezal, J. Neonatal glutaric aciduria type II: An X-linked recessive inherited disorder. *Hum. Genet.* 59 (1981) 263–265

Dusheiko, G., Kew, M., Jofee, B., Lewin, J., Mantagos, S. and Tanaka, K. Glutaric aciduria type II: A cause of recurrent hypoglycemia in an adult. *N. Engl. J. Med.* 301 (1979) 1405–1411

Goodman, S., Stene, D., McCabe, E., Norenberg, M., Shikes, R., Stumpf, D. and Blackburn, G. Glutaric acidemia type II: Clinical, biochemical, and morphologic considerations. *J. Pediatr.* 100 (1982) 946–950

Mantagos, S., Genel, M. and Tanaka, K. Ethylmalonic-adipic aciduria: *In vivo* and *in vitro* studies indicating deficiency of activities of multiple acyl CoA dehydrogenases. *J. Clin. Invest.* 64 (1979) 1580–1589

Przyrembel, H., Wendel, K., Becker, K., Bremer, H., Bruinvis, L., Ketting, D. and Wadman, S. Glutaric aciduria type II: Report of a previously undescribed metabolic disorder. *Clin. Chim. Acta* 66 (1976) 227–239

Rhead, W. and Amendt, B. Oxidation of [1-^{14}C]palmityl-CoA and [1-^{14}C]isovaleric acid by fibroblast mitochondria from individuals with glutaric aciduria, type II, and ethylmalonic–adipic aciduria. *Pediatr. Res.* 16 (1982) 263A

Rhead, W. and Tanaka, K. Demonstration of a specific mitochondrial isovaleryl-CoA dehydrogenase deficiency in fibroblasts from patients with isovaleric acidemia. *Proc. Natl. Acad. Sci. USA* 77 (1980) 580–583

Rhead, W., Amendt, B., Fritchman, K. and Felts, S. Dicarboxylic aciduria: Deficient [1-^{14}C]octanoate oxidation and medium chain acyl-CoA dehydrogenase activity in fibroblasts. *Science* 221 (1983) 73–75

Rhead, W., Mantagos, S. and Tanaka, K. Glutaric aciduria type II: *In vitro* studies on substrate oxidation, acyl-CoA dehydrogenases, and electron-transferring flavoprotein in cultured skin fibroblasts. *Pediatr. Res.* 14 (1980) 1339–1342

J. Inher. Metab. Dis. 7 Suppl. 2 (1984) 101–102

Short Communication

Glutaric Aciduria Type II: Multiple Defects in Isolated Muscle Mitochondria and Deficient β-Oxidation in Fibroblasts

P. D. Mooy, M. A. H. Giesberts and H. H. van Gelderen
Department of Pediatrics, University Hospital, Leiden, The Netherlands

H. R. Scholte and I. E. M. Luyt-Houwen
Department of Biochemistry I, Erasmus University, Rotterdam, The Netherlands

H. Przyrembel and W. Blom
Department of Pediatrics, Sophia's Children Hospital, Erasmus University, Rotterdam, The Netherlands

A further patient with glutaric aciduria type II (GA II, McKusick) is described. He seems to be the first reported patient with an intermediate form of this disease. A deficiency was found in the carnitine stimulated mitochondrial β-oxidation of isolated muscle mitochondria and fibroblasts. He responded to chronic treatment with carnitine and riboflavin.

CASE HISTORY

In a 6-week-old boy with severe hypoglycaemia and hypotonia the excretion pattern of organic acids was typical of GA II and sarcosine was present in plasma and urine. A diet, low in fat and protein and enriched in carbohydrates, was started, supplemented with riboflavin. The urinary excretion of most organic acids decreased; he was less hypotonic, but a tendency to hypoglycaemia persisted. At the age of 10 months, in a life-threatening condition due to intercurrent infections, additional treatment with carnitine and temporary insulin helped to overcome the serious situation. At the age of 22 months (December 1983) his growth is only mildly retarded but his development is somewhat hampered by hypotonia.

METHODS

At the age of 7 months a muscle biopsy was performed. Mitochondria were isolated from 209 mg freshly obtained skeletal muscle. Mg^{2+}-ATPase was determined in the presence of albumin. The dehydrogenase activities and antimycin-sensitive succinate-cytochrome c reductase were determined in freeze-thawed mitochondria; other enzyme activities were determined within a few hours after isolation. Antimycin-insensitive succinate-cytochrome c reductase was measured like succinate dehydrogenase but by assaying the reduction of 0.1 mmol/l cytochrome c, instead of INT^+. The blank contained extra 1.82 μmol/l of the site II inhibitor antimycin. Glutaryl CoA dehydrogenase was determined in principle according to Besrat *et al.* (1969), but in a volume of 0.1 ml and with extra addition of 0.04 mg catalase. Skin fibroblasts were grown according to standard procedures. Culture medium was decanted and

the vessel was thoroughly rinsed with 0.25 mol/l sucrose. The fibroblasts were collected and suspended in sucrose on a Vortex shaker. Malonyl CoA decarboxylase, a mitochondrial matrix enzyme, was determined by a method based on earlier work (Scholte, 1973).

The description or references of other methods are given in Barth *et al.* (1983).

RESULTS

Carnitine was decreased in serum: free carnitine 5 μmol/l (controls 40 ± 1.0, $n = 71$), total carnitine 26 μmol/l (controls 51 ± 1.7, $n = 37$). In muscle tissue total carnitine was 1.38 μmol/g weight (controls 4.0 ± 0.1, $n = 59$); creatine kinase was also about one third of the average activity in controls. The mitochondrial enzymes in the muscle tissue (palmitoyl CoA synthetase, carnitine-palmitoyltransferases I and II and succinate dehydrogenase) showed normal activity. The mitochondrial yield was normal: 5.6 mg protein/g wet weight. The isolated muscle mitochondria oxidized all substrates with reduced rates. The oxygen uptake with ascorbate decreased at 50% of oxygen saturation (the vessel was saturated with air). This indicates a decreased affinity for oxygen in the patient, compared with controls (deflection at less than 10% O_2 saturation). The P/O ratio with ascorbate was also decreased. The basal Mg^{2+}-ATPase was increased, but uncoupler stimulated its activity considerably to a value comparable with controls. Also the activities of succinate dehydrogenase and glycerol-3-P dehydrogenase (FAD) were in the control range. Ca^{2+} did not stimulate the latter enzyme, as in controls, which suggests that the enzyme is optimally stimulated by the Ca^{2+} present in the (freeze-thawed) mitochondrial preparation. Glutaryl CoA dehydrogenase was decreased compared to controls, but its activity was higher than in a patient with GAI, where 1.7 pmol/min per mg protein was found (Blom, Janssen, Luyt-Houwen and Scholte, unpublished results).

An adequate method of measuring the β-oxidation, also in the presence of respiratory chain lesions (Scholte, Busch, Luyt-Houwen *et al.*, unpublished results) is the assay of the conversion of $[U-^{14}C]$palmitate into

Journal of Inherited Metabolic Disease. ISSN 0141-8955. Copyright © SSIEM and MTP Press Limited, Queen Square, Lancaster, UK.

Table 1   Results of measurements in isolated muscle mitochondria and fibroblasts of a patient with
GAII

	Patient	Controls	
Muscle mitochondria (per mg protein)			
Pyruvate (+ malate) (nat O/min)	17	87 ± 8	(12)
Palmitoylcarnitine (+ malate) (nat O/min)	15	77 ± 7	(12)
Succinate (+ rotenone) (nat O/min)	21	121 ± 11	(12)
Ascorbate (+ TMPD) (nat O/min)	197	365 ± 17	(12)
P/O with ascorbate	0.36	0.94 ± 0.07	(12)
Mg^{2+}-ATPase (nmol/min)	252	63 ± 22	(9)
Mg^{2+}-ATPase + uncoupler (nmol/min)	790	605 ± 84	(9)
Succinate-cytochrome *c* reductase (antimycin-sensitive) (nmol *c*/min)	115	133 ± 17	(5)
Succinate dehydrogenase (nmol INT^+/min)	15	33 ± 5	(11)
Glycerol-3-P dehydrogenase (nmol INT^+/min)	1.99	1.48 ± 0.16	(7)
Glycerol-3-P dehydrogenase + 1 mmol/l Ca^{2+} (nmol INT^+/min)	1.57	3.21 ± 0.52	(5)
Glutaryl CoA dehydrogenase (pmol/min)	12	51 ± 29	(4)
[U-^{14}C]palmitate oxidation (nmol/min)	0.05	0.50 ± 0.16	(5)
[U-^{14}C]palmitate + 1 mmol/l KCN (nmol/min)	0.00	0.22 ± 0.03	(3)
[U-^{14}C]palmitate + 0.5 mmol/l L-carnitine (nmol/min)	0.19	1.93 ± 0.17	(5)
Fibroblasts (per mg protein)			
[U-^{14}C]palmitate oxidation (pmol/min)	19 ± 2	31 ± 5: 48 ± 4	
[U-^{14}C]palmitate + 1 mmol/l CN^- (pmol/min)	14 ± 2	31 ± 1; 44 ± 3	
[U-^{14}C]palmitate + 0.5 mmol/l L-carnitine (pmol/min)	22 ± 3	89 ± 11; 117 ± 11	
Malonyl CoA decarboxylase (pmol/min)	181 ± 12	163 ± 16; 187 ± 7	

The average values are given $\pm$ SE. Parentheses, the number of controls. The fibroblast values are from four subcultures $\pm$ SE

$^{14}CO_2$ and perchloric acid soluble products. Even in the presence of carnitine this activity was reduced to 10% of control. The cyanide-insensitive peroxisomal oxidation was undetectably low.

In fibroblasts, where the amount of $^{14}CO_2$ evolved is quite low, only the perchloric acid soluble products were measured. The mitochondrial β-oxidation was clearly deficient, while another mitochondrial enzyme, malonyl CoA decarboxylase, showed a normal activity. The peroxisomal oxidation was decreased in the fibroblasts too, but not completely deficient.

DISCUSSION

GAII is possibly caused by a defect in the electron transport from ETF to ubiquinone (Goodman *et al.*, 1980; Rhead *et al.*, 1980), leading to a multiple CoA dehydrogenase deficiency. However, the isolated muscle mitochondria of the present patient show more defects. The oxidation of pyruvate plus malate is also low. This may be due to a lack of intra-mitochondrial coenzyme-A or a lack of counter ions for pyruvate transport. A lesion in electron transport at the level of ubiquinone-cytochrome bc_1 is excluded by the normal activity of succinate-cytochrome *c* reductase. Counter ion deficiency may explain the reduction in succinate oxidation, which also could be caused by increased oxaloacetate in the mitochondrial matrix. Cytochrome *c*

oxidase is also affected, with its activity and properties changed.

These results are an interesting example of the destructive effects of one genetic defect on other mitochondrial enzyme activities.

References

Barth, P. G., Scholte, H. R., Berden, J. A., Van der Kley-Van Moorsel, J., Luyt-Houwen, I. E. M., Van 't Veer-Korthof, E.Th., Van der Harten, J. J. and Sobotka-Plojhar, M. An X-linked mitochondrial disease affecting cardiac muscle, skeletal muscle and neutrophyl leucocytes. *J. Neurol. Sci.* 62 (1983) 327–355

Besrat, A., Polan, C. E. and Henderson, L. M. Mammalian metabolism of glutaric acid. *J. Biol. Chem.* 244 (1969) 1461–1467

Goodman, S. F., McCabe, E. R. B., Fenessey, P. V. and Mace, J. W. Multiple acyl-CoA dehydrogenase deficiency (glutaric aciduria type II) with transient hypersarcosinaemia and sarcosinuria; possible inherited deficiency of an electron transfer flavoprotein. *Pediatr. Res.* 14 (1980) 12–17

Rhead, W., Mantagos, S. and Tanaka, K. Glutaric aciduria type II: *in vitro* studies on substrate oxidation, acyl-CoA dehydrogenases and electron transferring flavoprotein in cultured skin fibroblasts. *Pediatr. Res.* 14 (1980) 1339–1342

Scholte, H. R. Liver malonyl-CoA decarboxylase. *Biochim. Biophys. Acta* 309 (1973) 457–465

J. Inher. Metab. Dis. 7 Suppl. 2 (1984) 103–104

Short Communication

Glutaryl-CoA Dehydrogenase Activity Determined with Intact Electron-transport Chain: Application to Glutaric Aciduria Type II

E. CHRISTENSEN

Section of Clinical Genetics, Department of Pediatrics and Department of Obstetrics and Gynaecology, Rigshospitalet, University of Copenhagen, Blegdamsvej 9, 2100 Copenhagen, Denmark

Normal glutaric aciduria type II (GA II, McKusick 23168) is a fatal inborn error of metabolism with onset within the first days of life (Przyrembel *et al.*, 1976; Gregersen *et al.*, 1980). It is characterized by the urinary excretion of a number of organic acids that seem to be derived from substrates to a group of FAD containing acyl-CoA dehydrogenases. These dehydrogenases all transfer electrons to the electron-transport chain (ETC) through electron transfer flavoprotein (ETF) and ETF dehydrogenase (ETF DH).

Glutaryl-CoA dehydrogenase (GDH, EC 1.3.99.7) is one of the acyl-CoA dehydrogenases not functioning *in vivo*, although the *in vitro* GDH activity is normal when methylene blue (MB) is used as an artificial electron acceptor (EA) (Gregersen *et al.*, 1980).

When GDH is measured with the intact electron-transport system very low activity is found in fibroblasts from GA II patients. This enzymatic method is more specific for the diagnosis of GA II than the earlier reported methods that used the decreased oxidation of ^{14}C-labelled lysine, the branched-chain amino acids and fatty acids by intact fibroblasts (Przyrembel *et al.*, 1976; Dusheiko *et al.*, 1979).

METHODS

GDH activity was determined with two different methods. The first method was described earlier (Christensen, 1983). The other method is a modification where MB is omitted as an exogenous EA and instead a homogenizing procedure is employed that preserves the endogenous ETC which *in vivo* transfers electrons from GDH to molecular oxygen via ETF and ETF DH. This new GDH assay is thus dependent on normal GDH, ETF, ETF DH and ETC (from CoQ_{10} to O_2) for activity. A defect in any one of these components will be detected as diminished GDH activity.

RESULTS

The activities of GDH determined with the two different assay methods are shown in Table 1. The first method with MB as EA gives higher specific activities than the

Table 1 Glutaryl-CoA dehydrogenase activity in fibroblasts from patients with glutaric aciduria types I and II[1]

Fibroblast cell line	Glutaryl-CoA dehydrogenase activity (μmol h^{-1} (g protein)$^{-1}$)	
	With methylene blue as electron acceptor	*With intact ETC*
Normal homozygote	2.86	0.44
GA I heterozygote	1.34	0.24
GA I homozygote	0.00	0.00
GA II heterozygote, mother[2]	1.96	0.37
GA II heterozygote, father[2]	2.99	0.53
GA II homozygote I[2]	2.68	0.014
GA II homozygote II[3]	2.23	0.022
GA II homozygote III[4]	2.77	0.035
GA II homozygote IV[5]	3.17	0.070
GA II, adult type[6]	1.97	0.29
DCA (riboflavin responsive)[7]	2.92	0.59

[1] Two different methods have been used. One with methylene blue as electron acceptor and one without any exogenous electron acceptor but with the *in vivo* electron transport system preserved
[2] Gregersen *et al.*, 1980
[3] Coudé *et al.*, 1981
[4] Goodman *et al.*, 1982
[5] Sweetman *et al.*, 1980
[6] Dusheiko *et al.*, 1979
[7] Gregersen *et al.*, 1982

Journal of Inherited Metabolic Disease. ISSN 0141-8955. Copyright © SSIEM and MTP Press Limited, Queen Square, Lancaster, UK.

other method with intact ETC but both methods show half normal activity in GA I heterozygotes and no activity in GA I homozygotes. However, in GA II homozygotes a very low GDH activity is measured with intact ETC, whereas the GDH activity with MB as EA is normal. Normal GDH activity was found in two obligate GA II heterozygotes with both MB as EA and with intact ETC. A patient reported to have an adult type of GA II and a patient with riboflavin responsive dicarboxylic aciduria were also shown to have normal GDH activity with both methods.

DISCUSSION

A new GDH method has been developed that requires an intact ETC for activity. Although this assay method can be used for the diagnosis of GA I heterozygotes and homozygotes it is not as sensitive for that purpose as the method using MB as EA. However, GA II homozygotes have very little activity with this new method in contrast to the MB method indicating a defective electron transport in GA II. As the ETC from CoQ_{10} to O_2 seems to be normal in GA II a defect in ETF or ETF DH is most likely (Christensen *et al.*, 1984). Two obligate GA II heterozygotes have been shown to have normal GDH activity measured both with MB as EA and with intact ETC.

Disorders related to GA II with similar excretion pattern of organic acids seem to have normal GDH activities with intact ETC. Two examples are shown in Table 1: the adult type of GA II and riboflavin responsive dicarboxylic aciduria.

Prenatal diagnosis of GA II by the determination of GDH with intact ETC seems to be possible in view of the normal activity in GA II heterozygotes and the very low activity in GA II homozygotes (see Table 1). Thus the GDH method described looks very promising as a tool in both the pre- and postnatal diagnosis of GA II.

References

Christensen, E. Improved assay of glutaryl-CoA dehydrogenase in cultured cells and liver: Application to glutaric aciduria type I. *Clin. Chim. Acta* 129 (1983) 91–97

Christensen, E., Kølvraa, S. and Gregersen, N. Glutaric aciduria type II: Evidence for a defect related to the electron transfer flavoprotein or its dehydrogenase. *Pediatr. Res.* (1984). In press

Coudé, F. X., Ogier, H., Charpentier, C., Thomassin, G., Checoury, A., Amédée-Manesme, O., Saudubray, J. M. and Frézal, J. Neonatal glutaric aciduria type II: An X-linked recessive inherited disorder. *Hum. Genet.* 59 (1981) 263–265

Dusheiko, G., Kew, M. C., Joffe, B. I., Lewin, J. R., Path, F. F., Mantagos, S. and Tanaka, K. Recurrent hypoglycemia associated with glutaric aciduria type II in an adult. *N. Engl. J. Med.* 301 (1979) 1405–1409

Goodman, S. I., Stene, D. O., McCabe, E. R. B., Norenberg, M. D., Shikes, R. H., Stumpf, D. A. and Blackburn, G. K. Glutaric acidemia type II: Clinical, biochemical, and morphologic considerations. *J. Pediatr.* 100 (1982) 946–950

Gregersen, N., Kølvraa, S., Rasmussen, K., Christensen, E., Brandt, N. J., Ebbesen, F. and Hansen, F. H. Biochemical studies in a patient with defects in the metabolism of acyl-CoA and sarcosine: another possible case of glutaric aciduria type II. *J. Inher. Metab. Dis.* 3 (1980) 67–72

Gregersen, N., Wintzensen, H., Kølvraa, S., Christensen, E., Christensen, M. F., Brandt, N. J. and Rasmussen, K. C_6–C_{10}-Dicarboxylic aciduria: investigations of a patient with riboflavin responsive multiple acyl-CoA dehydrogenation defects. *Pediatr. Res.* 16 (1982) 861–868

Przyrembel, H., Wendel, U., Becker, K., Bremer, H. J., Bruinvis, L., Ketting, D. and Wadman, S. K. Glutaric aciduria type II: Report of a previously undescribed metabolic disorder. *Clin. Chim. Acta* 66 (1976) 227–239

Sweetman, L., Nyhan, W. L., Trauner, D. A., Merritt, A. and Singh, M. Glutaric aciduria type II. *J. Pediatr.* 96 (1980) 1020–1026

J. Inher. Metab. Dis. 7 Suppl. 2 (1984) 105–106

Short Communication

Medium Chain Acyl-CoA Dehydrogenase Deficiency: Apparent K_m and V_{max} Values for Fibroblast Acyl-CoA Dehydrogenase towards Octanoyl CoA in Patient and Control Cell Lines

N. Gregersen and S. Kølvraa

Research Laboratory for Metabolic Disorders, University Department of Clinical Chemistry, Aarhus Kommunehospital and Institute of Human Genetics, University of Aarhus, Aarhus, Denmark

Eight cases of hypoglycaemic, 'non-ketotic' dicarboxylic aciduria have been proved by specific enzyme assays to be caused by a defect in general (medium chain) acyl-CoA dehydrogenase (Kølvraa *et al.*, 1982; Divry *et al.*, 1983; Rhead *et al.*, 1983; Coates *et al.*, 1982). The acyl-CoA dehydrogenases are flavoenzymes and in one of the cases it was shown that the binding of FAD to the apoenzyme was normal, indicating very strongly that the site of defect is localized to the apoenzyme (Kølvraa *et al.*, 1982).

By improving the sensitivity and the precision of the product-formation assay described previously (Kølvraa *et al.*, 1982) it has been possible to determine the kinetic parameters (apparent K_m and V_{max}) for fibroblast acyl-CoA dehydrogenases towards octanoyl CoA, thus approaching an elucidation of the molecular nature of the defect.

MATERIALS AND METHODS

Skin fibroblasts were grown in Eagle's essential medium containing 10 % human serum. The enzyme assays were performed in cells which were cultured in less than five passages. The fibroblasts were grown for a week giving approximately 25×10^4 cells per bottle and harvested by trypsination. They were washed twice with PBS-buffer (phosphate buffered saline) before freeze-thawing four times in 0.1 mmol/l phosphate buffer (pH 7.5). The mixture was centrifuged $1000\,g$ for 10 min and the supernatant solution (approximately 1 mg protein/ml) was used immediately in assay. Incubations were performed at 37 °C for 15 min in a mixture consisting of:

400 µl potassium phosphate-buffer, 0.1 mmol/l (pH 7.5);
100 µl supernatant of fibroblast homogenate, 0.1 mg protein;
50 µl FAD, 5.0 µmol/ml phosphate-buffer (280 µmol/l assay);
50 µl cysteine, 25 µmol/ml phosphate-buffer (1.4 mmol/l assay);
60 µl crotonase, 0.9 µg protein;
200 µl phenazine methosulphate, 17.4 µmol/ml phosphate-buffer (3.9 mmol/l assay);
25 µl octanoyl CoA, dilution series from 27.7 µmol/ml (783 µmol/l assay).

The total incubation volume was 885 µl.

The reaction was stopped by adding 500 µl sodium hydroxide (0.1 mol/l) and 25 µl of a solution of 1.7 mmol 8-hydroxyoctanoic acid/l (internal standard for GC–MS), after which it was hydrolysed at 60 °C for 30 min. 50 µl hydrochloric acid (5 mol/l) was added (pH 1) and dilution to 2 ml was performed with water. The solution was mixed with 4 g silica gel (Silica Woelm TSC, Woelm Phama, GmbH and Co, Eschwege, GFR) and poured into a column from which the acids were extracted by 80 ml ethylacetate. The organic phase was mixed with 100 µl of a solution of sodium methoxide (0.5 g sodium/100 ml methanol) and evaporated in a stream of nitrogen. The residue was trimethylsilylated by 100 µl trimethylsilyltrifluoroacetamide/1 % trimethylchlorosilane at 100 °C for 30 min. The produced 3-hydroxyoctanoic acid was quantitatively determined by selected ion monitoring (SIM) GC–MS in the chemical ionization mode (CI) with methane as reaction gas. The monitored ions were $289.1\,m/z$ for 3-hydroxyoctanoic acid and $215.1\,m/z$ for 8-hydroxyoctanoic acid (int. std.).

RESULTS AND DISCUSSION

The activity curves in Figure 1 show clearly that the activity of fibroblast acyl-CoA dehydrogenases for

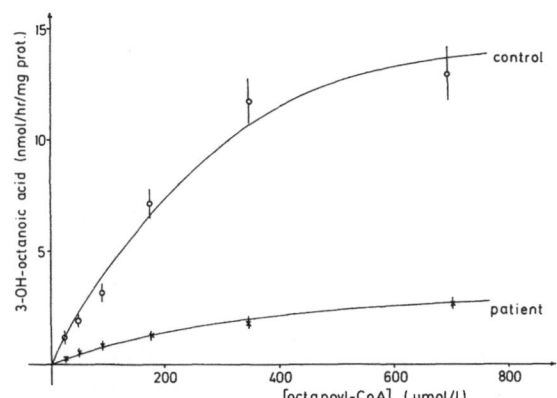

Figure 1 The amount of 3-hydroxyoctanoic acid produced, as measured by SIM, in reaction mixtures containing fibroblast homogenate (× patient and ○ control), crotonase, phenazinemethosulphate, FAD and varying amounts of octanoyl CoA. The bars represent a coefficient of variation of 10 %

105

Journal of Inherited Metabolic Disease. ISSN 0141-8955. Copyright © SSIEM and MTP Press Limited, Queen Square, Lancaster, UK.

octanoyl CoA is very low in the patient compared to the control cell lines. A kinetic analysis performed by use of the hyperbolic statistical computer program developed by Cleland (1979) revealed apparent K_m values of 312 ± 127 and 298 ± 68 µmol/l for patient and control respectively. The corresponding V_{max} values were 3.8 ± 0.7 nmol/h per mg protein for the patient dehydrogenases and 19 ± 2 nmol/h per mg protein for the control enzyme. The measured apparent K_m value is not a measure of the affinity of general (medium chain) acyl-CoA dehydrogenase for octanoyl CoA, but the affinity for the mixture of short chain, medium chain and long chain acyl-CoA dehydrogenases, which have overlapping affinities (Beinert, 1963; Furuta et al., 1981; Ikeda et al., 1983). The comparable K_m values for the control and patient enzymes indicate that the binding of substrate to all three acyl-CoA dehydrogenases, including the defective medium chain acyl-CoA dehydrogenase in the fibroblasts of the patient is not altered. On the other hand the low value of V_{max} for the patient enzyme compared to the control enzyme indicates that the enzyme deficiency is caused by decreased amounts of medium chain acyl-CoA dehydrogenase apoenzyme.

We thank technician Mrs Vibeke S. Winter for her contribution to the investigation, which was supported by The Danish Medical Research Council.

References

Beinert, H. Acyl-coenzyme A dehydrogenases. In Boyer, P. D., Lardy, H. and Myrback, K. (eds.) *The Enzymes*, 2nd Edn., Academic Press, New York, 1963, pp. 447–466

Cleland, W. W. Statistical analysis of enzyme kinetic data. In Purich, D. L. (ed.) *Methods in Enzymology*, Vol. 63, Academic Press, New York, 1979, 103–138

Coates, P. M., Stanley, C. A., Hale, D. E., Corkey, B. E., Hall, C. L. and Cortner, J. A. Fatty acid oxidation in fibroblasts of patients with medium-chain acyl-CoA dehydrogenase deficiency. *Am. J. Hum. Gen.* 34 (1982) 48A

Divry, P., David, M., Gregersen, N., Kølvraa, S., Christensen, E., Collet, J. P., Dellamonica, C. and Cotte, J. Dicarboxylic aciduria due to medium-chain acyl-CoA dehydrogenase defect: A cause of hypoglycemia in childhood. *Acta Paediatr. Scand.* 72 (1983) 943–949

Furuta, S., Miyazawa, S. and Hashimoto, T. Purification and properties of rat liver acyl-CoA dehydrogenases and electron transfer flavoprotein. *J. Biochem.* 90 (1981) 1739–1750

Ikeda, Y., Dabrowski, C. and Tanaka, K. Separation and properties of five distinct acyl-CoA dehydrogenases from rat liver mitochondria: Identification of a new 2-methyl branched chain acyl-CoA dehydrogenase. *J. Biol. Chem.* 258 (1983) 1066–1076

Kølvraa, S., Gregersen, N., Christensen, E. and Hobolth, N. *In vitro* fibroblast studies in a patient with C_6–C_{10}-dicarboxylic aciduria: Evidence for a defect in general acyl-CoA dehydrogenase. *Clin. Chim. Acta* 126 (1982) 53–67

Rhead, W. J., Amendt, B. A., Fritchman, K. S. and Felts, J. Dicarboxylic aciduria: Deficient 1-^{14}C-octanoate oxidation and medium-chain acyl-CoA dehydrogenase activity in fibroblasts. *Science* 211 (1983) 73–75

J. Inher. Metab. Dis. 7 Suppl. 2 (1984) 107–108

Short Communication

Mitochondrial Myopathy with Partial Cytochrome Oxidase Deficiency and Impaired Oxidation of NADH-Linked Substrates

H. S. A. SHERRATT

Department of Pharmacological Sciences, University of Newcastle upon Tyne, Newcastle upon Tyne NE1 7RU, UK

N. E. F. CARTLIDGE, M. A. JOHNSON and D. M. TURNBULL

Department of Neurology, University of Newcastle upon Tyne, Newcastle upon Tyne NE1 4LP, UK

Mitochondrial abnormalities in skeletal muscle are a feature of chronic progressive external ophthalmoplegia occurring in association with various craniosomatic abnormalities. Recently we have described a partial deficiency of cytochrome oxidase in seven of these patients (Johnson *et al.*, 1983). We describe a further case with an abnormality in the oxidation of NADH-linked substrates in addition to partial cytochrome oxidase deficiency.

CASE REPORT

This 49-year-old man had a 16-year history of progressive external ophthalmoplegia. Over the past 2 years he had developed slight slurring of speech and unsteadiness of gait. He was otherwise well apart from angina. General medical examination was normal. Examination of the fundi revealed bilateral pigmentary retinal change and decreased visual acuity on the right. There was bilateral ptosis and almost complete external opthalmoplegia. Left-sided sensorineural deafness was noted. Mild weakness of facial and proximal limb muscles was evident without significant wasting. There was mild limb and truncal ataxia. Deep tendon reflexes were normal, plantar responses bilaterally flexor and there was no sensory deficit. There was no family history of neurological disease. Routine haematology and biochemistry were normal except for creatinine kinase activity which was slightly increased at 232 µ/l (normal range <175). An electrocardiogram revealed widening of the QRS complex suggestive of an intraventricular conduction defect.

METHODS AND RESULTS

Skeletal muscle (3 g) was obtained at open biopsy from the patient or during hip replacement operations from the controls, and frozen in CF_2Cl_2 at $-150\,°C$ for cytochemistry or used to prepare mitochondrial fractions. Cytochemical and biochemical assays were performed as described by Johnson *et al.* (1983).

Muscle taken from the patient showed abnormal variation in fibre size but no muscle necrosis. There were, however, approximately 10% of muscle fibres with abnormal accumulations of mitochondria at the fibre periphery, seen most clearly by staining for succinate dehydrogenase activity. Virtually all these fibres gave a negative reaction for cytochrome oxidase activity. There were many other fibres without detectable morphological mitochondrial abnormalities which nevertheless had decreased cytochrome oxidase activity compared with the controls. All metabolic fibre types were affected, but the Type 1 and Type 2A fibres showed a greater decrease in cytochrome oxidase activity when measured by microdensitometry than the Type 2B fibres.

Total cytochrome oxidase activity in the skeletal muscle mitochondrial fraction from the patient was 706 nmol cytochrome c (II) oxidized min^{-1} (mg protein)$^{-1}$ (control values for six subjects 1058 ± 319). The cytochrome difference spectrum of the mitochondrial fraction revealed a marked deficiency of cytochrome aa_3 (about 30%) but with normal concentrations of cytochrome b and c (Table 1). Oxidations by the mitochondrial fraction were normal with succinate and DL-3-glycerophosphate as substrates, but the rates of oxidation of NADH-linked substrates were only about 10–15% of the control rates (Table 1).

DISCUSSION

Three forms of cytochrome oxidase deficiency in human skeletal muscle have been described: (1) fatal infantile myopathy with total cytochrome oxidase deficiency in skeletal muscle but not heart, liver or brain (Van Biervliet *et al.*, 1977), (2) severe but spontaneously resolving infantile myopathy characterized in the neonatal period by a low cytochrome oxidase activity in skeletal muscle which gradually increased over the next few months (DiMauro *et al.*, 1983) and (3) partial cytochrome oxidase deficiency in chronic progressive external ophthalmoplegia (Johnson *et al.*, 1983). In this paper we describe a new variant in which partial cytochrome oxidase deficiency is associated with impaired oxidation of NADH-linked substrates.

There have been four reports of defects in NADH-cytochrome b reductase activity (Morgan-Hughes *et al.*, 1979, 1982; Land *et al.*, 1981a,b). These cases showed normal rates of succinate oxidation but impaired oxidation of NADH-linked substrates. These authors

Journal of Inherited Metabolic Disease. ISSN 0141–8955. Copyright © SSIEM and MTP Press Limited, Queen Square, Lancaster, UK.

Table 1   Cytochrome concentrations in, and substrate oxidations by, skeletal muscle mitochondrial fractions

	Patient	Controls
Cytochrome concentrations (nmol (mg protein)$^{-1}$)		
Cytochrome aa_3	0.94	1.28 ± 0.16
Cytochrome b	0.53	0.57 ± 0.17
Cytochrome c	1.23	1.31 ± 1.23
Ratio $\dfrac{\text{Cytochrome } aa_3}{\text{Cytochrome } c}$	0.76	0.99 ± 0.11
Ratio $\dfrac{\text{Cytochrome } b}{\text{Cytochrome } c}$	0.40	0.44 ± 0.12
Substrate oxidations (nmol min^{-1} (mg of protein)$^{-1}$)		
10 mmol/l Succinate	209	216 ± 25
20 mmol/l D,L-Glycerolphosphate	63	61 ± 18
10 mmol/l Glutamate + 1 mmol/l malate	26	141 ± 30
10 mmol/l 2-Oxoglutarate + 1 mmol/l malate	13	156 ± 36

Concentrations of cytochromes reducible by 10 mmol/l succinate were measured for their reduced–oxidized difference spectra at $-190\,°C$. Substrate oxidations by intact mitochondria were measured at $30\,°C$ by following the reduction of Fe (CN)$_6^{3-}$ as final electron acceptor at 420–475 nm. Control values are expressed as means $\pm SD$ for six subjects.

also determined NADH-ferricyanide reductase activities and found normal values. However, NADH-ferricyanide reductase in crude mitochondrial preparations does not reflect the activity of NADH-cytochrome b reductase as exogenous NADH does not have access to NADH-dehydrogenase in intact mitochondria and NADH-dependent reduction of this artificial electron acceptor will also occur at NADH-cytochrome b_5 reductase, a flavoprotein tightly bound to the membranes of the endoplasmic reticulum and outer mitochondrial membrane (Mihara and Sato, 1978). More recently, a defect affecting both succinate cytochrome c reductase and rotenone sensitive NADH cytochrome c reductase has been described (Buist et al., 1983), but it is not known if there was an associated defect in cytochrome oxidase.

D.M.T. is in receipt of an MRC Training Fellowship. We thank Mr I. Pinder for providing the control muscle samples.

References

Buist, N., Darley-Usmar, V., Papadimitriou, A., Kennaway, N., DiMauro, S., S'Agostino, A. and Blank, N. Lactic acidosis and myopathy associated with ubiquinone cytochrome c reductase deficiency. *Pediatr. Res.* 17 (1983) 287A

DiMauro, S., Nicholson, J. F., Hayes, A. P., Eastwood, A. B., Papadimitriou, A., Koenigsberger, R. and De Vivo, D. C. Benign infantile mitochondrial myopathy due to reversible cytochrome c oxidase deficiency. *Ann. Neurol.* 14 (1983) 226–234

Johnson, M. A., Turnbull, D. M., Dick, D. A. and Sherratt, H. S. A. A partial deficiency of cytochrome c oxidase in chronic progressive external ophthalmoplegia. *J. Neurol. Sci.* 60 (1983) 31–53

Land, J. M., Hockaday, J., Hughes, J. T. and Ross, B. D. Childhood mitochondrial myopathy with ophthalmoplegia. *J. Neurol. Sci.* 51 (1981a) 371–382

Land, J. M., Morgan-Hughes, J. A. and Clark, J. B. Mitochondrial myopathy. Biochemical studies revealing a deficiency of NADH-Cytochrome b reductase activity. *J. Neurol. Sci.* 50 (1981b) 1–13

Mihara, K. and Sato, R. Detergent-solubilized NADH-cytochrome b_5 reductase. *Meth. Enzymol.* 52 (1978) 102–108

Morgan-Hughes, J., Darvenzia, P., Landon, D. M., Land, J. M. and Clark, J. B. A mitochondrial myopathy with a deficiency of respiratory chain NADH-CoQ reductase activity. *J. Neurol. Sci.* 43 (1979) 27–46

Morgan-Hughes, J. A., Hayes, D. J., Clark, J. B., Landon, D. N., Swash, M., Stark, R. J. and Rudge, P. Mitochondrial encephalomyopathies. Biochemical studies revealing defects in the respiratory chain. *Brain* 105 (1982) 553–582

Van Biervliet, J. P. G. M., Bruinvis, L., Ketting, D., de Bree, P. K., Van der Heiden, C., Wadman, S. K., Willems, J. L., Bookelman, H., Van Haelst, U. and Monnens, L. A. H. Hereditary mitochondrial myopathy with lactic acidaemia, a De-Toni–Fanconi–Debré Syndrome, and a defective respiratory chain in voluntary skeletal muscles. *Pediatr. Res.* 11 (1977) 1088–1093

J. Inher. Metab. Dis. 7 Suppl. 2 (1984) 109–110

Short Communication

L-Carnitine Insufficiency in Disorders of Organic acid Metabolism: Response to L-Carnitine by Patients with Methylmalonic Aciduria and 3-Hydroxy-3-methylglutaric Aciduria

R. A. CHALMERS, T. E. STACEY, B. M. TRACEY and C. DE SOUSA
Paediatric Research Group, MRC Clinical Research Centre, Watford Road, Harrow HA1 3UJ, UK

C. R. ROE and D. S. MILLINGTON
Pediatric Metabolism Division, Duke University Medical Center, Durham, NC 27710, USA

C. L. HOPPEL
Veterans' Administration Medical Center, Departments of Pharmacology and Medicine, Case Western Reserve University School of Medicine, Cleveland, OH 44106, USA

Recent publications have indicated the possibility of secondary carnitine deficiency and the need for supplemental L-carnitine in patients with disorders of organic acid metabolism (Roe and Bohun, 1982; Gregersen *et al.*, 1982; Roe *et al.*, 1983). L-Carnitine has a classical and important role in mediating the transport of long chain fatty acids into the mitochondrion for β-oxidation and additional and possibly equally-important roles have been proposed for the modulation of intramitochondrial acyl-CoA/CoA ratios and the availability of free CoA, and in the detoxification and facilitated removal of excess and potentially toxic acyl groups from the mitochondrion and cell as acylcarnitine esters (Chalmers *et al.*, 1983). Evidence for these roles has now been provided by our studies on patients with disorders of organic acid metabolism. In addition, the concept of a general approach to the treatment of patients with these disorders, that of L-carnitine therapy, has been developed from our observations.

METHODS

Urinary organic acids were determined quantitatively using established methods involving DEAE Sephadex extraction and capillary gas–liquid chromatography on fused silica columns (Chalmers and Lawson, 1982; Roe *et al.*, 1983). Plasma and urinary carnitine and acylcarnitines were determined using a radio-enzymatic assay (Brass and Hoppel, 1978) and urinary acyl-carnitines were identified using fast atom bombardment (FAB) mass spectrometry (Roe *et al.*, 1983). Acetyl-carnitine and propionylcarnitine were quantified in urine by isotope dilution analysis using FAB mass spectrometry (Millington *et al.*, 1984).

RESULTS AND DISCUSSION

We have studied 26 children with disorders of branched chain amino acid metabolism characterized by intra-mitochondrial accumulation of acyl-CoA intermediates, including patients with isovaleric acidaemia (McKusick 24350), multiple carboxylase deficiency (McKusick 21020, 21021), 3-hydroxy-3-methylglutaric aciduria, 'β-ketothiolase deficiency' (McKusick 20375), propionic acidaemia (McKusick 23200) and methylmalonic aciduria (McKusick 25100, 27740). The results of these studies, which are summarized elsewhere (Chalmers *et al.*, 1983), showed that in all cases, acylcarnitine excretion was greatly increased above normal and that the acylcarnitine/carnitine ratios were also greatly increased, although urinary free carnitines were within the normal range in the majority of patients. Our further observations, given below, on patients with disorders associated with a dicarboxylic aciduria, all of which are presumed to be associated with the intramitochondrial accumulation of acyl-CoA intermediates, have shown similar results. Concentrations of acylcarnitines observed, expressed in nmoles (mg creatinine)$^{-1}$ were: glutaric aciduria (glutaryl CoA dehydrogenase deficiency, McKusick 23167), 456, 328 ($n = 2$); multiple acyl-CoA dehydrogenase deficiency ('glutaric aciduria type 2', McKusick 23168), 590; dicarboxylic aciduria associated with suberylglycinuria, average 222 ($n = 3$); other undefined dicarboxylic acidurias associated with non-ketotic hypoglycaemia, average 321 ($n = 3$). Normal acylcarnitine excretion is 74 ± 40 nmol (mg creatinine)$^{-1}$. In all cases the acylcarnitine/carnitine ratios were greatly increased above the normal value of 2.0, with a range of 12.1–164. These results add support to the general concept of secondary carnitine insufficiency in such disorders of organic metabolism, where insufficient L-carnitine is available for the increased metabolic requirements of the patients secondary to their metabolic disorder, despite normal free carnitine in the circulation and urine.

Evidence for an increased requirement of this kind has been provided by the results of challenges of L-carnitine

Journal of Inherited Metabolic Disease. ISSN 0141–8955. Copyright © SSIEM and MTP Press Limited, Queen Square, Lancaster, UK.

given to patients with methylmalonic aciduria and with 3-hydroxy-3-methylglutaric aciduria. In the patient with methylmalonic aciduria for example, administration of a challenge dose of L-carnitine (Roe *et al.*, 1983) resulted in a dramatic increase in acylcarnitine excretion with concomitant decreases in methylmalonate and methylcitrate and a dramatic increase in hippurate (benzoylglycine) excretion. The major acylcarnitine was identified as propionylcarnitine and the increase in excretion of hippurate provided evidence for the underlying biochemical mechanisms involved; removal of accumulating propionyl groups as propionylcarnitine, releasing free CoA with consequent stimulation of key metabolic processes and of mitochondrial ATP synthesis (Chalmers *et al.*, 1983; Roe *et al.*, 1983).

Further evidence for the biochemical basis of the action of L-carnitine has been provided by results obtained during a severe ketotic episode in the same patient when L-carnitine was being administered (Figure 1). During this period, despite regular L-carnitine therapy ($100\,mg^{-1}\,kg\,day^{-1}$), methylmalonate excretion remained high and hippurate excretion was low, suggesting insufficient L-carnitine was available for her increased metabolic requirements arising from her ketosis. Increase of L-carnitine to $400\,mg\,kg^{-1}\,d^{-1}$ during one day resulted in a dramatic increase in propionylcarnitine excretion which was followed by a fall in methylmalonate and accompanied by an increase in hippurate excretion. Her ketosis was resolved without

recourse to intravenous therapy and only transient restriction of dietary protein was required. Hippurate excretion remained high despite cessation of carnitine therapy for other clinical reasons, and subsequently citrate excretion also increased markedly (Figure 1), indicating a return to normal metabolic function. Similar observations of the effect of L-carnitine have been made in two patients with 3-hydroxy-3-methylglutaric aciduria, a disorder caused by a defect in a different pathway of intermediary metabolism, supporting the concept that these observations are representative of a general phenomenon in all disorders in which there is intramitochondrial accumulation of acyl-CoA intermediates.

In conclusion, we believe L-carnitine will be of general and long-term benefit to these patients and may have a key role in their clinical and biochemical management, particularly during acute crises. Further studies on more patients with these disorders of organic acid metabolism, carried out in the detail outlined here, will, it is hoped, extend this concept of a general approach to their long-term management and treatment.

These studies were approved by the Ethical Committee of Northwick Park Hospital and Clinical Research Centre, Harrow, UK. The studies were supported in part by the National Reye's Syndrome Foundation, Bryan, Ohio, The Reye's Syndrome Research Fund – SFA (Duke University Medical Center), the National Institutes of Health (AM 15804) and the Muscular Dystrophy Association of the USA. We thank Mr D. A. Maltby, Miss M. Jones and Mrs J. Turkaly for their skilled assistance in this work.

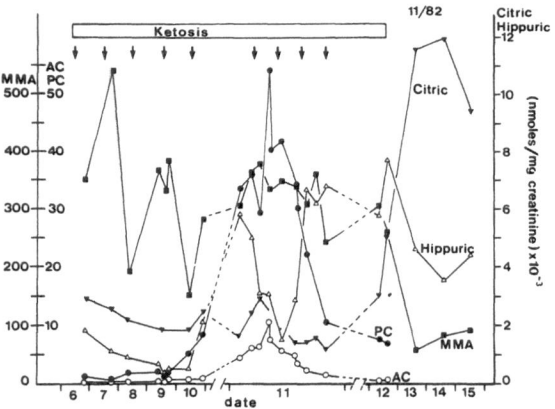

Figure 1 Urinary organic acid and acylcarnitine excretion by a patient with methylmalonic aciduria during a ketotic episode and L-carnitine therapy. The arrows indicate the administration of L-carnitine, 100 mg/kg body weight, with four equally-spaced doses being given on day 11. Abbreviations used are: MMA, methylmalonic acid; PC, propionylcarnitine; AC, acetylcarnitine. All units are in $(nmol/mg\ creatinine) \times 10^{-3}$. Despite L-carnitine therapy, during the increasing ketosis MMA excretion (■) remained high with a low hippurate (△) and citrate (▼) excretion. Administration of four times the normal dose of L-carnitine over one day produced a dramatic rise in propionylcarnitine (●) excretion, (accompanied by a small rise in acetylcarnitine (○) excretion) which was followed by a sustained rise in hippurate excretion and a delayed but marked increase in citrate excretion, with a return of methylmalonate to preketosis levels

References

Brass, E. P. and Hoppel, C. L. Carnitine metabolism in the fasting rat. *J. Biol. Chem.* 253 (1978) 2688–2693

Chalmers, R. A. and Lawson, A. M. *Organic Acids in Man. Analytical Chemistry, Biochemistry and Diagnosis of the Organic Acidurias.* Chapman & Hall, London, 1982

Chalmers, R. A., Roe, C. R., Tracey, B. M., Stacey, T. E., Hoppel, C. L. and Millington, D. S. Secondary carnitine insufficiency in disorders of organic acid metabolism: Modulation of acyl CoA/CoA ratios by L-carnitine *in vivo*. *Biochem. Soc. Trans.* 11 (1983) 724–725

Gregersen, N., Wintzensen, H., Kolvraa, S., Christensen, E., Christensen, M. F., Brandt, N. J. and Rasmussen, K. C_6–C_{10} dicarboxylic aciduria: Investigations of a patient with riboflavin responsive multiple acyl CoA dehydrogenation defects. *Pediatr. Res.* 16 (1982) 861–868

Millington, D. S., Roe, C. R. and Maltby, D. A. Application of high resolution fast atom bombardment and constant B/E ratio linked scanning to the identification and analysis of acylcarnitines in metabolic disease. *Biomed. Mass Spectrom.* (1984) in press

Roe, C. R. and Bohun, T. P. L-Carnitine therapy in propionic acidaemia. *Lancet* 1 (1982) 1411–1412

Roe, C. R., Hoppel, C. L., Stacey, T. E., Chalmers, R. A., Tracey, B. M. and Millington, D. S. Metabolic response to carnitine in methylmalonic aciduria: An effective strategy for elimination of propionyl groups. *Arch. Dis. Child.* 58 (1983) 916–920

J. Inher. Metab. Dis. 7 Suppl 2 (1984) 111–112

Short Communication

An Evaluation of Urine Lactate for Detection of Inborn Errors of Metabolism

D. B. DUNGER and J. V. LEONARD
Institute of Child Health, 30 Guilford Street, London WC1, UK

Lactic acidaemia is a feature of many inborn errors (Israels *et al.*, 1975; Leonard, 1982) but since blood lactate concentrations may be elevated for many other reasons (Braybrooke *et al.*, 1975; Eldridge and Salzer, 1967) it may be difficult to identify those children who require further study. We have investigated the value of quantitative urinary lactate estimations when screening for disorders of lactate metabolism.

METHODS

Blood and urinary lactate were assayed by an enzymatic method adapted for the autoanalyser (Gutmann and Wahlefield, 1974). The method was accurate, specific and the overall precision at a mean concentration of 1.3 mmol/l was 0.02 mmol/l (Dunger, 1982). Urinary creatinine was measured by the alkaline picrate method, and the urinary lactate concentration expressed as a lactate creatinine ratio (L/C).

Random urine samples were obtained from 176 normal children aged 2 weeks to 12 years at home or in hospital for minor surgical procedures. In addition simultaneous blood and urine specimens were obtained from 75 children who were being investigated for inborn errors.

RESULTS

In the random urines from normal children there was a linear correlation between lactate and creatinine concentrations (after logarithmic transformation of both variables, $r = 0.73$) (Figure 1). The mean L/C ratio was 0.078 with a range (± 2 SD) of 0.028–0.22.

Fifty of the 75 children who were being investigated for inborn errors had normal L/C ratios although in 17 of these corresponding blood lactates were elevated (> 2 mmol/l) on more than one occasion. Many of these children had frequent fits or spasticity but in none was any other evidence of disordered lactate metabolism detected on subsequent investigation. The elevated blood lactate levels were thought to be caused by difficulties with venepuncture or excessive muscular activity.

In the other 25 children, the L/C ratio was consistently raised and in 23 blood lactate was also elevated (Figure 1). The final diagnoses included congenital lactic acidosis, pyruvate carboxylase deficiency, fructose-1,6-diphosphatase deficiency, mitochondrial myopathy and glycogen storage disease types I and Ib. In the two remaining patients, gross lactic aciduria was not accompanied by a raised blood lactate and both had evidence of a Fanconi syndrome.

DISCUSSION

We have provided further confirmation that urinary lactate level is raised in patients with inborn errors that cause lactic acidaemia (Fernandes and Blom, 1976). In patients in whom the blood lactate is elevated secondary to convulsions, hyperventilation or muscle activity, the urinary lactate is not raised. Thus, urinary lactate appears to be a useful discriminant.

It has been suggested that lactate is freely filtered by the glomerulus and almost totally reabsorbed by the proximal tubule (Craig, 1946). The small amounts in normal urine represent the small fraction not absorbed and in addition lactate may diffuse into the distal tubule

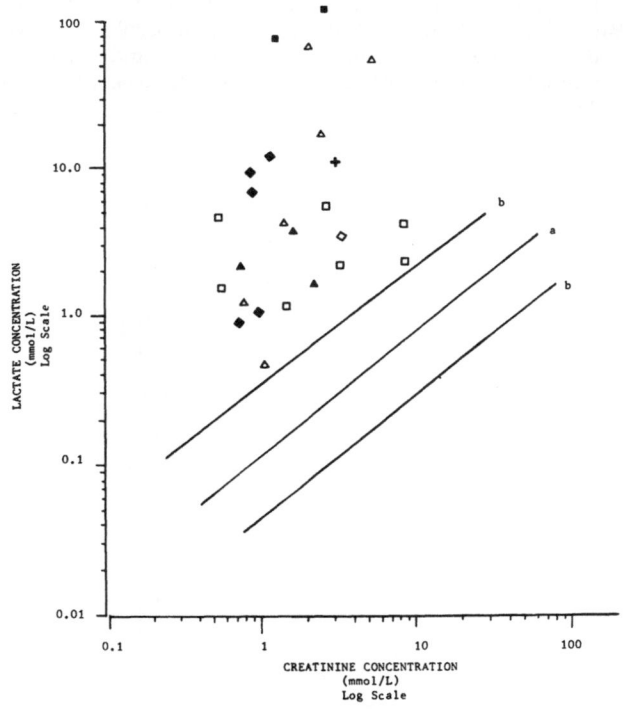

Figure 1 The relationship between the concentration of lactate and creatinine in random urine specimens. The values for 176 healthy children are represented by the regression line a ($\log_e [\text{lactate}] = -2.09 + 0.79 \log_e [\text{creatinine}]$). The lines marked b represent the 95% confidence limits. The symbols represent patients with raised urine lactate concentrations: □ glycogen storage disease type I and Ib; ◇ pyruvate carboxylase deficiency; ■ fructose-1,6-diphosphatase deficiency; △ congenital lactic acidosis; + Fanconi syndrome; ▲ undiagnosed neurodegenerative disorder (Leigh's syndrome); ◆ others

Journal of Inherited Metabolic Disease. ISSN 0141-8955. Copyright © SSIEM and MTP Press Limited, Queen Square, Lancaster, UK.

from the medulla where glycolytic activity is prominent (Dell and Winters, 1967). It has been suggested that there is a renal threshold for lactate (approximately 7.7 mmol/l) in man (Cohen and Woods, 1976) and that lactate would only be found in excessive amounts in the urine when this was exceeded. But in several of the children we studied, blood lactate concentrations were well below this (3–4 mmol/l) yet large quantities of lactate were excreted. This finding might support the hypothesis that tubular reabsorption of lactate is linked to removal of lactate by gluconeogenesis (Hohmann *et al.*, 1974), following a concentration gradient rather than obeying carrier mediated kinetics. Any inborn error affecting lactate metabolism, particularly those of gluconeogenesis would result in excessive lactate excretion in the urine. Tubular reabsorption of lactate may also be affected by conditions which affect proximal tubular function in a more general manner causing a Fanconi syndrome (Brenton *et al.*, 1981).

References

Brenton, D. P., Isenberg, D. A., Cusworth, D. C., Garrod, P., Krywawych, S. and Stamp, T. C. D. The adult presenting Fanconi syndrome. *J. Inher. Metab. Dis.* 4 (1981) 211–215

Braybrooke, J., Lloyd, B., Nattrass, M. and Alberti, I. G. M. M. Blood sampling techniques for lactate and pyruvate estimation: A reappraisal. *Ann. Clin. Biochem.* 12 (1975) 252–254

Cohen, R. D. and Woods, H. F. *Clinical and Biochemical Aspects of Lactic Acidosis.* Blackwell Scientific, Oxford, 1976

Craig, F. N. Renal tubular reabsorption, metabolic utilisation and isomeric fractionation of lactic acid in a dog. *Am. J. Physiol.* 146 (1946) 146–152

Dell, R. B. and Winters, R. W. Lactate gradients in the kidney of the dog. *Am. J. Physiol.* 213 (1967) 301–307

Dunger, D. B. Clinical and metabolic studies of hepatic glycogen storage disease. MD Thesis, London University, 1982

Eldridge, F. and Salzer, J. Effect of respiratory alkalosis on blood lactate and pyruvate in humans. *J. Appl. Physiol.* 22 (1967) 461–468

Fernandes, J. and Blom, W. Urinary lactate excretion in normal children and in children with enzyme defects of carbohydrate metabolism. *Clin. Chim. Acta* 66 (1976) 345–352

Gutmann, I. and Wahlefield, A. W. L-Lactate determination with lactate dehydrogenase and NAD. In Bergmayer, H. V. (ed.) *Methods of Enzymatic Analysis*, Vol 3. 2nd edn. Academy Press, New York, 1974, pp. 1465–1468

Hohmann, B., Frohnert, P. P., Kinne, R., Baumann, K., Papavassilou, F. and Wagner, M. Proximal tubular lactate transport in the rat kidney. A micropuncture study. *Kidney International* 5 (1974) 261–270

Israels, S., Haworth, J. C., Dunn, H. G. and Applegarth, D. A. Lactic acidosis in childhood. *Adv. Pediatr.* 22 (1975) 267–303

Leonard, J. V. Problems in the congenital lactic acidoses. In Porter, R. and Lawrenson, G. (eds) *Metabolic Acidosis. Ciba Foundation Symposium 87.* Pitman Books, London, 1982

J. Inher. Metab. Dis. 7 Suppl. 2 (1984) 113–114

Short Communication

Metabolic Acidosis versus a Compensation of Respiratory Alkalosis in Four Children with Leigh's Disease

E. PRONICKA and B. HALIKOWSKI

Department of Metabolic Disorders, Monument-Hospital Child Health Centre, Warszawa and Institute of Pediatrics, Pomeranian Medical Academy, Szczecin, Poland

Lactic acidaemia with increased serum pyruvate and alanine concentrations is characteristic for patients with subacute necrotizing encephalopathy (Leigh's disease) (Clayton *et al.*, 1967; Blass *et al.*, 1976). A decrease of pyruvate carboxylase activity (PC; EC 6.4.1.1) found in some of the patients can explain this biochemical picture. A primary importance of PC deficiency in initiation of brain impairment is controversial (Cooper *et al.*, 1973; Atkin *et al.*, 1979).

Accumulation of lactic and pyruvic acid is a part of respiratory alkalosis compensation (Kokot, 1976). In complete compensated respiratory alkalosis and metabolic acidosis only serum non-estimated anions concentration ('anion gap') and the degree of hydrogen excretion in kidney can show the direction of primary acid–base changes (Schwartz *et al.*, 1977).

Analysing acid–base disequilibrium in four patients with Leigh's disease we suggest that inhibition of PC activity in the patients could be secondary to chronic hyperventilation following brain degeneration.

PATIENTS AND METHODS

Leigh's disease was diagnosed in four patients on the basis of the clinical course and biochemical data. There was onset at 9–18 months, progressive course with periodic improvement and deterioration, vomiting, failure to thrive, hyperpnoea, discrete hirsutism and telangiectasiae, hypotonia, tremor, ataxia, strabismus, regression of motor development, normal or hyperactive deep tendon reflexes, and in two children central respiratory failure and death at ages 18 and 36 months. Autopsy performed on one case confirmed the diagnosis. Enzyme activity in tissues was not estimated.

In all patients, acid–base equilibrium was measured several times before and during ineffective vitamin B_1 treatment. 'Ion gap' was calculated from the formula $Na^+ - (Cl^- + HCO_3^-)$ (Gabow *et al.*, 1980). Urine hydrogen excretion was assayed in two patients under basal conditions.

Artificial respiration had to be applied in two children because of apnoeic attacks. They were kept under the respirator, for 2 weeks in one case and 5 months in the second, up to death. Acid–base equilibrium, lactate and pyruvate concentrations were systematically estimated during this period.

RESULTS

Acid–base equilibrium measurements in four patients showed a continuous decrease of base excess (BE) and carbon dioxide pressure (pCO_2) without marked changes in blood pH. In spite of this 'anion gap' was in the normal range in three out of four cases and urine hydrogen excretion in two patients studied was not elevated (Table 1). In two patients under artificial ventilation pCO_2 was 'artificially' kept within the physiological range. Then, without alkaline drugs complete normalization of BE occurred and lactate concentration had a tendency to decrease (Table 1).

Table 1 Biochemical data (mean values) in patients with Leigh's disease (a) before treatment, (b) under respirator

Case		pH	pCO_2 (mm Hg)	BE (mmol/1)	Lactate (mg %)	Pyruvate (mg %)	'Anion gap' (mmol/l)	Urine hydrogen excretion (μmol min^{-1} 1.73 m^{-2})
1	(a)	7.38	22.0	−9.9	57.2	1.7	13.6	—
	(b)	7.39	39.7	+0.1	27.8	1.2	—	—
2	(a)	7.35	30.6	−7.6	31.3	1.3	11.5–13.9	—
	(b)	7.33	46.8	−0.1	26.4	1.3	—	—
3	(a)	7.45	21.1	−6.2	37.9	1.5	5.4–12.0	23.7–26.5
4	(a)	7.35	26.6	−9.1	44.8	1.5	17.0–22.0	6.4–36.6
Normal		7.35–7.45	33.0–45.0	±2.5	8.0–18.0	0.6–1.1	<14.0	0–80.0

Journal of Inherited Metabolic Disease. ISSN 0141–8955. Copyright © SSIEM and MTP Press Limited, Queen Square, Lancaster, UK.

COMMENTS

Low 'anion gap', low urine hydrogen excretion and normalization BE during maintenance of normal pCO_2 under the respirator shows that respiratory acid–base changes (hyperventilation) could be primary in our patients.

We speculate that an increase of lactic acid, pyruvate and alanine in the patients is secondary to chronic hypocapnia and connected to compensatory inhibition of pyruvate carboxylase activity.

We conclude that primary chronic hyperventilation should be excluded in every patient with pyruvicaemia and lactic acidaemia.

References

Atkin, B., Buist, N., Utter, M., Leiter, A. and Banker, B. Pyruvate carboxylase deficiency and lactic acidosis in retarded child without Leigh's disease. *Pediatrics* 13 (1979) 109–116

Blass, J. P., Cederbaum, S. D. and Dunn, H. G. Biochemical abnormalities in Leigh's disease. *Lancet* 1 (1976) 1237–1238

Clayton, B., Dobbs, R. and Patrick, A. Leigh's subacute necrotising encephalopathy: clinical and biochemical study with special reference to therapy with lipoate. *Arch. Dis. Child.* 42 (1967) 467–478

Cooper, J. and Pincus, J. Thiamine triphosphate deficiency in Leigh's disease. In Hommes, E. and Van den Berg, C. (eds.) *Inborn Errors of Metabolism.* Academic Press, London, 1973, pp. 119–132

Gabow, P., Kaehny, W., Fennessey, P., Goodman, S., Gross, P. and Schrier, R. Diagnostic importance of an increased serum anion gap. *N. Engl. J. Med.* 303 (1980) 854–855

Kokot, F. *Gospodarka wodno-elektrolitowa i kwasowo-zasadowa w stanach fizjologii i patologii.* PZWL, Warszawa, 1976, pp. 133–139

Schwartz, A. Differential diagnosis of metabolic acidosis using anion gap. In Schwartz, A. and Lyons, H. (eds.) *Acid–base and Electrolyte Balance.* Grune & Stratton, New York, 1977, pp. 27–44

J. Inher. Metab. Dis. 7 Suppl. 2 (1984) 115–116

Short Communication

Chemical Diagnosis of Dihydrolipoyl Dehydrogenase Deficiency

T. Kuhara, Y. Inoue, T. Shinka, M. Matsumoto and I. Matsumoto

Institute of Human Genetics, Kanazawa Medical University, Uchinada, Kahoku-gun, Ishikawa 920-02, Japan

M. Yoshino

Department of Pediatrics, Kurume University School of Medicine, Kurume, Fukuoka 830, Japan

S. Okada

Department of Pediatrics, Osaka University School of Medicine, Osaka 553, Japan

Dihydrolipoyl dehydrogenase (E_3) deficiency (McKusick 24690) was first described by Haworth *et al.* (1976). Only a few cases of E_3 deficiency have been reported (Robinson *et al.*, 1977, 1981; Munnich *et al.*, 1982) and their diagnosis was based on E_3 activity in tissues or skin fibroblasts. The determination of E_3 activity in skin fibroblasts normally takes several weeks but an accurate diagnosis is required much sooner because the condition of the patient deteriorates rapidly once this late-onset disease manifests itself. E_3 is the third and common component of the pyruvate, 2-oxoglutarate and branched chain keto acid dehydrogenase complexes. Therefore patients with E_3 deficiency exhibit lactic aciduria, 2-oxoglutaric aciduria and branched chain ketonuria and a chemical diagnosis can thus be best made by the multicomponent analysis of urinary acids using gas chromatographic–mass spectrometric (GC–MS) techniques. This paper describes the chemical diagnosis of E_3 deficiency in two patients: a 6-month-old boy suspected to have atypical maple syrup urine disease (MSUD) and a 5-month-old child with Leigh's syndrome.

EXPERIMENTAL

Case 1

T.K. was the first child of healthy and unrelated Japanese parents. A neonatal screening test done at 5 days of age revealed an elevated leucine level in blood (0.46 mmol/l), but he developed normally on an ordinary diet until he experienced the first severe clinical episode at the age of 4 months. Development of his motor skills was delayed, and persistent metabolic acidosis was observed at the age of 6 months. GC–MS studies of urinary acids were strongly suggestive of an E_3 deficiency (Kuhara *et al.*, 1983). The serum levels of valine, leucine and isoleucine were distinctively elevated. Subsequent studies with skin fibroblasts showed complete lack of E_3 activity. The further enzyme studies with the liver and muscle from the patient will be published elsewhere (Matuda *et al.*, (1984).

Case 2

K.H., a boy, developed normally until 4 months of age. The blood level of leucine was normal by the neonatal mass screening test. At the age of $4\frac{1}{2}$ months, the child became acutely sick: he was very floppy and developed tonic–clonic convulsions in the upper extremities. The patient had metabolic acidosis (blood pH, 7.45; base excess, -8.5; bicarbonate, 13.9 mmol/l). He became lethargic, developed anuria and died at the age of 5 months. The serum amino acid levels of leucine, isoleucine, valine, proline, alanine and glutamine were greatly elevated. Computerized tomography revealed progressive loss of density of basal ganglia bilaterally, indicating that the patient suffered from Leigh's syndrome. The GC–MS analysis of urinary acids suggested that the child was deficient in E_3. Enzyme assay with lymphoblastoid cells showed that the E_3 activity was about 30% of the control.

The urinary organic acids were extracted with diethyl ether, converted to trimethylsilyl derivatives and analysed using the GC and GC–MS system as reported previously (Kuhara *et al.*, 1982).

RESULTS AND DISCUSSION

The reconstructed ion current and mass chromatograms of the urinary organic acids of the patient T.K. at 6 months of age are shown in Figure 1. Massive urinary excretion of lactate was found; 261 and 221 μmol/mg creatinine, 290 times and 246 times that of the control in T.K. and K.H. respectively. The 2-oxoglutarate levels in the two infants were also greatly elevated; 9.9 and 8.4 μmol/mg creatinine, 25 times and 21 times that of the control and the 2-hydroxyglutarate levels were 11 times and 13 times that of the control, respectively. The levels of 2-oxoisocaproate, 2-hydroxyisocaproate and 2-hydroxyisovalerate were greatly elevated compared to the controls; these branched chain acid levels were comparable to those of an intermediate MSUD.

There are many causes of chronic lactic acidosis: glucose-6-phosphatase deficiency, fructose 1,6-diphosphatase deficiency, pyruvate carboxylase deficiency, pyruvate dehydrogenase (E_1) deficiency, dihydrolipoyl transacetylase deficiency, cytochrome C oxidase deficiency, E_3 deficiency, etc. The urinary organic acid profiles of these two patients with E_3 deficiency were distinctly different from those with classical MSUD, intermediate MSUD, E_1 deficiency, Reye's syndrome and other lactic acidoses where we had determined the

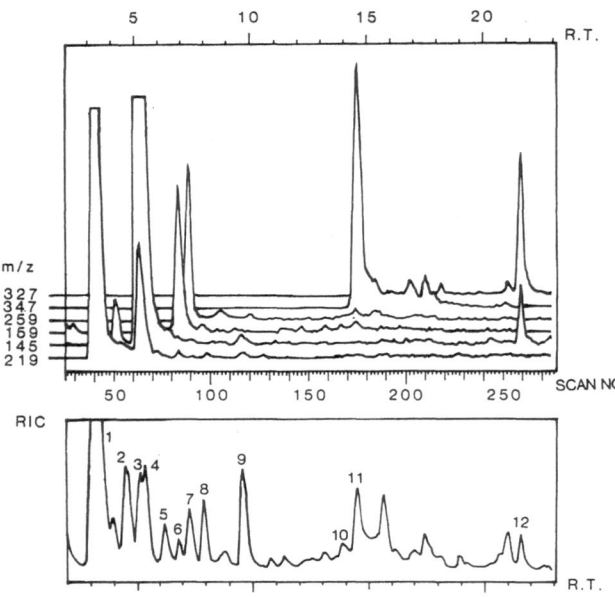

Figure 1 Reconstructed ion current (RIC) and mass chromatograms of trimethylsilyl derivatives of urinary acids (case I). 1, lactate; 2, 2-hydroxybutyrate; 3, 2-hydroxyiso-valerate; 4, 3-hydroxybutyrate; 5, 2-hydroxyisocaproate and 2-hydroxymethylbutyrate; 6, acetoacetate (isomer 1); 7, 2-oxoisocaproate; 8, acetoacetate isomer 2); 9, succinate and fumarate; 10, 2-hydroxyglutarate; 11, 2-oxoglutarate; 12, *n*-heptadecanoate (IS)

urinary organic acid profiles by GC–MS. The urinary acids which we found to be diagnostic for E_3 deficiency are lactate, 2-hydroxyisovalerate, 2-hydroxyisocapro-ate, 2-oxoisocaproate, 2-hydroxyglutarate and 2-oxoglutarate. Pyruvate, 2-oxoisovalerate and 3-methyl-2-oxovalerate would also be diagnostic but they would have to be converted to the oxime TMS esters or TMS-quinoxalonol derivatives prior to analysis. It appears that the urinary levels of the branched chain hydroxy acids are higher than those of their corresponding keto acids.

In one of our patients (T.K.) E_3 activity in fibroblasts was undetectable (control $7.0 \pm 2.2\,\mathrm{nmol\,min^{-1}\,(mg}$ protein$)^{-1}$), while in the other (K.H.) E_3 activity in lymphoblastoid cells was about 30% of normal. The E_3 activity in a patient reported by Munnich *et al.* (1982) was significantly higher than that in the other patients, 59% of the control in fibroblasts. However, the total activity of the pyruvate dehydrogenase complex was greatly reduced; 28% of the control. The clinical manifestations and other biological data of this patient were, however, very similar to that of a patient with

markedly decreased E_3 activity reported by Robinson *et al.* (1981). As Munnich *et al.* (1982) pointed out, there might be a mutation altering the structure of E_3 in such a way that the apparent E_3 activity is almost normal when measured using the free substrate. However, when the substrate has a strict spatial coordinate dictated by the binding of E_3 to E_2, then the mutation may have more dramatic effect in slowing down the overall working rate of the complex. It appears that the urinary acid profiles properly reflect the overall working rate of the complex.

A high-carbohydrate diet was recommended for a patient with E_3 deficiency (Robinson *et al.*, 1981). The patients with E_1 deficiency are treated with a diet comparatively rich in fat as they have a normal capacity for acetyl CoA metabolism through the TCA cycle. Thus it is important to distinguish E_3 deficiency from E_1 deficiency in order to prescribe a suitable diet.

We have shown that in patients suspected of having atypical MSUD, chronic lactic acidosis or Leigh's syndrome, E_3 deficiency can be rapidly and correctly diagnosed by a chemical analysis of the urinary acids. The more time-consuming enzyme studies should then be carried out to provide a better comparative data base.

References

Haworth, J. C., Perry, T. L., Blass, J. P., Hansen, S. and Urquhart, N. Lactic acidosis in three sibs due to defects in both pyruvate dehydrogenase and α-ketoglutarate dehydro-genase complexes. *Pediatrics* 58 (1976) 564–572

Kuhara, T., Shinka, T., Matsuo, M. and Matsumoto, I. Increased excretion of lactate, glutarate, 3-hydroxyiso-valerate and 3-methylglutaconate during clinical episodes of propionic acidemia. *Clin. Chim. Acta* 123 (1982) 101–109

Kuhara, T., Shinka, T., Inoue, Y., Matsumoto, M., Yoshino, M., Sakaguchi, Y. and Matsumoto, I. Studies of urinary organic acid profiles of a patient with dihydrolipoyl dehydrogenase deficiency. *Clin. Chim. Acta* 133 (1983) 133–140

Matuda, S., Kitano, A., Saheki, T., Sakaguchi, Y. and Yoshino, M. Pyruvate dehydrogenase subcomplex with lipoamide dehydrogenase deficiency in a patient with lactic acidosis and branched-chain ketonuria. *Clin. Chim. Acta* (1984) in press

Munnich, A., Saudubray, J. M., Taylor, J., Charpentier, C., Marsac, C., Rocchiccioli, F., Amédée-Manesme, O., Coudé, F. X., Frézal, J. and Robinson, B. H. Congenital lactic acidosis, α-ketoglutaric aciduria and variant form of maple syrup urine disease due to a single enzyme defect. *Acta Pediatr. Scand.* 71 (1982) 167–171

Robinson, B. H., Taylor, J. and Sherwood, W. G. Deficiency of dihydrolipoyl dehydrogenase. A cause of congenital chronic lactic acidosis infancy. *Pediatr. Res.* 11 (1977) 1198–1202

Robinson, B. H., Taylor, J., Kahler, S. G. and Kirkman, H. N. Lactic acidemia, neurologic deterioration and carbohydrate dependence in a girl with dihydrolipoyl dehydrogenase deficiency. *Eur. J. Pediatr.* 136 (1981) 35–39

J. Inher. Metab. Dis. 7 Suppl. 2 (1984) 117–118

Short Communication

3-Hydroxy-3-Methylglutaric, 3-Methylglutaconic and 3-Methylglutaric Acids can be Non-specific Indicators of Metabolic Disease

J. HAMMOND and B. WILCKEN
Oliver Latham Laboratory, N.S.W. Department of Health, P.O. Box 169, North Ryde 2113 (Sydney) Australia

Several cases of 3-hydroxy-3-methylglutaryl coenzyme A lyase deficiency (McKusick 24645: HMG-CoA lyase, EC 4.1.3.4) have been confirmed since the first report of Faull *et al.* (1976). Some reports which suggest HMG-CoA lyase deficiency have omitted enzyme information or recorded normal enzyme activity. This paper reports on three babies who excreted 3-hydroxy-3-methylglutaric (HMG), 3-methyl-glutaconic (MGC) and 3-methylglutaric (MGR) acids in different relative amounts. Two had normal HMG-CoA lyase activity and one was severely deficient. Details of Case 1 have been reported by Truscott *et al.* (1979).

CASE REPORTS

Case 1, L.S., the first child of 4th cousin Italian parents, became ill on day 3 with vomiting and coma. The blood ammonia level was 1200 µmol/l and plasma amino acids were abnormal, with elevated glutamine, alanine and lysine. In liver tissue obtained shortly before death at 5 days, carbamoyl-phosphate synthetase I (CPS) activity was 9% of control, ornithine carbamoyltransferase (OCT) 12%, argininosuccinate synthetase 100%, argininosuccinate lyase 16%, and arginase 100%. Activity of HMG-CoA lyase in cultured skin fibroblasts kindly assayed by L. Sweetman was normal. Quantitation of urinary organic acids showed elevated levels of HMG, MGC and MGR acids (Truscott *et al.*, 1979).

Her sister, G. S., became hyperammonaemic on day 3, before protein feeding. Plasma glutamine was elevated at 12 h but her urinary organic acids were normal Urinary orotic acid excretion was not increased. Treatment included sodium benzoate by mouth, and a low protein diet. She grew well, but had considerable developmental delay, and died aged 17 months. CPS activity was 16–28% of control, and OCT activity 155% in a liver biopsy obtained during life.

Case 2, M. D., male, was born to first cousin Turkish parents. A sister was healthy, but two male double first cousins had died in the first week of life of unknown cause. The baby developed metabolic acidosis at 24 h. He had increased plasma tyrosine (1026 µmol/l) and excreted tyrosine metabolites in the urine. His urinary organic acid profile also revealed increased lactic acid, 3-hydroxybutyric acid and small increases in HMG, MGC, MGR, 3-hydroxyisovaleric (HIV) and adipic acids. After 10 days he could tolerate normal protein feeds, and his organic acid profile became normal except that he continued to excrete the leucine catabolites at low levels (Figure 1b). The levels increased when a protein challenge was given and after an 11-h fast when glutaric, adipic and 3-hydroxyisobutyric acids also appeared. Blood ammonia was never elevated. Activity of HMG-CoA lyase in cultured skin fibroblasts assayed by S. Wysocki was in the normal range. He had microcephaly, delayed growth and development, and bilateral nerve deafness. He died at 10 months. Post-mortem examination revealed bronchopneumonia. The brain showed zones in the basal ganglia where normal tissue had been replaced by large numbers of capillaries and reactive glial tissue, appearances resembling those of Leigh's disease.

Case 3, P. N., is a Chilean girl of unknown parentage. She was well until three months of age, when she had vomiting, with rapid onset of coma, profound hypo-glycaemia and hepatomegaly. The urinary organic acid profile (Figure 1a) was typical of HMG-CoA lyase deficiency. Plasma ammonia and amino acids were normal. Activity of HMG-CoA lyase in cultured skin fibroblasts, assayed by L. Sweetman, was 1% of normal. Protein withdrawal was followed by rapid recovery. She was maintained on milk feeds plus a supplement, tolerating $2 \, g \, kg^{-1} \, day^{-1}$ of protein which included 120 mg/kg of leucine. Although she progressed well for some months, she had episodes of metabolic acidosis at 5, 8 and 10 months. Bilateral nerve deafness was diagnosed at 10 months, but at 18 months she is progressing well.

DISCUSSION

Case 3. P. N., clearly exhibits all the biochemical indicators of HMG-CoA lyase deficiency. These include severe hypoglycaemia and metabolic acidosis without ketosis, grossly increased urinary excretion of HMG, MGC, and MGR as well as HIV and moderate excretion of adipic and glutaric acids. Enzyme activity in cultured skin fibroblasts confirmed the diagnosis.

Case 1, L. S., on the other hand had hyperammonaemia, mildly increased urinary HMG, MGC and MGR and none of the other features. It is assumed that she and her sister had a primary defect of carbamoylphosphate

Journal of Inherited Metabolic Disease. ISSN 0141-8955. Copyright © SSIEM and MTP Press Limited, Queen Square, Lancaster, UK.

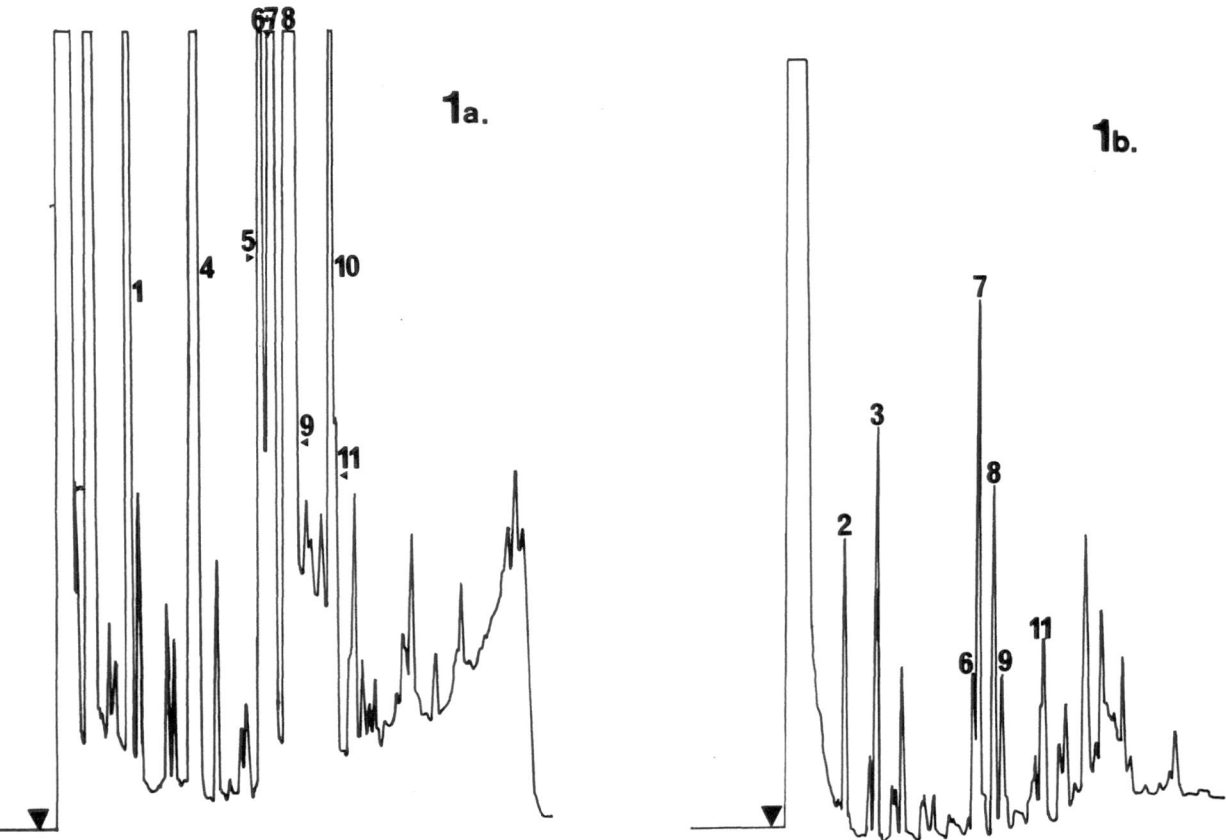

Figure 1   Gas liquid chromatograms of urinary organic acids (a) in Case 3 during acute illness and (b) Case 2 during a non-acute period. An ethyl acetate extraction was followed by derivatization with BSTFA/1 % TMCS. A volume of derivative corresponding to 40 nmol urinary creatinine was injected onto 3 % SE-30 and temperature programmed from 80°C to 240°C at 6°C/min. Peak identifications, kindly supplied by L. Hick, Wollongong University are: 1, unknown; 2, lactic acid; 3, 3-hydroxyisobutyric acid; 4, 3-hydroxyisovaleric acid; 5, glutaric acid; 6, 3-methylglutaric acid; 7 and 8, 3-methylglutaconic acid; 9, adipic acid; 10, 3-hydroxy-3-methylglutaric acid and 11, 4-hydroxyphenylacetic acid

synthetase I (EC 6.3.4.16) but a defect of *N*-acetylglutamate synthetase (EC 2.3.1.1.) cannot be excluded. The similarity of this patient with that reported by Applegarth *et al.* (1979) who also had CPS deficiency suggests that HMG-CoA lyase may be inhibited by some as yet undefined metabolite in this disorder.

Case 2, M. D., cannot be so easily defined. His mild and persistent increase in urinary MGC and MGR was accompanied by similar levels of HMG, HIV, adipic and glutaric acids at times, and either 3-hydroxybutyric or 3-hydroxyisobutyric acids were present occasionally. Hypoglycaemia and hyperammonaemia were not a feature of his stormy neonatal period, but his progressive neurological disease somewhat resembled that of two patients described by Greter *et al.* (1978). They excreted slightly elevated levels of MGC and MGR but no HMG. or HIV. No enzyme results were presented.

It appears that grossly elevated levels of HMG, MGC and MGR acids in urine usually indicate HMG-CoA lyase deficiency. Moderately elevated levels may result from secondary inhibition of the enzyme or severe metabolic stress in a heterozygote (Duran *et al.*, 1979).

Assays of enzyme activity are required to confirm each diagnosis.

References

Applegarth, D. A., MacLeod, P. N., Toone, J. R., Kirby, L. T., MacLean, J. R., Mamer, O. A. and Montgomery, J. A. Organic acids and Reye's Syndrome. *Lancet* ii (1979) 1147

Duran, M., Schutgens, R. B. H., Ketel, A., Heymans, H., Berntssen, W. J. M., Ketting, D. and Wadman, S. K. 3-Hydroxy-3-methylglutaryl coenzyme A lyase deficiency: postnatal management following prenatal diagnosis by analysis of maternal urine. *J. Pediatr.* 95 (1979) 1004–1007

Faull, K., Bolton, P., Halpern, B., Hammond, J., Danks, D. M., Hähnel, R., Wilkinson, S. P., Wysocki, S. J. and Masters, P. L. Patient with a defect in leucine metabolism. *N. Engl. J. Med.* 294 (1976) 1013

Greter, J., Hagberg, B., Steen, G. and Söderhjelm, U. 3-Methylglutaconic aciduria: Report on a sibship with infantile prograssive encephalopathy. *Eur. J. Pediatr.* 129 (1978) 231–238

Truscott, R. J. W., Halpern, B., Wysocki, J., Hähnel, R. and Wilcken, B. Studies on a child suspected of having a deficiency in 3-hydroxy-3-methylglutaryl-CoA lyase. *Clin. Chim. Acta* 95 (1979) 11–16

J. Inher. Metab. Dis. 7 Suppl. 2 (1984) 119–120

Short Communication

Different Organic Acid Patterns in Urine and in Cerebrospinal Fluid in a Patient with Biotinidase Deficiency

M. Di Rocco, A. Superti-Furga, P. Durand, R. Cerone and C. Romano
3rd Pediatric Division and Pediatric Clinics, Istituto 'G. Gaslini', Via 5 Maggio 39, 16148 Genova, Italy

C. Bachmann
Chemisches Zentrallabor, Insespital, Bern, Switzerland

R. Baumgartner
Metabolic Unit, Basler Kinderspital, Basel, Switzerland

Multiple carboxylase deficiency (MCD) is characterized by decreased activities of the biotin-dependent carboxylases and a specific urinary organic acid pattern. The early-onset form is due to a defect of holocarboxylase-synthetase (Sweetman, 1981) while deficient biotinidase activity leads to the late-onset form (Wolf *et al.*, 1983). Both forms are responsive to administration of biotin in pharmacological dosage. We report preliminary results of original studies carried out on the cerebrospinal fluid (CSF) of a new case of biotinidase-deficient MCD.

CASE REPORT

The patient, a girl born to healthy, unrelated parents, was well until 14 months of age, when neurological deterioration began. At the age of 18 months she exhibited myoclonic seizures, truncal ataxia, hypotonia, mild optic atrophy and hyperpnoea with laryngeal stridor. No conjunctival or cutaneous lesions were observed. Venous pH was 7.38, HCO_3^- 15 mmol/l, sodium 137 mmol/l, chloride 112 mmol/l, anion gap 10 mEq/l, pCO_2 was 22 mm Hg, plasma lactate 4.5 mmol/l and pyruvate 85 µmol/l. Lactate concentration in CSF was 9.8 mmol/l, pyruvate 370 µmol/l.

The diagnosis of MCD, based on an abnormal metabolite excretion pattern, led us to instigate biotin treatment (10 mg/day *per os*) which resulted in normalization of the CSF lactate and pyruvate and was followed by remission of the hyperpnoea and marked neurological improvement. After 10 days of therapy the CSF concentrations of lactate and pyruvate had returned to 1.9 mmol/l and 101 µmol/l, respectively.

SPECIAL INVESTIGATIONS

Plasma and CSF amino acids were determined by ion-exchange chromatography. (We thank Mr Ubaldo Caruso, Pediatric Clinics R.) Organic acids were analysed by gas chromatography and mass spectrometry (GC–MS). Plasma biotinidase activity was estimated by measuring biotinyl–PABA cleavage with a colorimetric assay (Knappe *et al.*, 1963).

The urinary organic acid pattern was consistent with MCD. In the CSF the lactate level was very high, but only traces of other organic acids were found, the presence of 3-hydroxyisovalerate being abnormal (Table 1).

Plasma biotinidase activity was 0.071 $nmol\,min^{-1}\,ml^{-1}$ (controls 5.82 ± 0.37, $n = 20$).

Blood amino acid levels were normal; in the CSF aspartate was low (2 µmol/l; controls 3.7–6.9 µmol/l; $n = 5$), as well as glutamate (2 µmol/l; 9.5–29) and glutamine (266 µmol/l; 535–869), while alanine was increased (54 µmol/l; 21.7–31.7); we found only traces of ornithine (controls 23–30 µmol/l). Gamma-aminobutyric acid was below the sensitivity of the method (5 µmol/l for GABA) in the patient and in controls.

DISCUSSION

The different organic acid pattern in the urine and in CSF may indicate that impairment of pyruvate carboxylase activity has a functionally predominant role in the central nervous system (CNS). However, the consequences of a defective pyruvate carboxylase activity at the CNS level are still not entirely clear. Lactate accumulation may result in marked acidosis of the CSF, owing to its low buffering capacity; a direct toxic action of lactate on cerebellum has also been postulated (Sanders *et al.*, 1980).

It has been suggested that neurological symptoms in pyruvate carboxylase deficiency are caused by impaired

Table 1   Organic acids in the MCD patient

	Urine (mmol/mmol creat.)	CSF (mmol/l)
Lactate	0.28	9.4
2-OH-butyrate	—	traces
3-OH-isovalerate	0.98	traces
3-OH-propionate	0.07	traces
3-CH_3-crotonylglycine	traces	—
Methylcitrate	traces	—

119

Journal of Inherited Metabolic Disease. ISSN 0141-8955. Copyright © SSIEM and MTP Press Limited, Queen Square, Lancaster, UK.

synthesis of the putative neurotransmitters aspartate (through decreased oxaloacetate formation), glutamate and gamma-aminobutyric acid, rather than by inadequate production of ATP and other high-energy compounds (Blass, 1983). In agreement with this hypothesis, we found a CSF amino acid pattern consistent with a Krebs cycle depletion and possibly consequent impaired synthesis of these neurotransmitters. However, CSF amino acids might not entirely reflect the intraneuronal amino acid levels, and certainly not differences between glial and neuronal cells.

We think that the application of GC–MS and amino acid chromatography to the study of the metabolic profile of the CSF in the different organic acidurias may yield valuable information concerning their pathogenetic mechanism.

References

Blass, J. P. Inborn errors of pyruvate metabolism. In Stanbury, J. B., Wyngaarden, J. B., Fredrickson, D. S., Goldstein, J. L. and Brown, M. S. *The Metabolic Basis of Inherited Disease*, 5th edn., McGraw-Hill, New York, 1983, pp. 193–203

Knappe, J., Brunner, W. and Bederbick, K. H. Reinigung und Eigenschaften der Biotinidase aus Schweinenieren und Lactobacillus Casei. *Biochem. Z.* 338 (1963) 599–613

Sanders, J. E., Malamud, N., Cowan, M. J., Packman, S., Amman, A. J. and Wara, D. W. Intermittent ataxia and immunodeficiency with multiple carboxylase deficiencies: a biotin-responsive disorder. *Ann. Neurol.* 8 (1980) 544–547

Sweetman, L. Two forms of biotin-responsive multiple carboxylase deficiency. *J. Inher. Metab. Dis.* 4 (1981) 53–54

Wolf, B., Grier, R., Parker, W. D., Goodman, S. I. and Allen, R. J. Deficient biotinidase activity in late-onset multiple carboxylase deficiency. *N. Engl. J. Med.* 308 (1983) 161

J. Inher. Metab. Dis. 7 Suppl. 2 (1984) 121–122

Short Communication

Biotinidase Deficiency: The Possible Role of Biotinidase in the Processing of Dietary Protein-bound Biotin

B. Wolf, G. S. Heard, J. R. Secor McVoy and H. M. Raetz
Departments of Human Genetics and Pediatrics, P.O. Box 33 MCV Station, Medical College of Virginia, Richmond, VA 23298, USA

Biotinidase (EC 3.5.1.12) cleaves covalently-bound biotin from partially degraded carboxylases and from biocytin, thereby recycling biotin. We have recently demonstrated that the activity of biotinidase is deficient in serum from children with late-onset multiple carboxylase deficiency (Wolf *et al.*, 1983a, b). Using a newly developed, sensitive radioassay, we have shown that biotinidase activity is also deficient in peripheral blood leukocytes and fibroblasts of affected patients (Wolf and McVoy, 1984). The enzyme activities in the parents of these children are intermediate between deficient and normal values. These findings indicate that the primary enzyme defect in late-onset multiple carboxylase deficiency is in biotinidase activity and that the disorder is inherited as an autosomal recessive trait. Children lacking biotinidase activity are unable to recycle biotin and depend on exogeneous biotin to prevent the clinical and biochemical features of biotin deficiency. Although previous reports have described 'impaired' intestinal absorption of free biotin in patients with late-onset multiple carboxylase deficiency, the absorption of free biotin was found to be normal in one of these patients when loading studies were repeated while her tissues were not biotin-depleted. Moreover, this patient was found to be biotinidase deficient (Thoene and Wolf, 1983). Because there is considerable clinical variability in this disorder (Wolf *et al.*, 1983c) and the concentrations of free and protein-bound biotin in foods are variable, biotinidase may also play a critical role in the processing of dietary protein-bound biotin.

MATERIALS AND METHODS

Blood, obtained by cardiac puncture, kidneys and small intestines were taken from 300 g Sprague–Dawley rats. The mucosa was scraped from the intestine using a microscope slide. Brush-border membranes (microvilli) from kidney and intestines were isolated as described elsewhere (Booth and Kenny, 1974; Kessler *et al.*, 1978). Bile and pancreatic juices were obtained via catheters placed in the bile ducts and common ducts of anesthetized rats. Serum biotinidase activity was determined colorimetrically (Wolf *et al.*, 1983b). Biotinidase activities in tissue, bile and pancreatic juice were determined using a radioassay which measures the liberation of *p*-amino-$[^{14}C]$benzoate from biotinyl-*p*-amino-$[^{14}C]$benzoate (Wolf and McVoy, 1984). Alkaline phosphatase activity was determined colorimetrically by measuring the formation of 4-nitrophenolate from 4-nitrophenolphosphate (Malamy and Horecker, 1966). Soluble protein was determined by the method of Bradford (1976).

RESULTS

The mean activity of biotinidase ($\pm$ SD) in rat serum is 6100 ± 1000 pmol min^{-1} ml^{-1} (range 4400–7400; $n = 6$) or 118 ± 10 pmol min^{-1} (mg protein)$^{-1}$ (range 107–127). The biotinidase activities in homogenates of rat renal and intestinal mucosa (Table 1) were similar to those reported previously (Pispa, 1965). The activity of

Table 1 Biotinidase activity in renal and intestinal brush-border membranes

Tissue	Fraction	Alkaline phosphatase activity[1]	Biotinidase activity[2]
Kidney	Homogenate	0.217	92.9
	Brush border	5.518	24.4
	Fold-enrichment	25.4	0.26
Intestines	Homogenate	0.305	31.8
	Brush border	7.416	3.2
	Fold-enrichment	24.3	0.10

[1] μmoles of 4-nitrophenolate formed min^{-1} (mg protein)$^{-1}$
[2] pmoles of *p*-aminobenzoate formed min^{-1} (mg protein)$^{-1}$

Journal of Inherited Metabolic Disease. ISSN 0141–8955. Copyright © SSIEM and MTP Press Limited, Queen Square, Lancaster, UK.

alkaline phosphatase, an enzyme known to be in the brush-border membrane, is enriched in brush-border fractions from kidney and intestines when compared to that in homogenates, whereas the activity of biotinidase is not enriched (Table 1). Mucosa from separate sections of the small intestine showed little difference in activity. The mean activities (pmol min^{-1} (mg protein)$^{-1}$) were 49 ± 2 (range 46–51; $n = 4$), 59 ± 15 (range 49–76; $n = 3$), and 52 ± 17 (range 32–68; $n = 4$) in the mucosa of duodenum, jejunum and ileum, respectively. Biotinidase activity was not detectable in rat bile but was present in pancreatic juice, the mean activity being 316 ± 189 pmol min^{-1} ml^{-1} (range 129–507; $n = 3$).

DISCUSSION

The presence of considerable biotinidase activity in homogenate and limited activity in brush-border membranes of kidney suggests that the major role of the enzyme in this organ is the recycling biotin and not reabsorption of biocytin or biotin-containing peptides. This seems likely because any bound biotin secreted into the blood would be expected to be rapidly hydrolysed by serum biotinidase before reaching the kidney.

Mammals cannot synthesize biotin and therefore must derive the vitamin from two major sources: the pool of biotin-containing enzymes (holocarboxylases) on which biotinidase acts, and the gut, from which biotin of dietary and microbial origin may be absorbed. However, most of the biotin in foods such as meats and cereals is protein-bound (Pispa, 1965). In the intestines, protein-bound biotin can be hydrolysed by biotinidase from several sources including bile, pancreatic juice, secretions of the intestinal glands, synthetic or metabolic products of bacterial flora, and the brush-border microvilli.

Our results indicate that there is biotinidase activity in the pancreatic juice and in intestinal mucosa, but not in the intestinal brush-border membranes or bile. The biotinidase in the pancreatic juice together with various secreted proteases may liberate protein-bound biotin. Biotinidase in the intestinal mucosa may originate in the columnar or specialized glandular cells. It is also possible that proteases located in the brush-border membrane hydrolyse dietary, biotin-containing proteins to yield biocytin or biotin-containing peptides which enter the mucosal cells and are cleaved subsequently to release free biotin for utilization. Regardless of whether all or some of these mechanisms operate, it is very likely

that biotinidase plays a critical role in the processing of protein-bound biotin. If biotinidase production by intestinal flora is insignificant, then patients with biotinidase deficiency would have no mechanism for liberating biotin from protein-bound sources in food. Furthermore, if, as some studies have suggested, the contribution of the microflora to the free biotin pool is small, then these patients would depend entirely on free biotin to meet their requirements for the vitamin. These conditions would further aggravate biotin deficiency in such individuals and emphasize the importance of considering the form in which the dietary biotin is provided and the necessity of using free biotin in the treatment of the disorder.

References

Booth, A. G. and Kenny, A. J. A rapid method for the preparation of microvilli from rabbit kidney. *Biochem. J.* 142 (1974) 575–581

Bradford, M. M. A rapid and sensitive method for the quantitation of microgram quantities of protein utilizing the principle of protein-dye binding. *Anal. Biochem.* 72 (1976) 248–254

Kessler, M., Acuto, O., Storelli, C., Murer, H., Muller, M. and Semenza, G. A modified procedure for the rapid preparation of efficiently transporting vesicles from small intestinal brush border membranes. *Biochem. Biophys. Acta* 506 (1978) 136–154

Malamy, M. and Horecker, B. L. Alkaline phosphatase. *Meth. Enzymol.* 9 (1966) 639

Pispa, J. Animal biotinidase. *Ann. Med. Exp. Biol. Fenn.* 43 Suppl 5 (1965) 5–39

Thoene, J. and Wolf, B. Biotinidase deficiency in juvenile multiple carboxylase deficiency. *Lancet* 2 (1983) 398

Wolf, B., Grier, R. E., Parker, W. D., Goodman, S. I. and Allen, R. J. Deficient serum biotinidase activity in late-onset multiple carboxylase deficiency. *N. Engl. J. Med.* 308 (1983a) 161

Wolf, B., Grier, R. E., Allen, R. J., Goodman, S. I. and Kien, C. L. Biotinidase deficiency: the enzymatic defect in late-onset multiple carboxylase deficiency. *Clin. Chim. Acta* 131 (1983b) 273–281

Wolf, B., Grier, R. E., Allen, R. J., Goodman, S. I., Kien, C. L., Parker, W. D., Howell, D. M. and Hurst, D. L. Phenotypic variation in biotinidase deficiency. *J. Pediatrics* 103 (1983c) 233–237

Wolf, B. and McVoy, J. S. A sensitive radioassay for biotinidase activity: deficient activity in tissues of serum biotinidase-deficient individuals. *Clin. Chim. Acta* 135 (1984) 275–281

J. Inher. Metab. Dis. 7 Suppl. 2 (1984) 123–125

Short Communication

Biotin-responsive Multiple Carboxylase Deficiency (MCD): Deficient Biotinidase Activity Associated with Renal Loss of Biotin

E. R. Baumgartner, T. Suormala and H. Wick
University Children's Hospital, 4005 Basel, Switzerland

J. P. Bonjour
Hoffmann-La Roche & Co., 4005 Basel, Switzerland

Biotin-responsive multiple carboxylase deficiencies (MCD) are inherited disorders characterized biochemically by the accumulation of a typical pattern of organic acids, caused by decreased activity of the three mitochondrial biotin-containing enzymes: propionyl CoA carboxylase (PCC, EC 6.4.1.3), 3-methylcrotonyl CoA carboxylase (MCC, EC 6.4.1.4) and pyruvate carboxylase (PC, EC 6.4.1.1). Clinically this disorder exists in at least two forms, namely an early-onset (neonatal) and a late-onset (juvenile) form. Both types of the disorder respond to high doses of biotin. In most instances, the neonatal form appears to be caused by deficient holocarboxylase synthetase activity due to an elevated K_m for biotin (Burri et al., 1981), while in some patients with late-onset MCD the primary biochemical defect has recently been found to be a deficiency in the activity of biotinidase, the enzyme regenerating biotin from endogenous biocytin (Wolf et al., 1983).

We have investigated five patients from three unrelated families with late-onset MCD. Plasma biotinidase activity was decreased to 1–2% of normal in all patients. In addition, renal clearance studies showed increased renal excretion of biotin, whereas intestinal absorption of biotin was found to be normal. Renal loss of biotin explains, at least in part, the high biotin requirement in these patients.

CASE REPORTS

Case 1. S.M., female, born 6.1.1978. First symptoms at age 7 weeks: seizures, muscular hypotonia, seborrhoic dermatitis, conjunctivitis, metabolic acidosis, peculiar odour. Diagnosis and initiation of biotin therapy at age 10 weeks (Lehnert et al., 1979).

Case 2. S.T., male, born 26.11.1982. Sibling of S.M. The mother was treated with biotin during her pregnancy. Increased plasma biotin concentrations and carboxylase activities in lymphocytes of cord blood. Treatment with biotin since birth. Diagnosis at age 5 months by assaying serum biotinidase activity.

Case 3. H.D., male, born 7.11.1978. Diagnosis and beginning of treatment at age 6 months after a febrile episode accompanied by seizures, muscular hypotonia, skin rash and hepatosplenomegaly (Baumgartner et al., 1981).

Case 4. C.G., female, born 19.11.1981. Diagnosis was made at age 3 months after the child had presented with seizures, muscular hypotonia, developmental retardation, alopecia and metabolic acidosis since the age of 2 months.

Case 5. C.K., female, born 10.11.1982. Sibling of C.G. The mother received no supplementation of biotin during pregnancy. Normal biotin concentrations and carboxylase activities in cord blood. At 8 days of age increased irritability and discreet abnormalities in e.e.g. Diagnosis at 12 days of age by finding decreased carboxylase activities in lymphocytes and subnormal biotin plasma concentration.

With continuous biotin supplementation (2.5–40 mg/daily) all patients developed normally both physically and mentally except for S.M. who has a sensory-neural hearing loss.

METHODS

PCC, MCC and PC activities in cultured skin fibroblasts and peripheral lymphocytes were measured with slight modifications of published methods. Biotinidase activity was measured in plasma by the method of Knappe et al. (1963). Biotin was determined microbiologically with *Lactobacillus plantarum* (Frigg and Brubacher, 1976).

In the patients, renal biotin clearance studies were performed after cessation of biotin therapy, when biotin plasma levels had reached normal concentrations. In controls they were performed both while on a normal diet and during prolonged supplementation with daily biotin doses of 35 and 150–200 µg/kg.

Intestinal biotin absorption was tested after an overnight fast with 1.5 µg/kg oral biotin, in the patients when plasma biotin levels were at or below 1 nmol/l. The absorption test was repeated in the patients with 100 µg/kg when biotin supplementation had been withheld for an even longer period of time and carboxylase activities in lymphocytes had decreased to 6–49% of normal

RESULTS AND DISCUSSION

PCC, MCC and PC activities in cultured skin fibroblasts of all patients were in the normal range, even when grown in biotin-depleted medium or in the presence of avidin, excluding a defect of holocarboxylase synthetase. Biotinidase activity in plasma was reduced to 1–3% in all patients and to 38–63 % of normal in the parents (Table 1) and in some male and female siblings.

The following observations demonstrated increased biotin requirement, increased renal excretion, and normal intestinal absorption of biotin in the patients (Table 1).

(1) Withholding biotin treatment resulted in a rapid fall of plasma biotin to subnormal concentrations within 3–14 days and reappearance of abnormal metabolites, decreased carboxylase activities in lymphocytes and discreet clinical symptoms (alopecia, periocular and perioral rash) within 2 weeks to $3\frac{1}{2}$ months depending on the biotin dose administered beforehand (2.5–40 mg daily).

(2) The patients needed a much higher biotin supplementation than controls to maintain similar biotin plasma concentrations.

(3) At similar biotin plasma concentrations, renal biotin excretion was 3–6-fold higher in the patients than in controls as long as plasma biotin levels were in or above the normal range but fell to subnormal concentrations when plasma biotin became subnormal.

(4) At normal biotin plasma concentrations the ratio of renal biotin clearance to creatinine clearance was ≥ 1 in the patients, whereas in adult controls it ranged between 0.4 and 0.64, in nine healthy children (3–13 years), the mean ratio was 0.33 (range 0.14–0.76). With increasing plasma biotin concentrations during prolonged biotin supplementation in healthy adults, the ratio increased and almost reached 1.0 at a biotin plasma concentration of ~ 70 nmol/l.

(5) Intestinal absorption of a single dose of biotin (1.5 µg/kg) was similar to that of controls, i.e. a maximal increase in plasma biotin of 2–6-fold was observed 45–60 min after ingestion of biotin (Baumgartner *et al.*, 1982). In some experiments, when the patients were in a state of severe biotin depletion (carboxylase activities in lymphocytes 20–30 % of normal), the postabsorptional plasma biotin peak was less marked, but instead the carboxylase activities increased 6–22 % within 2 hours. After an oral biotin load of 100 µg/kg, the decreased carboxylase activities in lymphocytes became normal within 45 min in all three patients tested.

Our findings confirm biotinidase deficiency as the probable primary defect in five patients with late-onset MCD as originally described by Wolf *et al.* (1983). In addition, renal clearance studies in three of our patients clearly demonstrate a renal loss of biotin (biocytin is not measured by our method). Our biotin absorption studies indicate normal intestinal absorption and transport of biotin to the mitochondrial apoenzymes.

Table 1   Biotinidase activity and biotin concentrations in plasma and urine of patients and controls

Biotin supplementation	Time after last biotin administ.	Biotin in plasma nmol/l[†]	Biotin/creat. in urine, nmol/mmol[†]	Clearance ml/min × 1.73 m²[†] Biotin	Creatinine	Biotinidase activity nmol/min per ml plasma[†]
Healthy adults						
n.s. ($n = 8$)	—	1.9 ± 0.6	10 ± 6	49 ± 20	124 ± 16	6.00 ± 0.79
35 µg/kg ($n = 8$)	12 h	20 ± 5	192 ± 75	110 ± 25	127 ± 32	($n = 5$)
150–200 µg/kg ($n = 6$)	12 h	74 ± 13	907 ± 300	118 ± 26	120 ± 6	
Healthy children						
3–13 y, n.s. ($n = 9$)	—	2.3 ± 1.6	17 ± 15	32 ± 11	98 ± 43	5.52 ± 0.79 ($n = 15$)
Patients						
S.M., 2 × 2.5 mg/d	12 h	22	678	158	134	0.11
(~ 260 µg/kg/d)	68 h	2.7	92			
	84 h	0.45	0.27			
	11 d	<0.4*	3.5			
H.D., 2 × 5 mg/d	24 h	2.3	77	136	105	0.08
(~ 220 µg/kg per day)	8 d	<0.4*	3.2			
C.G., 2.5 mg/d	15 h	71	4150	121	97	0.15
(~ 900 µg/kg per day)	39 h	15	775			
	86 h	2.8	104			
	96 h	<0.4*	1.6			
Parents						
Mother of C.G., n.s.‡	—	1.3	3.1	11	89	3.52
Father of C.G., n.s.‡	—	3.6	23	60	107	2.52

* Limit of detection: 0.4 nmol/l; † Control values expressed as $\bar{X} \pm SD$; ‡ n.s., on normal diet, without biotin supplementation

The mechanism by which biotinidase deficiency leads to renal loss of biotin and to increased biotin requirement remains to be investigated. Inhibition of holocarboxylase synthetase by biocytin seems unlikely since decreased carboxylase activities in patient S.M. and C.K. were partially restored within 45 min after a single administration of oral biotin (1.5 µg/kg) at plasma biotin concentration of 2.9 (S.M.) and 0.8 (C.K.) nmol/l. Conceivably biotinidase might play a role in renal handling of biotin or as a specific biotin-binding protein in plasma, or alternatively, biocytin might interfere with renal reabsorption of biotin.

References

Baumgartner, R., Suormala, T., Wick, H., Geisert, J. and Lehnert, W. Infantile multiple carboxylase deficiency: evidence for normal intestinal absorption but renal loss of biotin. *Helv. Paediatr. Acta* 37 (1982) 499–502

Baumgartner, R., Suormala, T., Wick, H., Bachmann, C. and Jaggi, K. H. Biotin dependency causing multiple carboxylase deficiency *in vivo. Pediatr. Res.* 15 (1981) 1189

Burri, B. J., Sweetman, L. and Nyhan, W. L. Evidence for the enzyme defect in early infantile biotin-responsive multiple carboxylase deficiency. *J. Clin. Invest.* 68 (1981) 1491–1495

Frigg, M. and Brubacher, G. Biotin deficiency in chicks fed a wheat-based diet. *Int. J. Vitam. Nutri. Res.* 46 (1976) 314–321

Knappe, J., Brümmer, W. and Biederbick, K. Reinigung und Eigenschaften der Biotinidase aus Schweineniere und Lactobacillus casei. *Biochem. Z.* 338 (1963) 591–613

Lehnert, W., Niederhoff, H., Junker, A., Saule, H. and Frasch, W. A case of biotin-responsive 3-methyl-crotonylglycin- and 3-hydroxy-isovaleric aciduria. *Eur. J. Pediatr.* 132 (1979) 107–114

Wolf, B., Grier, R. E., Parker, W. D., Goodman, S. J. and Allen, R. J. Deficient biotinidase activity in late-onset multiple carboxylase deficiency. *N. Engl. J. Med.* 308 (1983) 161

J. Inher. Metab. Dis. 7 Suppl. 2 (1984) 126

Short Communication

Organic Acids in Urine: Sample Preparation for GC/MS

C. BACHMANN, R. BÜHLMANN and J. P. COLOMBO

Department of Clinical Chemistry, Inselspital, University of Berne, 3010 Berne, Switzerland

A rapid diagnosis is important for the successful treatment of organic acidurias. The determination of organic acids in urine is usually done by gas chromatography, preferably coupled with mass spectrometry (GC/MS). For sample preparation, extraction of the acids into organic solvents (e.g. ether/ethylacetate) is not quantitative for several metabolites (Goodman and Markey, 1981), while elution from anion exchange columns is rather time consuming. We present a rapid and reliable method derived from gradient liquid chromatography as described by Sweetman (1974) and from our experience with short-chain fatty acid determinations (Bachmann *et al.*, 1979).

METHODS

To 700 µl of urine 100 µl of internal standard (tricarballate 12.5 mmol/l) and 100 µl of HCl (6 mol/l) are added, and applied to a ready-made column (9 × 40 mm) of Extrelute® (Merck No. 15371) . After 30 min absorption time the organic acids are eluted with 15 ml of chloroform/2-methylbutan-2-ol (1:1, v/v). The acids are extracted from the eluate into 2 ml of aqueous ammonia (1 mol/l) and dried down under N_2 at 45°C. The residue is derivatized with 150 µl BSTFA (containing 1 % TMCS, Pierce). For evaluation of the method 11 critical metabolites were added to urine. The GC conditions were: injector 220°C, detector 290°C, oven program 80 to 250°C at 4°C/min, column 2 mm × 2 m, SE 30 or Dexsil 400, N_2: 25 ml/min (MS: He 18 ml/min); integrator Sigma 10. Mass spectrometry was performed on a HP 5990A with jet separator.

RESULTS

Table 1 shows precision and recovery of the metabolites. The total time elapsing up to GC injection was 2 h. In comparison with the method presented, ether/ethylacetate extraction showed very variable recoveries of 3-hydroxypropionate (10–27%) and 3-hydroxyisovalerate (13–22%) and consistently low recoveries of citrate (17%) and methylcitrate (52%). The contribution of direct injection of standards into the GC on the coefficient of variation (CV) was 3%. The method is linear from at least 0.1 mmol/l to 30 mmol/l as assessed with the four metabolites just mentioned.

DISCUSSION

The method is rapid enough to allow prompt and specific treatment in children with acute symptoms. Its

Table 1 Recovery and precision (seven replicates)

Metabolite	Addition (µmol)	Recovery (%)	CV (%)
3-Hydroxypropionate	3.15	96	14
3-Hydroxyisovalerate	1.33	84	18
Methylmalonate	1.15	96	3.2
Ethylmalonate	1.06	93	9.3
Glutarate	0.98	97	2.7
o-Hydroxyphenylacetate	0.96	94	2.3
p-Hydroxyphenylacetate	0.82	94	3.3
Propionylglycine	1.04	116	5.6
Isovalerylglycine	1.76	84	3.9
Citrate	1.89	95	4.2
Methylcitrate	0.77	101	6.7

precision is sufficient to follow up the biochemical parameters quantitatively, even if low concentrations are to be quantitated (e.g. biotinidase deficiency: 3-hydroxyisovalerate at 0.1 mmol/l). An alkaline pH is essential during evaporation of the extract in order to prevent losses, e.g. of 3-hydroxypropionate or 3-hydroxyisovalerate. Pyridine should be avoided during derivatization to obtain reliable results with methylmalonate. The present method has proven its effectiveness during the last 5 years, allowing us to detect patients with the following acidurias: 2-methyl-3-hydroxybutyric (1 patient), propionic (12), methylmalonic (8), isovaleric (1), 3-hydroxy-3-methylglutaric (1), glutaric type II (1), pyroglutamic (1) and late-onset multiple carboxylase deficiencies (3). These patients were detected during the work-up of hyperammonaemia. In addition we found two tyrosinaemias with succinylacetone excretion and a glyceroluric family.

References

Bachmann, C., Colombo, J. P. and Berueter, J. Short chain fatty acids in plasma and brain: quantitative determination by GC. *Clin. Chim. Acta* 92 (1979) 153–159

Goodman, S. I. and Markey, S. P. *Diagnosis of Organic Acidemias by Gas Chromatography–Mass Spectrometry.* Alan R. Liss, New York, 1981

Sweetman, L. Liquid partition chromatography and GC/MS in identification of acid metabolites of aminoacids. In Nyhan, W. L. (ed.) *Heritable Disorders of Aminoacid Metabolism*, New York, 1974, pp. 730–751

Journal of Inherited Metabolic Disease. ISSN 0141-8955. Copyright © SSIEM and MTP Press Limited, Queen Square, Lancaster, UK.

J. Inher. Metab. Dis. 7 Suppl. 2 (1984) 127–128

Short Communication

Experience with Prenatal Diagnosis of Propionic Acidaemia and Methylmalonic Aciduria

A. H. FENSOM and P. F. BENSON
Paediatric Research Unit, Guy's Hospital Medical School, London, SE1 9RT, UK

R. A. CHALMERS, B. M. TRACEY and D. WATSON
Paediatric Research Group and Mass Spectrometry Section, MRC Clinical Research Centre, Harrow, HA1 3UJ, UK

G. S. KING and B. R. PETTIT
Department of Chemical Pathology, Bernhard Baron Memorial Research Laboratories, Queen Charlotte's Maternity Hospital, London, W6 0XG, UK

C. H. RODECK
Department of Obstetrics and Gynaecology, King's College Hospital, London, SE5, UK

The prenatal diagnosis of disorders of organic acid metabolism by enzymology on cultured amniotic cells obtained by amniocentesis at 15–18 weeks' gestation has been applied to an increasing number of these disorders during the past 10 years, including propionic acidaemia and methylmalonic aciduria (see e.g. Chalmers and Lawson, 1982; Sweetman *et al.*, 1982). The prenatal diagnosis of the latter two metabolically-related disorders is now carried out routinely by measurement of incorporation of label from [1-^{14}C]propionate into cell protein in cultured cells or, more rarely, by direct measurement of activity of propionyl-CoA carboxylase (EC 6.4.1.3) or methylmalonyl-CoA metabolism. Methods involving cell culture are time-consuming because of the requirement for sufficient cells for assay and potentially unreliable because of the possibility of failed cultures and the rare occurrence of overgrowth by maternal fibroblasts (Buchanan *et al.*, 1980). The direct chemical analysis of cell-free amniotic fluid for metabolites excreted by the fetus offers the considerable advantages of rapid and early diagnoses and repeatable and reliable assays (see, e.g. Chalmers and Lawson, 1982). Propionic acidaemia and methylmalonic aciduria can be diagnosed in this way by measurement of methylcitrate or of methylmalonate and methylcitrate respectively. We report here our experience of monitoring 12 pregnancies at risk for these diseases using a combination of enzymology and direct chemical methods. Ambiguous results in one pregnancy at risk for propionic acidaemia necessitated enzymology of fetal leucocytes to resolve the diagnosis.

PATIENTS AND METHODS

The index case in all of the 10 families under study had previously been diagnosed by the characteristic organic aciduria and confirmed wherever possible by enzymology on cultured skin fibroblasts. Amniocentesis was carried out in all cases at between 15 and 17 weeks' gestation.

Amniotic cell and fibroblast cultures were initiated by standard techniques and grown in Dulbecco's MEM supplemented with 20% fetal calf serum for enzyme studies. Measurement of incorporation of label from [1-^{14}C]propionate into cell protein was used as the general method in laboratories A and C, with direct measurement of propionyl-CoA carboxylase in cell extracts by measurement of propionyl-CoA-dependent fixation of NaH^{14}CO$_3$ in laboratory C where necessary. Organic acid extracts were prepared from cell-free fluid supernatant and analysed using either capillary gas–liquid chromatography and GC–MS (laboratory A) or by isothermal GC–MS on packed columns (laboratory B). Both laboratories used selected ion monitoring (SIM) for quantification and operated independently with results being compared only at the conclusion of the analyses.

RESULTS

Results obtained for five pregnancies at risk for propionic acidaemia and four pregnancies at risk for methylmalonic aciduria were all within the normal ranges for amniotic fluid metabolite concentrations and amniotic cell enzyme activities. In all cases, continuation of the pregnancies resulted in unaffected babies with no clinical or biochemical evidence for the disorders concerned.

In one pregnancy at risk for propionic acidaemia and in one at risk for methylmalonic aciduria, amniotic fluid methylcitrate concentrations and methylcitrate with methylmalonate concentrations respectively were greatly increased above the normal values for both laboratories (Table 1), consistent with the diagnosis of an affected fetus. The diagnosis was confirmed by enzymology on cultured amniotic cells (Table 1) and the pregnancies were terminated in both cases. No follow-up was possible on one fetus, but cultured fetal fibroblasts from the second case showed a rate of incorporation of label from [1-^{14}C]propionate into cell protein of 82

Journal of Inherited Metabolic Disease. ISSN 0141–8955. Copyright © SSIEM and MTP Press Limited, Queen Square, Lancaster, UK.

Table 1   Results of prenatal diagnosis for methylmalonic aciduria and propionic acidaemia[1]

	Gestation (weeks)	Amniotic fluid metabolites (µmol/l)				Enzyme activities in cultured cells	
		Methylcitrate		Methylmalonate		$[1-^{14}C]propionate$ incorporation into protein (patom (mg protein)$^{-1}$h^{-1})	Propionyl CoA carboxylase (nmol (mg protein)$^{-1}$h^{-1})
		Lab.A[2]	Lab.B	Lab.A	Lab.B		
Patient							
Cra.[3]	16	3.9,3.6	6.8	—	—	22	0.41
Cla.[4]	16	2.4	4.6	31.8	42.0	18	—
Sab.[3] (a)	15	2.4	2.6	—	—	302	5.52
(b)	22	0.6	1.3	—	—	267	5.63
Normal values	15–20	<0.5	<1.0	<0.5	<0.8	341 134–963 (n = 25)	24.1 12.1–45.5 (n = 8)

[1] Results on five pregnancies at risk for propionic acidaemia and for four pregnancies at risk for methylmalonic aciduria were all within the normal values shown. Results for three other pregnancies are given separately
[2] Sum of the 2S,3S and 2S,3R isomers of methylcitrate observed
[3] At risk for propionic acidaemia
[4] At risk for methylmalonic aciduria

patom (mg protein)$^{-1}$h^{-1} compared to a simultaneous control of 875.

A further pregnancy at risk for propionic acidaemia showed results on amniocentesis at 15 weeks' gestation that were ambiguous: methylcitrate concentrations were above normal (Table 1) but not of the values expected for pregnancies with an affected fetus. Enzymology on cultured cells showed intermediate activities (Table 1) consistent with a heterozygous fetus. In order to clarify the diagnosis and after full parental consultation 2 ml of fetal blood was obtained at 22 weeks' gestation for direct assay of fetal leucocyte propionyl-CoA carboxylase activity: an activity of 113 pmol (mg protein)$^{-1}$h^{-1} was observed compared to fetal controls of 220 and 317, again consistent with a heterozygous fetus. Amniotic fluid obtained at the same time showed a much reduced methylcitrate concentration and similar enzyme activities of cultured cells to those obtained previously (Table 1). The pregnancy was allowed to continue and the mother was delivered of a normal healthy female baby.

CONCLUSIONS

Our experience with prenatal diagnosis of propionic acidaemia and methylmalonic aciduria by direct chemical analysis of amniotic fluid is similar to that of Sweetman and his colleagues (Naylor *et al.*, 1980; Sweetman *et al.*, 1982). However, the results obtained in the pregnancy at risk for propionic acidaemia with a probably heterozygous fetus indicate the caution required in the interpretation of methylcitrate concentrations and the need to establish amniotic cells in culture for supportive enzymology if required in cases of doubt. Assay of fetal leucocyte propionyl-CoA carboxylase activity may be used to resolve the most difficult cases. In general, however, the use of direct chemical analysis for prenatal diagnosis of these conditions, particularly methylmalonic aciduria, appears reliable and may be used as the primary diagnostic method.

These prenatal diagnoses were all carried out for the clinical care of the families at risk for the diseases concerned: we are grateful to the many physicians, clinical geneticists, cytogeneticists and biochemists who have been responsible for the co-ordination and referral of these cases to us. R.A.C. is indebted to Dr S. Brandänge, Arrhenius Laboratory, University of Stockholm, Sweden, for the gifts of the 2S,3S and 2S,3R isomers of methylcitric acid for use as standards.

References

Buchanan, P. D., Kahler, S. G., Sweetman, L. and Nyhan, W. L. Pitfalls in the prenatal diagnosis of propionic acidaemia. *Clin. Genet.* 18 (1980) 177–183

Chalmers, R. A. and Lawson, A. M. *Organic Acids in Man. Analytical Chemistry, Biochemistry and Diagnosis of the Organic Acidurias.* Chapman & Hall, London, 1982, pp. 221–229

Naylor, G., Sweetman, L., Nyhan, W. L., Hornbeck, C., Griffiths, J., Mörch, L. and Brandänge, S. Isotope dilution analysis of methylcitric acid in amniotic fluid for the prenatal diagnosis of propionic and methylmalonic acidaemia. *Clin. Chim. Acta* 107 (1980) 175–183

Sweetman, L., Naylor, G., Ladner, T., Holm, J., Nyhan, W. L., Hornbeck, C., Griffiths, J., Mörch, L., Brandänge, S., Gruenke, L. and Craig, J. C. Prenatal diagnosis of propionic and methylmalonic acidaemia by stable isotope dilution analysis of methylcitric and methylmalonic acids in amniotic fluid. In Schmidt, H.-L., Förstel, H. and Heinzinger, K. (eds.) *Stable Isotopes*, Elsevier, Amsterdam, 1982, pp. 287–293

J. Inher. Metab. Dis. 7 Suppl. 2 (1984) 129–130

Short Communication

Methylmalonic Aciduria with Homocystinuria

A. RIBES, M. A. VILASECA, P. BRIONES, A. MAYA and J. SABATER
Instituto de Bioquímica Clínica, Apartado 145, Cerdanyola (Barcelona), Spain

P. PASCUAL, L. ALVAREZ, J. ROS and E. GONZALEZ PASCUAL
Hospital de San Juan de Dios, Barcelona, Spain

Methylmalonic aciduria with homocystinuria (McKusick 27740) is a disorder of the cytosolic metabolism of cobalamin (Levy *et al.*, 1970) which involves an impaired synthesis of the two cobalamin forms 5′-deoxyadenosyl-cobalamin (AdoCbl) and methyl-cobalamin (MeCbl), which act as coenzymes in the two cobalamin-dependent reactions demonstrated conclusively in mammalian systems. AdoCbl is a cofactor in the intramitochondrial isomerization of methylmalonyl-CoA to succinyl-CoA, by methyl-malonyl-CoA mutase (EC 5.4.99.2). Methyl-Cbl is a cofactor in the remethylation of homocysteine to methionine, which is a cytosolic reaction catalysed by *N*-methyltetrahydrofolate-homocysteine-methyl transferase (EC 2.1.1.13). The defect, not precisely identified, may affect one or more of the first reduction steps of OHCbl, subsequent to its cellular uptake and common to the synthesis of both coenzymes. This Cbl disorder implies some biochemical abnormalities: methylmalonic aciduria with homocystinuria, cystathioninuria and hypomethioninaemia, with normal values of serum cobalamin. The ten affected patients known at present (Baumgartner *et al.*, 1979a; Levy *et al.*, 1970; Dillon *et al.*, 1974; Goodman *et al.*, 1970) have been classified by Rosenberg (Willard *et al.*, 1978) into two genetic complementation groups Cbl C and Cbl D, the patients of Cbl C group being more severely affected clinically and biochemically. We describe a possible new case of the Cbl C type and present the clinical and biochemical evolution in parallel with the treatment and protein intake.

CASE REPORT

H. M., a male infant born at term after an uncomplicated pregnancy, was the second child born alive (after one abortion) from young, healthy and unrelated parents. Delivery was normal. Neonatal antecedents were: Apgar score: 9/10; length: 49 cm; head circumference: 35 cm; weight: 3100 g. The patient suffered physiological jaundice throughout five days. The child was admitted to hospital at the age of 6 weeks owing to feeding difficulties with sporadic vomiting, failure to thrive, drowsiness and developmental retardation.

The patient presented moderate metabolic acidosis (pH: 7.24; pCO_2: 27; anion gap: 21), hyper-ammonaemia: 194 µg% (normal 50–70), hypochromic anaemia (Hb 9.8 g%) and tubulopathy (Ca excretion 20 mg kg^{-1} day^{-1} but normal ionogram), glycaemia and T_4. Amino acid analysis revealed homocystinuria

(132 µmol/24 h), hypomethioninaemia (0.01 µmol/ml), and cystathioninuria (26.4 µmol/24 h). Methylmalonic aciduria was suspected and confirmed by GC–MS with levels as high as 1375 µmol/24 h. Lactate, 3-hydroxybutyrate, 3-hydroxypropionate, 3-hydroxyisovalerate and 3-hydroxy-*n*-valerate were also excreted in large amounts. Total serum cobalamins were normal at 707 pg/ml (normal 200–1000) but serum folate was slightly high at 35.7 µg/ml (normal 3–16).

METHODS

Amino acids were quantified by ion-exchange chromatography with a Rank Hilger Chromaspek autoanalyser. Organic acids were analysed as TMS-derivatives on 10% OV-101 on 80–100 mesh GasChrom Q in a 2 m × 3 mm column. The temperature was programmed from 80°C to 280°C at 4°C/min with a Hewlett-Packard GC–MS model 5992. Serum total cobalamins were determined by a radioisotopic method.

RESULTS

Intravenous administration of 1 mg OH-Cbl daily resulted in a dramatic clinical response and a marked decrease in urinary methylmalonate (97.0%), homocystine (96.9%), and cystathionine (97.4%), paralleled by a reduction of blood ammonia (78.3%), after 7 days of treatment. However, serum methionine was observed only in trace amounts. From 2 to 6 months of age the patient gained weight regularly, in spite of some sporadic episodes of vomiting and diarrhoea accompanied by an increased excretion of methylmalonic acid and homocystine. Owing to these fluctuations and a stationary body weight at about the age of 6 months, the dose of OH-Cbl was doubled but the excretion of methylmalonic acid and homocystine did not decrease significantly. Therefore, 600 mg of vitamin B6 and 6 mg of folic acid daily were added to the treatment in order to stimulate the trans-sulphuration pathway (Baumgartner *et al.*, 1979b). After 10 days folic acid was omitted without apparent biochemical changes. Treatment with 600 mg B6 and 2 mg OH-Cbl was continued, which achieved a marked decrease in the methylmalonic acid and homocystine levels. Nevertheless, hypomethioninaemia was a constant finding. This therapy also led to an obvious improvement in the patient's clinical state which allowed normal oral feeding and treatment which continues at present without problems. Now the child is 9 months old and is normal on physical examination

Journal of Inherited Metabolic Disease. ISSN 0141-8955. Copyright © SSIEM and MTP Press Limited, Queen Square, Lancaster, UK.

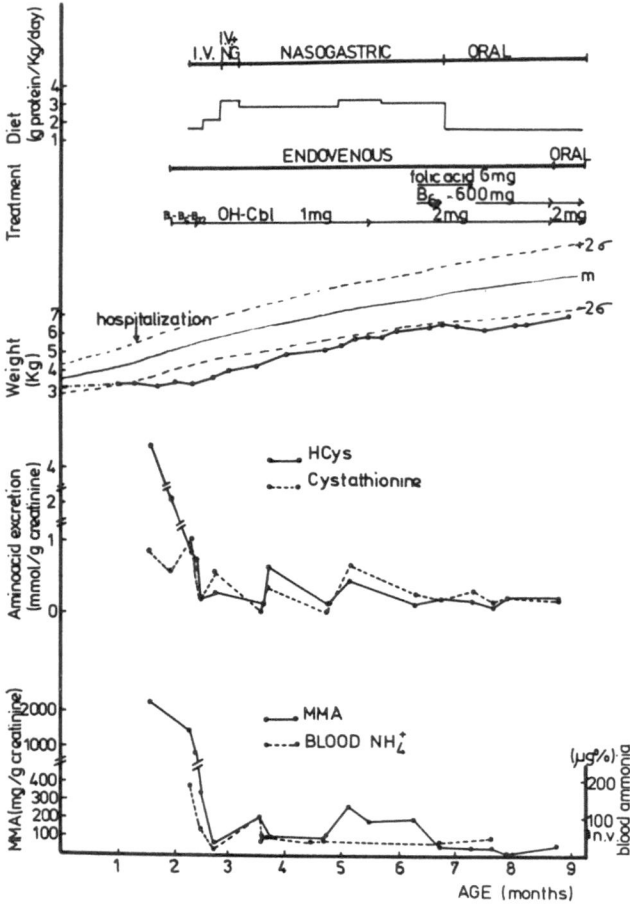

Figure 1 Changes in the levels of methylmalonic acid, ammonia, homocystine, cystathionine and body weight related to the treatment and diet

except for slight microcephaly (42.5 cm head circumference) and nystagmus. He presents psychomotor retardation.

DISCUSSION

Owing to the severe clinical and biochemical features and neonatal onset we suggest that this is a new case of methylmalonic aciduria due to a derangement in the first steps of B12 metabolism which might be included in the Cbl C group (Willard *et al.*, 1978). Further biochemical studies are in progress to confirm this hypothesis. The response to B12 therapy in this case is evident, but although B6 helped to improve the patient's evolution, additional treatment will have to be included to correct the hypomethioninaemia and, if possible, to further reduce methylmalonic and homocystine levels.

References

Baumgartner, E. R., Wick, H., Maurer, R., Egli, N. and Steinmann, B. Congenital defect in intracellular cobalamin metabolism resulting in homocystinuria and methylmalonic aciduria. I. Case report and histopathology. *Helv. Paediatr. Acta* 34 (1979a) 465–482

Baumgartner, E. R., Wick, H., Linnell, J. C., Gaull, G. E., Bachmann, C. and Steinmann, B. Congenital defect in intracellular cobalamin metabolism resulting in homocystinuria and methylmalonic aciduria. II. Biochemical investigations. *Helv. Paediatr. Acta* 34 (1979b) 483–496

Dillon, M. I., England, J. M., Gompertz, D., Goodey, P. A., Grant, D. B., Hussein, H. A. A., Linnell, J. C., Matthews, D. M., Mudd, S. H., Newns, G. H., Seakins, J. T. W., Uhlendorf, B. V. and Wise, I. J. Mental retardation, megaloblastic anaemia, methylmalonic aciduria and abnormal homocystine metabolism due to an error in vitamin B12 metabolism. *Clin. Sci. Mol. Med.* 47 (1974) 43–61

Goodman, S. I., Mol, P. G., Hammond, K. B., Mudd, S. H. and Uhlendorf, B. W. Homocystinuria with methylmalonic aciduria: Two cases in a sibship. *Biochem. Med.* 4 (1970) 500–515

Levy, H. L., Mudd, S. H., Schulman, J. D., Dreyfus, P. M. and Abeles, R. H. A derangement in B12 metabolism associated with homocystinemia, cystathioninemia, hypomethioninemia and methylmalonic aciduria. *Am. J. Med.* 48 (1970) 390–397

Willard, H. F., Mellman, I. S. and Rosenberg, L. E. Genetic complementation among inherited deficiencies of methylmalonyl-CoA mutase activity: Evidence for a new class of human cobalamin mutant. *Am. J. Hum. Genet.* 30 (1978) 1–13

J. Inher. Metab. Dis. 7 Suppl. 2 (1984) 131–132

Short Communication

Two Cases of β-Ketothiolase Deficiency: A Comparison

B. MIDDLETON
Department of Biochemistry, University Medical School, Queen's Medical Centre, Nottingham NG7 2UH, UK

R. G. F. GRAY
Sub-Department of Medical Genetics, University of Sheffield, Sheffield S10 5DN, UK

M. J. BENNETT
Department of Chemical Pathology, Sheffield Children's Hospital, Sheffield S10 2TH, UK

At least three isoenzymes of β-ketothiolase exist in human fibroblasts: (1) a mitochondrial 'branched chain' β-ketothiolase (MBK) (EC 2.3.1.9) which can thiolyse 2-methylacetoacetyl CoA and acetoacetyl CoA, (2) a mitochondrial 'straight chain' β-ketothiolase (MSK) (EC 2.3.1.16) which can thiolyse long and medium straight-chain 3-ketoacyl CoAs and, to a lesser extent, acetoacetyl CoA and (3) a cytosolic β-ketothiolase (CK) (EC 2.3.1.9) specific for acetoacetyl CoA.

Inherited defects of CK (De Groot *et al.*, 1977) and MBK (McKusick 20375) (Schutgens *et al.*, 1982) have been described associated with differing clinical and biochemical phenotypes. We report a comparison of metabolic and enzymological investigations in one case each of these disorders.

METHODS AND PATIENTS

Fibroblasts were cultured under standard conditions and screened for mycoplasmas. Cell homogenates were assayed for β-ketothiolases (using various substrates as in Middleton and Bartlett, 1983) and succinyl-CoA:3-ketoacyl-CoA transferase (Williamson *et al.*, 1971). Fatty acid and sterol synthesis rates were measured by incubation of confluent monolayers of fibroblasts for 17–24 h at 37 °C in Eagle's minimum essential medium containing [1-^{14}C]acetate (3 mmol/l at 0.221 Ci/mol) with or without 10 % fetal calf serum. Cells were digested in 2 mol/l NaOH and saponified at 80° for 1 h. Sterols were extracted into petroleum ether and isolated by thin layer chromatography. Fatty acids were similarly extracted after acidification of the saponification medium. All rates were expressed per mg cell protein which was measured by the method of Sedmak and Grassberg (1977).

J.C. is a male child who presented with progressive mental retardation and hypotonia. He was placed on a low fat diet, but has not significantly improved. A.K. is a female child who presented with pyrexia, vomiting and dehydration. Her diet was exceptionally high in protein and she is now doing well on a normal protein intake.

RESULTS AND DISCUSSION

Organic acid analysis of urine from J.C. and A.K. by gas chromatography–mass spectrometry revealed an excess of 3-hydroxybutyrate and acetoacetate. In A.K. this ketonuria was intermittent whilst in J.C. it was persistent (until treatment was started) and increased postprandially. A.K. (but not J.C.) also excreted in urine increased amounts of 2-methylacetoacetic and 2-methyl-3-hydroxybutyric acids, especially after a high protein meal.

In fibroblasts of J.C. and A.K. succinyl-CoA:3-ketoacid transferase activity of 8.2 and 11.9 nmol (mg protein)$^{-1}$ min^{-1} respectively was within the control range (14.0 ± 7.3 nmol (mg protein)$^{-1}$ min^{-1} ($n = 3$)) indicating normal ketone body activation. β-Ketothiolase measured with 3-ketohexanoyl CoA (Table 1) indicated normal MSK activity. However, in both patients β-ketothiolase activity with acetoacetyl CoA was reduced to approximately half normal levels (Table 1). Cells from A.K. showed no detectable activity towards 2-methylacetoacetyl CoA and no stimulation by K$^+$ (Table 1) indicting a gross deficiency of MBK activity. J.C., however, showed normal activities in these assays suggesting, by inference, that his cells were deficient in CK activity. The residual activity towards acetoacetyl CoA in cells from J.C. can be accounted for solely by the presence of MSK and MBK isoenzymes, suggesting that the deficiency of CK activity is pronounced.

Since β-ketothiolase catalyses the first committed step of *de novo* cholesterol synthesis (2-acetyl-CoA → acetoacetyl-CoA in cytosol) this process was assayed in J.C. fibroblasts. When assayed in the presence of serum-borne cholesterol his cells showed 36 % (29 pmol (mg protein)$^{-1}$ h^{-1}) of the normal rate of 81 ± 26 pmol (mg protein)$^{-1}$ h^{-1} ($n = 5$). After derepression for 24 h in serum-free medium the normal cells showed a 4.3-fold increase in sterol synthesis; a similar rate increase was found in J.C.'s cells but the sterol synthesis was still only 20 % of the normal rate (Table 1).

Journal of Inherited Metabolic Disease. ISSN 0141-8955. Copyright © SSIEM and MTP Press Limited, Queen Square, Lancaster, UK.

Table 1 β-Ketothiolase activities and rates of sterol and fatty acid synthesis in fibroblasts

	β-Ketothiolase activity with different substrates nmol 3-ketoacyl-CoA removed (mg protein)$^{-1}$ min^{-1}			Sterol synthesis rate	Fatty acid synthesis rate	Ratio of synthesis rates
				pmol *acetate incorp.* (mg protein)$^{-1}$ h^{-1}		$\dfrac{Sterol}{fatty\ acid}$
	C_4*	C_5*	C_6*			
Patient J. C.	25.7 (3.9)†	54.1	51.5	147	1086	0.14
Patient A.K.	24.8 (1.0)	0.6	46.6	729	1637	0.45
Normals (5)	50.1 (3.0)	55.3	59.9	346	1026	0.34
± SD	± 6.9 (±0.6)	±13.8	±16.3	±97	±106	±0.12

* C_4, C_5, C_6 = acetoacetyl, 2-methylacetoacetyl and 3-ketohexanoyl CoA respectively
† In parentheses: stimulation (-fold) by K^+ with C_4 substrate

Fatty acid synthesis was normal in J.C.'s cells whilst cells from A.K. showed enhanced fatty acid and sterol synthesis. This latter result may reflect a cell response to restricted supply of acetyl CoA due to the MBK deficiency.

The defect in cholesterol synthesis in J.C.'s cells may produce the severe neurological symptoms associated with this disorder by impairing myelination, altering membrane function and reducing steroid hormone levels – particularly under conditions of high sterol requirement as in the neonate. Furthermore, it could lead to deficiencies in essential isoprene-derived substances such as dolichols. In future cases of CK deficiency it will be important to investigate levels of sterol metabolites and, if abnormalities are found, to consider whether supplementation is required.

References

De Groot, C. J., Luit-de Haan, G., Mulstaert, C. E. and Hommes, F. A. A patient with severe neurological symptoms and acetoacetyl-CoA thiolase deficiency. *Pediatr. Res.* 11 (1977) 1112–1116

Middleton, B. and Bartlett, K. The synthesis and characterization of 2-methylacetoacetyl-CoA and its use in the identification of the site of the defect in 2-methylacetoacetic and 2-methyl-3-hydroxybutyric aciduria. *Clin. Chim. Acta* 128 (1983) 291–305

Schutgens, R. B. H., Middleton, B., v.d. Blij, J. F., Oorthuys, J. W. E., Veder, H. A., Vulsma, T. and Tegelaers, W. H. H. β-Ketothiolase deficiency in a family confirmed by *in vitro* enzymatic assays in fibroblasts. *Eur. J. Pediatr.* 139 (1982) 39–42

Sedmak, J. J. and Grassberg, S. E. A rapid, sensitive and versatile assay for protein using Coomassie Brilliant Blue G-250. *Anal. Biochem.* 79 (1977) 544–552

Williamson, D. H., Bates, M. W., Page, M. A. and Krebs, H. A. Activities of enzymes involved in acetoacetate metabolism in adult mammalian tissues. *Biochem. J.* 121 (1971) 41–47

J. Inher. Metab. Dis. 7 Suppl. 2 (1984) 133–134

Short Communication

L-Glyceric Aciduria (Primary Hyperoxaluria Type 2) in Siblings in Two Unrelated Families

R. A. Chalmers, B. M. Tracey and J. Mistry
Paediatric Research Group, MRC Clinical Research Centre, Watford Road, Harrow, HA1 3UJ, UK

K. D. Griffiths and A. Green
Department of Clinical Chemistry, The Children's Hospital, Ladywood Middleway, Birmingham, B16 8ET, UK

M. H. Winterborn
Department of Paediatrics, The Children's Hospital, Ladywood Middleway, Birmingham, B16 8ET, UK

L-Glyceric aciduria (primary hyperoxaluria type 2; McKusick 26000) was originally reported in four patients, three of whom were siblings, by Williams and Smith (1968), the disease being characterized by oxalate renal calculi with haematuria (Williams and Smith, 1968; Dent and Stamp, 1970). The disorder is distinguished from primary hyperoxaluria 'type 1' (glycollic aciduria) by the greatly increased excretion of L-glycerate into the urine in addition to raised oxalate excretion, with normal glycollate excretion (Chalmers and Lawson, 1982). It occurs because of deficient activity of D-glycerate dehydrogenase (EC 1.1.1.29) (Williams and Smith, 1968). Since the original report no further cases have occurred in the literature suggesting, by comparison with the more than 150 cases of the type 1 form (glycollic aciduria), that this form of primary hyperoxaluria is very rare. We present here a report of four previously-unidentified cases in two unrelated families, suggesting that the type 2 disorder may be more common and indicating the need for careful classification of patients with hyperoxaluria.

METHODS

Organic acids were determined in urine and ultrafiltered blood plasma using anion exchange extraction on to DEAE Sephadex and gas–liquid chromatography on fused silica capillary columns by established methods (Chalmers and Lawson, 1982; Tracey *et al.*, 1983). Identifications of acids were confirmed using capillary GC–MS. Oxalic acid concentrations in urine were also determined using an established enzymatic spectrophotometric assay based on oxalate decarboxylase and formate dehydrogenase (Chalmers, 1980). D-(R)- and L-(S)-glycoric acids were separated and characterized using capillary gas–liquid chromatography of their O-acetyl-L-menthyl esters essentially using the method of Kamerling *et al.* (1977). The activity of D-glycerate dehydrogenase (hydroxypyruvate:NAD oxidoreductase) was determined in leucocyte preparations using D-glycerate as substrate in the presence of hydrazine sulphate and monitoring the formation of NADH spectrophotofluorometrically.

PATIENTS AND RESULTS

In family 1 (Mag.), the propositus (G.Mag.) presented originally at 7 years of age with renal calculi, was diagnosed as having oxalate stones and hyperoxaluria and treated with magnesium hydroxide and high fluid intake. His urine was examined in the present study for organic acids at the age of 10 years and showed greatly increased amounts of glyceric acid in the presence of increased oxalate and normal glycollate concentrations (Table 1). The glycerate was shown to have the L-configuration and a diagnosis of L-glyceric aciduria (type 2 primary hyperoxaluria) was made. Study of the family showed that his elder brother (W.A.Mag.) also had L-glyceric aciduria and hyperoxaluria (Table 1). Both siblings showed increased concentrations of glycerate in blood plasma. Their parents and three other siblings showed normal urinary and plasma organic acids. The pedigree of the family was consistent with an autosomal recessive mode of inheritance. D-Glycerate dehydrogenase activity in the propositus was 10 nmol glycerate oxidized per mg protein per h compared to activities of 21 and 24 in his parents and 41 ± 9 in normal control subjects. Further studies are in progress on the enzyme activities in other family members and those of family 2 described below.

In family 2 (Mar.), the propositus (N.Mar.) had originally presented with oxalate stones in his left kidney at 2 years of age, these being removed surgically. He required further surgery at 8 years to remove stones from his right kidney and at 11 years required a right nephrectomy. Primary hyperoxaluria had been diagnosed and he was treated with magnesium hydroxide. His renal function was reduced (GFR 59 ml min^{-1} 1.73 m^{-2}). Examination of his urine for organic acids in the present study when he was 20 years of age, showed he excreted increased amounts of L-glyceric acid (Table 1) and he was diagnosed as having type 2 primary

Journal of Inherited Metabolic Disease. ISSN 0141–8955. Copyright © SSIEM and MTP Press Limited, Queen Square, Lancaster, UK.

Table 1 Urinary and plasma organic acids in four previously-unidentified patients with primary hyperoxaluria type 2

Patient	Urine						Plasma		
	mmol/mol creatinine			mmol/24 h			μmol/l		
	Oxalic	L-Glyceric[1]	Glycollic	Oxalic	L-Glyceric	Glycollic	Oxalic	Glyceric	Glycollic
G.Mag.	58.4	1345	57.6	0.811	10.8	0.46	4.4	101	10.5
W.A.Mag.	44.0	286	12.4	1.114	2.82	0.09	23.3	133	26.3
N.Mar.	135.6	1130	37.3	1.522	13.6	0.45	21.1	226	23.7
R.Mar.	56.5	418	41.8	1.100	7.05	0.68	11.1	264	7.9
Control data (within family) Mag.	15.1– 85.4	ND[3]– 9.6[2]	25.3– 163.6	0.222– 0.333	ND– 0.12[2]	0.47– 0.67	3.3– 23.3	5.7– 15.1[2]	6.6– 32.9
Mar.	13.8– 25.1	ND– 3.2[2]	26.8– 72.9	0.177– 0.288	ND– 0.04[2]	0.26– 0.79	13.3– 18.9	8.5– 16.0[2]	11.8– 28.9

[1] Demonstrated as L-glyceric acid using capillary gas–liquid chromatography of the O-acetyl-L-menthyl esters
[2] Probably D-glycerate in controls
[3] ND = not detected

hyperoxaluria. An elder brother (R.Mar.) had a history of calcium stones having been removed at 19 years of age and examination of his urine also revealed L-glyceric aciduria and hyperoxaluria (Table 1). Both brothers showed increased amounts of glycerate in blood plasma. Their parents and three siblings showed normal urinary and plasma organic acids with their pedigree being consistent with an autosomal recessive mode of inheritance.

CONCLUSIONS

Two of the four patients identified in this study as having L-glyceric aciduria and hyperoxaluria had a well-known history of renal calculi with hyperoxaluria and their two affected siblings also had a history of renal calculi and associated clinical problems. Although only four previous cases are recorded in the literature in one report (Williams and Smith, 1968; Dent and Stamp, 1970), the present findings suggest that the type 2 form of hyperoxaluria may be more common than previously believed. Patients with primary hyperoxaluria need to be carefully classified by examination of urine and plasma organic acids because of the potentially different prognosis and treatment of the two major forms of this disorder. Family studies may reveal other cases and a full study of this kind is necessary in order to produce the optimum clinical care to the families concerned.

References

Chalmers, R. A. The enzymatic spectrophotometric determination of oxalate in blood and urine, In Rose, G. A., Robertson, W. G. and Watts, R. W. E. (eds.) *Oxalate in Human Biochemistry and Clinical Pathology*. The Wellcome Foundation, London, 1980, pp. 61–66

Chalmers, R. A. and Lawson, A. M. *Organic Acids in Man. Analytical Chemistry, Biochemistry and Diagnosis of the Organic Acidurias*. Chapman & Hall, London, 1982, pp. 20–23; 409–414

Dent, C. E. and Stamp, T. C. B. Treatment of primary hyperoxaluria. *Arch. Dis. Child.* 45 (1970) 735–745

Kamerling, J. P., Gerwig, G. J., Vliegenthart, J. F. G., Duran, M., Ketting, D. and Wadman, S. K. Determination of the configurations of lactic and glyceric acids from human serum and urine by capillary gas–liquid chromatography. *J. Chromatogr.* 143 (1977) 117–123

Tracey, B. M., Stacey, T. E. and Chalmers, R. A. Urinary and plasma organic acids in dizygotic twin siblings with 3-hydroxy-3-methylglutaric aciduria, studied by gas chromatography and mass spectrometry using fused silica capillary columns. *J. Inher. Metab. Dis.* 6 Suppl. 2 (1983) 125–126

Williams, H. E. and Smith, L. H. L-Glyceric aciduria. A new genetic variant of primary hyperoxaluria. *N. Engl. J. Med.* 278 (1968) 233–239

J. Inher. Metab. Dis. 7 Suppl. 2 (1984) 135–136

Short Communication

The Antenatal Diagnosis and Aid to the Management of Hereditary Tyrosinaemia by Use of a Specific and Sensitive GC–MS Assay for Succinylacetone

B. R. Pettit, F. MacKenzie and G. S. King
Queen Charlotte's Maternity Hospital, Goldhawk Road, London W6 0XG, UK

J. V. Leonard
Institute of Child Health, Guilford Street, London WC1 1EH, UK

Succinylacetone (SA, 4,6-diketoheptanoic acid) is elevated both in the urine of patients with hereditary tyrosinaemia type 1 (McKusick 27670) (Berger *et al.*, 1981; Grenier *et al.*, 1982), and in the amniotic fluid of pregnancies with affected fetuses (Gangné *et al.*, 1982). This results from the abnormally low activity of fumarylacetoacetase (EC 3.7.1.2), probably the primary enzyme defect (Lindblad *et al.*, 1977). Existing methods for the analysis of SA were not sufficiently sensitive to establish normal amniotic fluid concentrations, nor sufficiently accurate or precise to enable rapid diagnosis and monitoring of SA excretion during treatment. Current methods using trimethylsilyl derivatives (Christensen *et al.*, 1981; Grenier *et al.*, 1982) are prone to 'carry over', a problem made worse by the wide range of concentrations analysed within one assay. This problem is caused by the silylating reagent, in which the sample is dissolved, passing through the syringe and over the injection region of the column, and reacting with partially derivatized material deposited there, thus causing the observation of erroneously elevated peak heights. We have therefore developed a new assay using combined gas chromatography–mass spectrometry (GC–MS) to make possible the measurement of SA in amniotic fluid and urine.

METHODS

The internal standard, 2 µg of glutarylacetone (5,7-diketo-octanoic acid), and 1 mg of hydroxylamine were added to urine (0.25 ml), and the mixture heated to form the isoxazole derivative (Christensen *et al.*, 1981). After acidification, the urine was absorbed onto dry silica gel, and the products extracted with ethyl acetate. The pentafluorobenzyl (PFB) ester was prepared using a mixture of PFB bromide, potassium hydroxide and triethylamine in ethanol. After removal of excess of reagent under a stream of dry nitrogen and partitioning between ethyl acetate and water, the upper organic layer was ready for analysis. The sample preparation for amniotic fluid was similar except that 0.5 ml was used together with 2 ng of glutarylacetone and 1 mg of hydroxylamine.

GC–MS was performed on a VG7070H mass spectrometer coupled to a VG2250 datasystem and fitted with a Hewlett Packard 5700 series GC. For urine analyses, a 2 m Silar 10C packed column was used at 260 °C. For amniotic fluid analyses, to gain extra

sensitivity, a 25 m WBOT BP1 bonded phase vitreous silica capillary column was used in conjunction with the Hewlett Packard on-column injector. The molecular ions of the SA and glutarylacetone derivatives were monitored. SA concentrations were extrapolated from a standard curve.

RESULTS AND DISCUSSION

With this method the SA concentration in amniotic fluid from unaffected pregnancies can be measured, and is less than 6 nmol/l. Amniotic fluid from pregnancies complicated by fetal hereditary tyrosinaemia type 1 have been reported to contain SA concentrations greater than 100 nmol/l (Gangné *et al.*, 1982). Using our method we have undertaken two antenatal diagnoses for pregnancies at risk for this disease, with the Québec group (Grenier *et al.*, 1982) performing their assay in parallel. One of these was for a subsequent pregnancy of the mother of one of the children under investigation (L.V.). Both laboratories found low levels of SA, and both mothers have subsequently delivered normal healthy children. The parents were aware that these assays were experimental.

Urine samples from 11 patients, in whom hereditary tyrosinaemia was suspected because of amino acid disturbances and severe liver disease, have been examined; four had concentrations above 5 mmol/mol creatinine and the remaining seven had less than 0.4 mmol/mol, a value consistent with those observed for children without amino acid disturbances and no liver disease (see Figure 1). We have been unable to demonstrate raised SA concentrations in any disorder other than hereditary tyrosinaemia. We have monitored the treatment of one child (L.V.), and examined the possibility of reducing the activity of their *p*-hydroxyphenylpyruvic acid oxidase (EC 1.13.11.27) by administration of precursors of specific inhibitors, such as *m*-tyrosine; the rationale being that a reduced flux would decrease the accumulation of toxic metabolites by lowering the substrate concentration for fumarylacetoacetase. However, no reduction has been observed, because the *m*-tyrosine is excreted mainly as *m*-hydroxyphenylacetic acid, with very little *m*-hydroxyphenyl-lactate. This is presumably due to the absence of amino-oxidation in the presence of active decarboxylation.

The measurement of SA in urine is of value in the

Journal of Inherited Metabolic Disease. ISSN 0141–8955. Copyright © SSIEM and MTP Press Limited, Queen Square, Lancaster, UK.

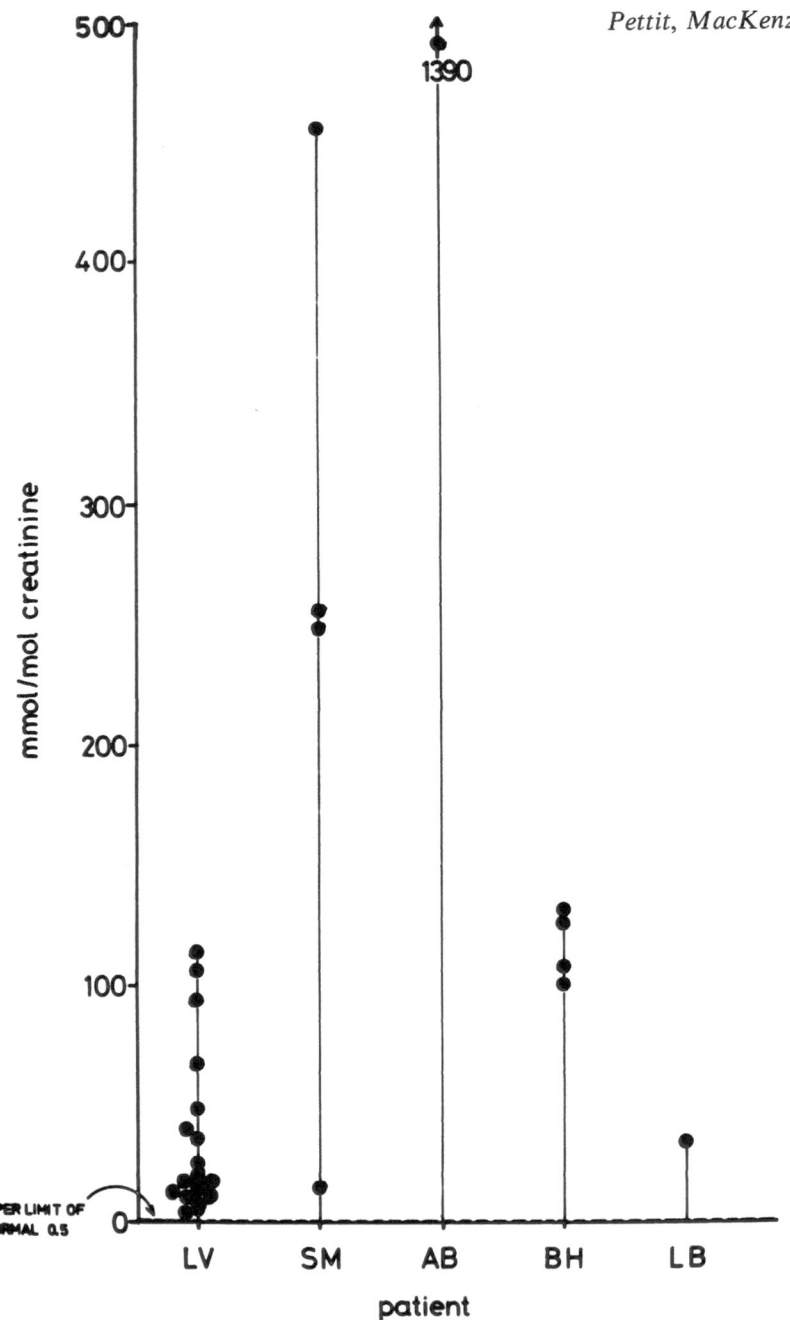

Figure 1   Urinary succinylacetone in five patients. Values in normal urine are less than 0.5 mmol/mol creatinine

differential diagnosis of tyrosinaemia. This would provide a sound basis on which to undertake an antenatal diagnosis of hereditary tyrosinaemia during a subsequent pregnancy.

References

Berger, R., Smit, G. P. A., Stoker-de Vries, S. A., Duran, M., Ketting, D. and Wadman, S. K. Deficiency of fumaryacetoacetase in a patient with hereditary tyrosinemia. *Clin. Chim. Acta* 114 (1981) 37–44

Christensen, E., Brock Jacobsen, B., Gregersen, N., Hjeds, H., Pedersen, J. B., Brandt, N. and Baeckmark, U. B. Urinary excretion of succinylacetone and delta-aminolevulinic acid in patients with hereditary tyrosinemia. *Clin. Chim. Acta* 116 (1981) 331–341

Gangné, R., Lescault, A., Grenier, A., Laberge, C., Mélançon, S. B. and Dallaire, L. Prenatal diagnosis of tyrosinaemia: Measurement of succinylacetone in amniotic fluid. *Prenat. Diag.* 2 (1982) 185–188

Grenier, A., Lescault, A., Laberge, C., Gangné, R. and Mamer, O. Detection of succinylacetone and the use of its measurement in mass screening for hereditary tyrosinemia. *Clin. Chim. Acta* 123 (1982) 93–99

Lindblad, B., Lindstedt, S. and Steen, G. On the enzymic defect in hereditary tyrosinemia. *Proc. Natl. Acad. Sci. USA* 74 (1977) 4641–4645

J. Inher. Metab. Dis. 7 Suppl. 2 (1984) 137–138

Short Communication

The Enzyme Defects in Hereditary Tyrosinaemia Type I

N. Furukawa, T. Hayano, N. Sato, F. Inoue, Y. Machida, A. Kinugasa, S. Imashuku, T. Kusunoki and T. Takamatisu*

Department of Pediatrics and Department of Pathology*, Kyoto Prefectural University of Medicine, Kawaramachi, Hirokoji, Kamikyo-Ku, Kyoto, Japan 602

Two cases of hypertyrosinaemia accompanied by a defect of fumarylacetoacetate fumarylhydrolase (FAH, EC 3.7.12) are described. The deficient FAH activities were found in the liver of one case and in the kidney of another case, indicating the possible heterogeneity among patients.

The aetiology of hereditary tyrosinaemia (HT) type I (McKusick 27670) is not clearly understood, although multiple biochemical abnormalities have been identified in the patients. Recently, it has been suggested that the primary defect resides in the enzyme FAH (Lindblad *et al.*, 1977). Actual deficiency of hepatic FAH activity has been confirmed by Gray *et al.* (1981) and Kvittingen *et al.* (1981). In this study, we determined several enzyme activities related to tyrosine metabolism, including FAH, in HT type I patients (case 1, died at 28 days of age and case 2, died at 9 months of age) and compared the data with those of age-matched controls to reconfirm the hypothesis of Lindblad *et al.*

MATERIALS AND METHODS

Urinary organic acids were measured by GC–MS. Liver and kidney tissues from case 1, liver tissue only from case 2 and control tissues from age-matched infants who died of unrelated diseases were obtained at autopsy. Activities of tyrosine aminotransferase (TAT, EC 2.6.1.5), p-hydroxyphenylpyruvate oxidase (p-HPPA oxidase, EC 1.14.2.2), and FAH in tissues were assayed according to the methods of Granner and Tomkins (1970), Fellman *et al.* (1972), and Edwards *et al.* (1955), respectively.

RESULTS

Both cases of HT type I excreted abnormally high amount of tyrosyl compounds in urine, p-hydroxy-phenyl-lactate being 230–310 times normal. TAT activities in cases 1 and 2 were not different from controls, both in liver and kidney (Table 1). In case 1,

Table 1 Enzyme activities† in liver and kidney of the patients with tyrosinaemia type I patients and controls

		Age	TAT Liver	TAT Kidney	p-HPPA oxidase Liver	p-HPPA oxidase Kidney	FAH Liver	FAH Kidney
Control	1	1 d					13.13	4.43
Control	2	2 d			0.23			
Control	3	4 d	4.92	0.47	1.18	0.02	11.04	5.21
Control	4	13 d	2.51	0.39	2.08	0.15	9.23	6.55
Control	5	29 d			0.82		7.35	5.14
Median			3.72	0.43	1.00	0.09	10.14	5.18
Patient	1	28 d	1.68	0.51	1.40	0.27	11.01	1.05
Control	6	4 months						6.22
Control	7	4 months	2.34	0.79	6.79	0.53		
Control	8	9 months					16.95	
Control	9	12 months					21.81	8.54
Control	10	1½ y			3.56			
Control	11	1½ y	3.10	0.71	5.56	1.20	26.19	12.20
Control	12	3½ y	19.04		4.41		24.00	
Median			3.10		4.99		22.91	
Patient	2	9 months	2.48		0.46		5.00	

† Enzyme activities are expressed as nmol/min per mg protein

Journal of Inherited Metabolic Disease. ISSN 0141-8955. Copyright © SSIEM and MTP Press Limited, Queen Square, Lancaster, UK.

activities of hepatic *p*-HPPA oxidase, FAH and renal *p*-HPPA oxidase were comparable to control values, whereas renal FAH activity was remarkably decreased. K_m values of these enzymes for corresponding substrates were not different from those of controls. In case 2, *p*-HPPA oxidase and FAH in liver were both decreased. K_m value of *p*-HPPA oxidase for *p*-HPPA was not different from controls, however FAH had high K_m for fumarylacetoacetate (case 2: 8.7 μmol/l vs. controls: 1.3 ± 0.6 μmol/l, $n = 10$).

DISCUSSION

Our results reported here made it difficult to conclude that the primary defect of HT type I was in FAH in liver alone. In fact, in case 1, the defect was in renal FAH, while in case 2, hepatic FAH demonstrated decreased activity, with high K_m value. Hepatic *p*-HPPA oxidase was also decreased in case 2. Clinically, case 2 survived longer than case 1 whose hepatic *p*-HPPA oxidase activity was not decreased. This finding may be compatible with the statement of Lindblad that patients with a low activity of *p*-HPPA oxidase have a more protracted form of the disease whereas those with a high residual activity die young.

The developmental change of *p*-HPPA oxidase and FAH in liver and kidney is worth considering in studying enzyme defect in HT type I. *p*-HPPA oxidase was shown to be induced after birth, whereas FAH exists in considerable amount even before birth. Thus, Kvittingen *et al.* (1983) and Gagne *et al.* (1982) proposed that prenatal diagnosis of this inborn error of metabolism is possible by studying amniotic fluid. However, consider-

ing from the probable heterogeneity as shown here, caution should be exercised in evaluation of such prenatal diagnosis.

References

Edwards, S. W. and Knox, W. E. Enzymes involved in conversion of tyrosine to acetoacetate. In Colowick, S. P. and Kaplan, N. O. (eds.) *Methods in Enzymology*, Vol. 2, Academic Press, New York, 1955, p. 298

Fellman, J. H., Fujita, T. S. and Roth, E. S. Assay, properties and tissue distribution of *p*-hydroxyphenylpyruvate hydroxylase. *Biochim. Biophys. Acta* 284 (1972) 90–100

Gagne, R., Lescault, A., Grenier, A., Laberge, C., McLacon, S. B. and Dallaire, L. Prenatal diagnosis of hereditary tyrosinemia: measurement of succinylacetone in amniotic fluid. *Prenat. Diag.* 2 (1982) 185–188

Granner, D. K. and Tomkins, G. M. Tyrosine aminotransferase (rat liver) In Tabor, H. and Tabor, C. W. (eds.) *Methods in Enzymology*, Vol. 17A, Academic Press, New York, 1970, p. 633

Gray, R. G. F., Patrick, A. D., Preston, F. E. and Whitefield, M. F. Acute hereditary tyrosinaemia type I: Clinical biochemical and haematological studies in twins. *J. Inher. Metab. Dis.* 4 (1981) 37–40

Kvittingen, E. A., Jellum, E. and Stokke, O. Assay of fumarylacetoacetate fumarylhydrolase in human liver – deficient activity in a case of hereditary tyrosinemia. *Clin. Chim. Acta* 115 (1981) 311–319

Kvittingen, E. A., Halvorsen, S. and Jellum, E. Deficient fumarylacetoacetate fumarylhydrolase activity in lymphocytes and fibroblasts from patients with hereditary tyrosinemia. *Pediatr. Res.* 14 (1983) 541–544

Lindblad, B., Lindstedt, S. and Steen, G. On the enzymic defects in hereditary tyrosinemia. *Proc. Natl. Acad. Sci. USA* 74 (1977) 4641–4645

J. Inher. Metab. Dis. 7 Suppl. 2 (1984) 139–140

Short Communication— Noel Raine Award

The Possibility for Prenatal Diagnosis of PKU by Linkage Analyses based on Phenylalanine Hydroxylase Locus Specific DNA-Polymorphisms

S. L. C. WOO and J. H. ROBSON
Howard Hughes Medical Institute, Baylor College of Medicine, Houston, TX 77007, USA

F. GÜTTLER
The John F. Kennedy Institute, DK-2600 Glostrup, Denmark

Thanks to Asbjørn Fölling's most important discovery 50 years ago (Fölling, 1934), millions of newborn infants all over the world are screened today for phenylketonuria (PKU, McKusick 26160) and many thousand early-treated children and young persons with PKU are happy that they are bright and completely normal.

However, we are still confronted with a number of open questions concerning PKU. Nobody knows at what age it might be safe to discontinue the highly artificial and unpalatable diet required for phenylalanine restriction (Woolf, 1979). There are a number of biochemical candidates for the clinical features of 'late-onset phenylalanine intoxication' (Curtius *et al.*, 1981; Sandler, 1982; Pratt, 1982). The problem is more serious for the female child with PKU, in whom concern for future pregnancies must be a consideration (Lenke and Levy, 1980).

Since phenylalanine hydroxylase (EC 1.14.16.1) is a hepatic enzyme and not present in serum or fibroblast cells, there is currently no available methodology for prenatal diagnosis of PKU. We wish to report on the use of human liver phenylalanine hydroxylase *c*DNA fragments to analyse classical PKU by restriction fragment length polymorphisms in the phenylalanine hydroxylase gene. The analyses demonstrate the possibility for both prenatal diagnosis of the genetic disorder and identification of heterozygous trait carriers. Thus, PKU has happened to be the first inborn error of amino acid metabolism where genetic services can be provided based on analysis of locus specific DNA-polymorphisms.

METHODS

Rat liver phenylalanine hydroxylase *m*RNA was purified by polysome immunoprecipitation and used for synthesis and cloning of its *c*DNA as reported previously (Robson *et al.*, 1982). The rat liver *c*DNA was capable of hybridizing with human phenylalanine hydroxylase *m*RNA (Robson *et al.*, 1982) and used for screening of a human liver *c*DNA library comprising 40 000 independent transformants. Specific hybridization signals were obtained from the phenylalanine hydroxylase *c*DNA clones. The length of the largest inserted human phenylalanine hydroxylase *c*DNA fragment was 1.4 kb (Woo *et al.*, 1983). Partial DNA sequence analysis

indicated that the extent of sequence homology between the rat and human phenylalanine hydroxylase *c*DNA clones was in excess of 90 % (Robson *et al.*, unpublished results). Genomic DNAs isolated from random Caucasians were digested by a battery of restriction enzymes and three enzymes (*Sph* I, *Msp* I, and *Hind* III) were identified that by Southern blot analyses yielded polymorphic patterns in the phenylalanine hydroxylase locus (Woo *et al.*, 1983).

MATERIALS

Lymphocytes from seven Danish PKU-families with one or two affected children and unaffected siblings were analysed by restriction fragment length polymorphism. The classical type of PKU of the probands in these families was ensured by frequent adjustments and recalculations of the phenylalanine intake (Güttler, 1980). The combined phenotype of the parents based on phenylalanine loading tests was consistent with the prediction that their child should have classical PKU (Güttler, 1980).

RESULTS

Kindred analysis of seven Danish PKU-families by restriction fragment length polymorphisms using the enzymes *Sph* I, *Msp* I, and *Hind* III revealed 12 theoretical genotypic alleles of the human phenylalanine hydroxylase gene, each with a characteristic haplotype.

In all the families analysed it was possible to establish association of the restriction fragment pattern with the PKU-gene of the family (cf. Figure 1). In a family with two PKU-children the segregation of the PKU-alleles and disease state were concordant. Two unaffected siblings in the family have inherited different alleles from the parents. Allelic segregation between the proband and unaffected siblings was discordant in all families analysed. The powerful tool of haplotype analysis of the PKU-gene was documented in two Danish families.

COMMENTS

The present data based on the cloned human phenylalanine hydroxylase *c*DNA probe and three restriction enzymes suggest that prenatal diagnosis can

Journal of Inherited Metabolic Disease, ISSN 0141–8955. Copyright © SSIEM and MTP Press Limited, Queen Square, Lancaster, UK.

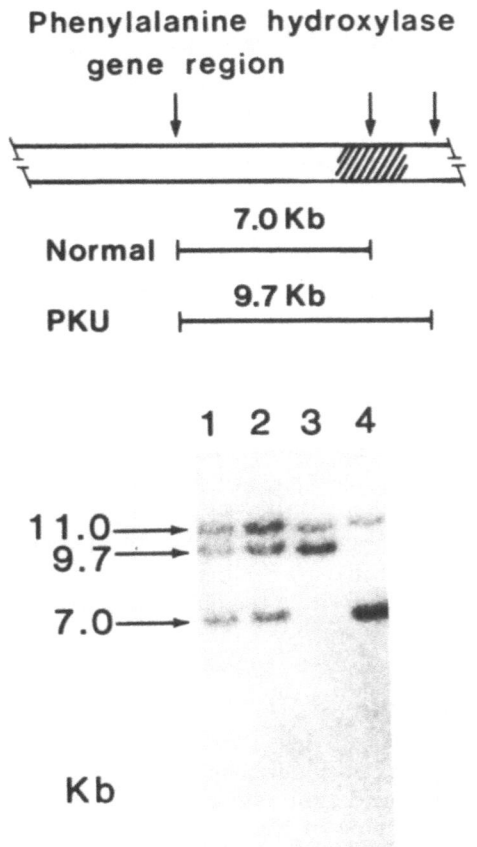

Figure 1 Analysis of restriction fragment length polymorphisms at the human phenylalanine hydroxylase locus using a cloned ^{32}P-labelled human liver phenylalanine hydroxylase gene cDNA-sequence as the probe and the restriction enzyme *Sph* I for digestion of DNA isolated from the leucocytes of (1) the father, (2) the mother, (3) the PKU-child and (4) an unaffected sibling who appears to be a normal homozygote. ↓ indicates the cleavage sites for the restriction enzyme *Sph* I. ■ indicates a base exchange which prevents hydrolysis by the restriction enzyme at this point of the gene region segregating with the PKU-allele

be performed for 75 % of random PKU-families. This is optimal estimates in that the haplotypes of all four phenylalanine hydroxylase genes in a particular family may not be identifiable by comparison with the proband alone. The probability at present would depend also on the availability of an additional unaffected sibling or grandparents.

Genetic services will improve in the future with the identification of additional restriction fragments associated with PKU-alleles. Consequently, prenatal diagnosis of PKU and carrier detection should become a reality for a majority of the PKU-families in the general population.

This work was partially supported by a March of Dimes Birth Defects Foundation Grant and NIH Grant to S.L.C.W. and by grants to F.G. from the Danish Medical Research Council and the Danish Health Insurance Foundation.

References

Curtius, H.-Ch., Niederwieser, A., Viscontini, M., Leimbacher, W., Wegmann, H., Blehova, B., Rey, F., Schaub, J. and Schmidt, H. Serotonin and dopamine synthesis in phenylketonuria. In Harper, B., Gabay, S., Issidorides, M. R. and Alivisates, S. G. A. (eds.) *Serotonin: Current Aspects of Neurochemistry and Function.* Plenum, New York, London, 1981, pp. 277–291

Fölling, A. Über Ausscheidung von Phenylbrenztraubensäure in Harn als Stoffwechselanomalie in Verbindung mit Imbezellität. *Hoppe-Seylers Z. Physiol. Chem.* 227 (1934) 169–176

Güttler, F. Hyperphenylalaninemia: Diagnosis and classification of the various types of phenylalanine hydroxylase deficiency in childhood. *Acta Paediatr. Scand.* 280 Suppl. 280 (1980) pp. 1–80

Lenke, R. R. and Levy, H. L. Maternal phenylketonuria and hyperphenylalaninemia: An international survey of the outcome of untreated and treated pregnancies. *N. Engl. J. Med.* 303 (1980) 1202–1208

Pratt, O. E. Transport inhibition in the pathology of phenylketonuria and other inherited metabolic diseases. *J. Inher. Metab. Dis.* 5 Suppl. 2 (1982) 75–81

Robson, J. H., Chandra, T., MacGillivray, R. T. A. and Woo, S. L. C. Polysome immunoprecipitation of phenylalanine hydroxylase mRNA from rat liver and cloning of its cDNA. *Proc. Natl. Acad. Sci. USA* 79 (1982) 4701–4705

Sandler, M. Inborn errors and disturbances of central neurotransmission (with special reference to phenylketonuria). *J. Inher. Metab. Dis.* 5 Suppl. 2 (1982) 65–70

Woo, S. L. C., Lidsky, A. S., Güttler, F., Chandra, T. and Robson, J. H. Cloned human phenylalanine hydroxylase gene allows prenatal diagnosis and carrier detection of classical phenylketonuria. *Nature* 306 (1983) 151–155

Woolf, L. I. Late onset phenylalanine intoxication. *J. Inher. Metab. Dis.* 2 (1979) 19–20

J. Inher. Metab. Dis. 7 Suppl. 2 (1984) 141–142

Short Communication

Complementation between Argininosuccinate Synthetase-deficient and Argininosuccinate Lyase-deficient Fibroblasts Depends on Intercellular Communication

J. S. DAVIDSON and E. H. HARLEY
Department of Chemical Pathology, University of Cape Town Medical School, Observatory 7925, Cape Town, South Africa

The autosomal recessive disorders, citrullinaemia (McKusick 21570) and argininosuccinic aciduria (McKusick 20790) result from deficiencies of argininosuccinate synthetase (ASS; EC 6.3.4.5) and argininosuccinate lyase (ASL; EC 4.3.2.1) respectively (Walser, 1983) and fibroblasts from these patients show decreased rates of incorporation of [^{14}C]citrulline into protein (Tedesco and Mellman, 1967). Here we report that incorporation of [^{14}C]citrulline by co-cultures of these mutant fibroblasts depends on intercellular communication and provides a model for the study of intercellular junctions.

METHODS

ASS-deficient and ASL-deficient fibroblast lines were established from skin biopsies from two neonates who died in the first week of life from citrullinaemia and argininosuccinic aciduria respectively. Fibroblast suspensions were obtained by trypsinization and the ASS-deficient and ASL-deficient cells were mixed in a 1:1 ratio, except where indicated. After re-attachment to the substratum, cultures were incubated for 5 h in serum-free Eagle's basal medium with [*ureido*-^{14}C]citrulline (0.5 µCi/ml, 0.01 mmol/l) and [^{3}H]leucine (0.5 µCi/ml, 0.2 mmol/l) except where indicated. The cells were then washed, trypsinized, treated with 10% trichloroacetic acid (TCA), and the precipitate was washed and counted for ^{3}H and ^{14}C radioacitivity.

RESULTS AND DISCUSSION

Both ASS-deficient and ASL-deficient cells showed very low rates of incorporation of [^{14}C]citrulline relative to [^{3}H]leucine when cultured separately. The ^{14}C/^{3}H dpm ratios were 4.7×10^{-4} ($\pm 1.9 \times 10^{-4}$) for the ASS-deficient cells and 7.8×10^{-4} ($\pm 3.2 \times 10^{-4}$) for ASL-deficient cells, but the ratio rose by 130-fold to 8.3×10^{-2} ($\pm 3.0 \times 10^{-2}$) when the cells were co-cultured (mean $\pm$ SD, $n = 7$). This rate of citrulline incorporation is similar to that obtained in normal fibroblasts ($9.0 \times 10^{-2} \pm 2.3 \times 10^{-2}$).

By mixing the two cell types in varying proportions, the ^{14}C/^{3}H dpm ratios plotted against percentage of cell type gave a curve which showed maximum complementation with 25% ASS-deficient and 75% ASL-deficient cells (Figure 1a). The curve was skewed to the right,

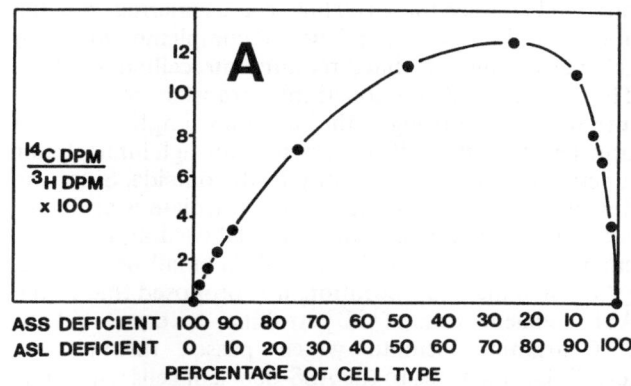

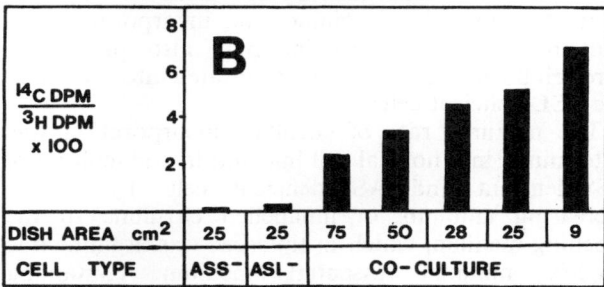

Figure 1 (A) Complementation between ASS-deficient and ASL-deficient fibroblasts as a function of the proportion of each cell type in the co-culture; (B) dependence of complementation on cell density

indicating that the admixture of as little as 4% ASS-deficient cells with ASL-deficient cells restored citrulline incorporation by the co-culture to half-maximal levels.

When the same volume of a mixed cell suspension was plated into dishes of different sizes, complementation increased with increasing cell density (Figure 1b).

To test whether complementation was due to the release of a metabolic intermediate into the medium, ASS-deficient and ASL-deficient cells were plated into adjacent halves of dishes divided by partitions. Other dishes were seeded with a mixed suspension of the two cell types. After the cells had attached to the dishes, the partitions were removed from some of the dishes and the cells were incubated with labelling medium. The ^{14}C/^{3}H dpm ratios were as follows (mean $\pm$ SD): cells separate, media separate: 0.08×10^{-2} ($\pm 0.01 \times 10^{-2}$); cells separate, common medium: 0.11×10^{-2}

Journal of Inherited Metabolic Disease. ISSN 0141–8955. Copyright © SSIEM and MTP Press Limited, Queen Square, Lancaster, UK.

($\pm 0.04 \times 10^{-2}$); co-culture: 10.2×10^{-2} ($\pm 0.10 \times 10^{-2}$). This indicates that complementation is not due to release of a metabolic intermediate into the medium.

The addition of a large amount of unlabelled argininosuccinate to the labelling medium caused only a small decrease in [^{14}C]citrulline incorporation by co-cultures. The ^{14}C/^{3}H dpm ratio in the absence of argininosuccinate was 9.4×10^{-2} ($\pm 0.1 \times 10^{-2}$) and in the presence of argininosuccinate (1 mmol/l) was 8.4×10^{-2} ($\pm 0.1 \times 10^{-2}$). A similar small decrease was seen in a normal cell line.

A likely mechanism for the complementation observed between these cell lines can be inferred from the above results. The dependence of complementation on cell density suggests that it requires intercellular contact. The absence of demonstrable transfer of labelled intermediates through the medium implies that if transfer of a metabolite occurs, it is through intercellular junctions which are not leaky to the outside. Since the obvious candidate for such an intermediate is argininosuccinate, and large amounts of unlabelled argininosuccinate in the medium caused only a small decrease in [^{14}C]citrulline incorporation, it is proposed that in the ASL-deficient cells [^{14}C]citrulline is converted to [^{14}C]argininosuccinate which passes through intercellular junctions to the ASS-deficient cells where it is converted into [^{14}C]arginine, and incorporated into protein. Some [^{14}C]arginine may also pass back through the junctions to be incorporated into protein in the ASL-deficient cells.

The maximal rate of citrulline incorporation was determined in a normal cell line and in a co-culture of ASS-deficient and ASL-deficient cells by adding increasing amounts of unlabelled citrulline to the labelling medium, which in this case was arginine-free Eagle's minimal essential medium containing 0.25 μCi/ml of [^{14}C]citrulline. Both the normal cells and the co-culture showed saturable kinetics, with half-maximal citrulline incorporation at a citrulline concentration of about 0.2 mmol/l. At a citrulline con-

centration of 2 mmol/l the normal cells incorporated 0.451 ± 0.011 and the co-cultures 0.471 ± 0.013 nmol citrulline (10^6 cells)$^{-1}$ h^{-1}, indicating that even at this maximal rate, the flux of citrulline to arginine was not limited by the capacity of the intracellular junctions to transmit argininosuccinate.

Serial measurements at varying times after mixing the cell suspensions showed that intercellular junctions were well established within the first hour of co-culture (data not shown).

Since intercellular junctions are involved in the complementation mechanism, the term metabolic co-operation may be applied to this system (Hooper, 1982). Several different systems, using cultured cells, have been used to study metabolic co-operation (Hooper, 1982; Loewenstein, 1979). The system described here has the advantages that it is simple and rapid to perform and the results are accurately quantifiable. Because incorporation of isotope into TCA-precipitable material can occur only as a result of metabolic co-operation, the background measurement is very low. This system should therefore prove useful in the study of the mechanisms of junction formation and factors which influence junctional permeability.

References

Hooper, M. L. Metabolic co-operation between mammalian cells in culture. *Biochim. Biophys. Acta* 651 (1982) 85–103

Loewenstein, W. R. Junctional intercellular communication and the control of growth. *Biochim. Biophys. Acta* 560 (1979) 1–65

Tedesco, T. A. and Mellman, W. J. Argininosuccinate synthetase activity and citrulline metabolism in cells cultured from a citrullinemic patient. *Proc. Natl. Acad. Sci. U.S.A.* 57 (1967) 829–834

Walser, M. Urea cycle disorders and other hereditary hyperammonemic syndromes. In Stanbury, J. B., Wyngaarden, J. B., Fredrickson, D. S., Goldstein, J. L. and Brown, M. S. (eds.) *The Metabolic Basis of Inherited Disease*, 5th Edn., McGraw-Hill, New York, 1983, pp. 402–438

J. Inher. Metab. Dis. 7 Suppl. 2 (1984) 143–144

Short Communication

Molecular Lesion of Non-ketotic Hyperglycinaemia

K. Tada and K. Hayasaka

Department of Pediatrics, Tohoku University Medical School, Sendai 980, Japan

Non-ketotic hyperglycinaemia (McKusick 23830) is an inborn error of metabolism in which large amounts of glycine are found in body fluids. Most patients with this disorder develop rapidly progressing neurological symptoms such as lethargy, muscular hypotonia, respiratory distress or convulsions in the neonatal period and die within a few weeks, whereas the survivors are handicapped with severe psychomotor retardation.

In 1969, our group demonstrated that the glycine cleavage system was defective in the liver from hyperglycinaemia patients (Tada *et al.*, 1969, 1974). Glycine cleavage system is composed of four protein components: P-protein, a pyridoxal phosphate-dependent glycine decarboxylase; H-protein, a lipoic acid-containing protein; T-protein, a tetrahydrofolate-requiring protein; and L-protein, a lipoamide dehydrogenase (Kikuchi, 1973). Therefore, the disturbance in the glycine cleavage system could be a defect in any of these four components. However, which particular component is defective in non-ketotic hyperglycinaemia has been obscure.

Recently we had the opportunity to investigate the individual components of the glycine cleavage system in liver and brain obtained from two autopsied cases and in liver biopsied from a case of non-ketotic hyperglycinaemia.

MATERIALS AND METHODS

The liver and brain were obtained at autopsy of two patients with non-ketotic hyperglycinaemia who died on the 12th day and 20th day of life. A liver specimen was biopsied from another patient with non-ketotic hyperglycinaemia at the age of 6 months. The specimens were frozen immediately and stored at $-80°C$ until analysed. Clinical and laboratory findings of the patients have been described elsewhere (Hayasaka *et al.*, 1983).

The activity of the glycine cleavage reaction was determined essentially by the method of Sato *et al.* (1969). Activities of P-protein and H-protein were assayed by the $^{14}CO_2$-glycine exchange reaction according to Motokawa and Kikuchi (1969). For the assay of P-protein activity, the assay mixture was supplemented with an excess of chicken-liver H-protein, and for the assay of H-protein activity, with an excess of chicken-liver P-protein. The activity of T-protein was assayed by measuring glycine cleavage activity in the reaction system supplemented with an excess of chicken-liver P-protein and H-protein and was also assayed by measuring the synthesis of glycine from methylene-

tetrahydrofolate, ammonium chloride and [^{14}C]bicarbonate in the reaction system supplemented with chicken liver P-protein and H-protein, according to the method of Okumura-Ikeda *et al.* (1982). The activity of L-protein was determined spectrophotometrically by measuring the lipoamide-dependent oxidation of NADH according to the method of Koike and Hayakawa (1972).

P-protein and H-protein were purified from chicken liver mitochondria by the method of Hiraga and Kikuchi (1980). P-protein purified to homogeneity from chicken-liver mitochondria was used to immunize white rabbits using the standard procedure. Antisera were collected and purified as IgG. The antibody against chicken-liver P-protein reacted similarly with P-protein of human liver and the P-protein of chicken liver.

RESULTS

The overall activities of the glycine cleavage system in the livers and brains of the patients with non-ketotic hyperglycinaemia were found to be extremely low (Table 1). Examination of the activities of the individual components revealed that the activity of P-protein was undetectable in the liver and brain from Patient 1 and in the liver from Patient 3. The activities of the other components were not significantly different from those of controls. On the other hand, in Patient 2 the activity of T-protein was undetectable in the brain and was extremely low in the liver. The activities of the other components of glycine cleavage system in Patient 2 did not differ significantly from those of controls.

To investigate whether the lack of activity of P-protein in Patient 1 was a consequence of absence of the enzyme protein, immunotitration and Ouchterlony double diffusion analysis of P-protein were carried out using antibody prepared against purified chicken-liver P-protein. Extracts of control livers gave single precipitin bands in Ouchterlony double diffusion analysis, but the liver extracts of the Patient 1 did not show any precipitin band. The results of the immunotitration revealed that the liver extract of Patient 1 does not contain protein which is reactive with the antibody against P-protein; suggesting that the lack of P-protein activity in Patient 1 represents an absence of the enzyme protein.

DISCUSSION

The present study clearly indicates a fundamental defect in the glycine cleavage system in the liver and brain of

Journal of Inherited Metabolic Disease. ISSN 0141-8955. Copyright © SSIEM and MTP Press Limited, Queen Square, Lancaster, UK.

Table 1   Activities of the glycine cleavage system and its individual enzyme components in the liver and brain of three patients with non-ketotic hyperglycinaemia

Source of tissue	*Activity* (μmol of product (g protein)$^{-1}$h^{-1})					
	Glycine cleavage	P-protein	H-protein	T-protein[1] A	B	L-protein[2]
Liver						
Patient 1	0.3	0	16.1	72.2	7.3	69.8
Patient 2	0.4	7.4	16.2	0.1	0.3	59.1
Patient 3	0.4	0	18.6	54.0	—	72.7
Control 1	5.2	5.7	18.3	77.9	7.7	78.8
Control 2	4.4	4.8	15.3	66.2	7.0	64.6
Control 3	3.8	4.5	14.6	52.1	7.3	62.8
Brain						
Patient 1	0.2	0	3.2	1.4		
Patient 2	0.1	0.6	4.2	0		
Patient 3	—	—	—			
Control 1	0.6	0.3	3.2	4.0		
Control 2	0.9	0.2	6.1	3.4		
Control 3	0.5	0.2	3.9	2.1		

[1]Column A, determined by the glycine cleavage reaction; column B, determined by the synthesis of glycine
[2]L-protein activity was expressed as μmol (g protein)$^{-1}$min^{-1}

patients with non-ketotic hyperglycinaemia. In two of the patients the abnormality of the glycine cleavage system was found to be due to a defect in the activity of P-protein. Immunochemical analysis indicated that the defect was due to an absence of the enzyme protein. In another patient, a specific defect in T-protein activity was found. Thus non-ketotic hyperglycinaemia may result from a defect in either P-protein or T-protein. This may be similar to the situation that obtains in the pyruvate dehydrogenase complex which is composed of at least three individual enzyme components, and where for at least two components patients with an isolated single component defect have been described (Robinson *et al.*, 1980).

The present data also suggest that the individual protein components involved in the glycine cleavage system in the brain and in the liver may be identical, and the syntheses of individual protein components may be controlled by the same genes in both organs.

The authors are indebted to Professor W. L. Nyhan, Department of Pediatrics, University of California, San Diego, for giving us the opportunity to investigate the specimens from the patients. This work was supported by grants from the Ministry of Education, Science and Culture and the Ministry of Health and Welfare, Japan.

References

Hayasaka, K., Tada, K. and Kikuchi, G. Nonketotic hyperglycinemia: two patients with primary defect of P-protein or T-protein, respectively, in the glycine cleavage system. *Pediatr. Res.* 17 (1983) 967–970
Hiraga, K. and Kikuchi, G. The mitochondrial glycine cleavage system: purification and properties of glycine decarboxylase from chicken liver mitochondria. *J. Biol. Chem.* 225 (1980) 11664–11670
Kikuchi, G. The glycine cleavage system: composition, reaction mechanism and physiologic significance. *Mol. Cell Biochem.* 1 (1973) 169–187
Koike, M. and Hayakawa, T. Purification and properties of lipoamide dehydrogenase from pig heart α-keto acid dehydrogenase complexes. In McCormick, D. B. and Wright, L. D. (eds.) *Methods in Enzymology*, Vol. 18, Academic Press, New York, 1972, pp. 298–307
Motokawa, T. and Kikuchi, G. Glycine metabolism by rat liver mitochondria IV. Isolation and characterization of hydrogen carrier protein, as essential factor for glycine metabolism. *Arch. Biochem. Biophys.* 135 (1969) 402–409
Okumura-Ikeda, K., Fujiwara, K. and Motokawa, Y. Purification and characterization of chicken liver T-protein, a component of the glycine cleavage system. *J. Biol. Chem.* 257 (1982) 135–139
Robinson, B. H., Taylor, J. and Sherwood, W. G. The genetic heterogeneity of lactic acidosis: occurrence of recognizable inborn errors of metabolism in a pediatric population with lactic acidosis. *Pediatr. Res.* 14 (1980) 956–962
Sato, T., Kochi, H., Sato, N. and Kikuchi, G. Glycine metabolism by rat liver mitochondria. III. The glycine cleavage and the exchange of caboxyl carbon of glycine with bicarbonate. *J. Biochem.* 65 (1969) 77–83
Tada, K., Corbeel, L. M., Eckels, R. and Eggermont, E. A block in glycine cleavage reaction as a common mechanism in ketotic and nonketotic hyperglycinemia. *Pediatr. Res.* 8 (1974) 721–723
Tada, K., Narisawa, K., Yoshida, T., Konno, T., Yokoyama, Y., Nakagawa, H., Tanno, K., Mochizuki, K., Arakawa, T., Yoshida, T. and Kikuchi, G. Hyperglycinemia: A defect in glycine cleavage reaction. *Tohoku J. Exp. Med.* 98 (1969) 289–296

J. Inher. Metab. Dis. 7 Suppl. 2 (1984) 145–146

Short Communication

Prolidase Deficiency: Detection of Cases by a Newborn Urinary Screening Programme

B. LEMIEUX, C. AURAY-BLAIS, R. GIGUERE and D. SHAPCOTT
Réseau de Médecine Génétique, Centre Hospitalier Universitaire de Sherbrooke, Département de Pédiatrie, Sherbrooke, Québec, Canada, J1H 5N4

Prolidase deficiency (EC 3.4.3.7) is a very rare inborn error of metabolism associated with severe dermatological manifestations and iminodipeptiduria. Previous cases were confirmed on the basis of their phenotype and only recently have been detected by newborn screening (Naughten *et al.*, 1982). We report on our experience related to prolidase deficiency in the newborn period in our Urinary Mass Screening Program of the Québec Network for Genetic Medicine.

Over the last decade, we have analysed newborn urine samples impregnated on filter paper, collected at 3 weeks of age by parents. This service to the population is government funded and is part of the Network for Genetic Medicine which is oriented towards preventive medicine. The Urinary Screening Program is voluntary and since 1981 the parents contribute directly to the cost of the programme by paying for postage of the samples. The co-operation of parents has always been good, attaining more than 90% of all the families in Québec. To increase the cost benefit ratio we have made a self-criticism of our programme over the years. The main modifications were: (1) to orientate our newborn screening towards the detection of disorders that can cause severe clinical problems and necessitate immediate medical intervention; (2) to modify our thin layer chromatography (TLC) technique by performing a combined TLC of amino acids and methylmalonic acid which has substantially reduced the cost per analysis.

MATERIALS AND METHOD

Urine samples are processed and prepared for TLC according to Auray-Blais *et al.* (1983). Ion-exchange chromatography with a Technicon TSM Amino Acid Analyzer, was used to identify x-pro-dipeptides (Figure 1). The resin is a DC-IA (Dionex Co.). The volume of urine analysed was calculated according to the concentration of 10 µg urinary α-amino-nitrogen, and this amount was mixed with an equal volume of 9% sulphosalicylic acid and 10 µmol of norleucine, the internal standard. The urine sample was hydrolysed by adding to it an equal volume of 6N HCl and heating at 110°C for 6–10 h. Enzymatic determinations were performed in Dr Charles Scriver's laboratory, Montreal.

RESULTS AND DISCUSSION

After spraying the plates with ninhydrin, we noticed a definite difference in the colour and migration of amino acids between the prolidase deficiency cases and the

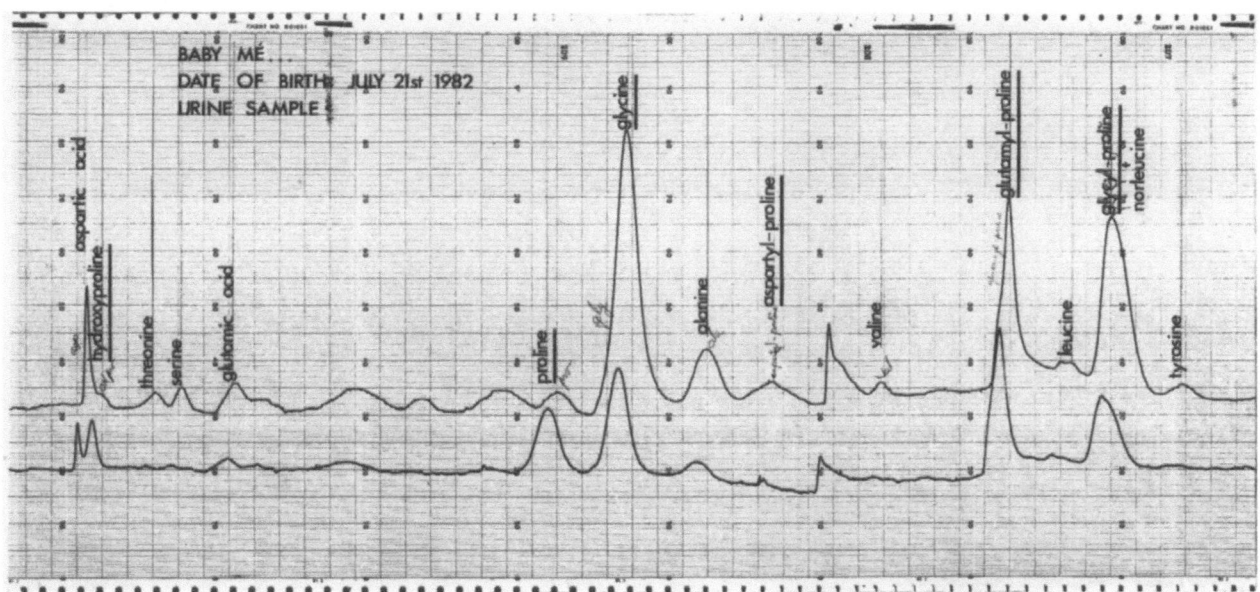

Figure 1 Ion-exchange chromatogram of urinary amino acids and x-pro-dipeptides of a confirmed prolidase deficiency patient

Journal of Inherited Metabolic Disease. ISSN 0141-8955. Copyright © SSIEM and MTP Press Limited, Queen Square, Lancaster, UK.

usual iminoglycinuria (R_f 0.58) pattern. The brownish yellow spot in the prolidase deficiency cases appeared very near glycine with a R_f of 0.54.

Subsequently, these abnormal samples were run on the amino acid analyser and three intense x-pro-dipeptide peaks were present: the major one was glycyl-proline followed by glutamyl-proline and aspartyl-proline. A confirmatory test was performed on the amino acid analyser by hydrolysing the urine sample permitting us to notice a considerable increase in proline and hydroxyproline.

In one of the two cases, enzymatic confirmation was performed on the baby as well as the parents. The baby was found to have a definite enzymatic deficiency; the erythrocyte prolidase activity was below 5 % of normal. Manganese ion did not restore the activity *in vitro*. The parents were confirmed as heterozygotes with intermediate values (Scriver, personal communication, 1983).

Considering that most patients are usually detected in childhood or in later years when clinical symptoms have appeared, it is evidently useful to be able to detect this disorder during the early stages of life by an increase of a specific biochemical marker. In our study, neither of the children has presented any clinical manifestation (they are now both 1 year old). In the study of Naughten *et al.* (1982), the children again presented no clinical manifestations when detected. Isemura *et al.* (1979)

report cases where both siblings presented a prolidase deficiency with one exhibiting clinical symptoms; the other was without clinical symptoms. He thus suggests that possibly the prolidase deficiency might not be responsible for pathogenesis of the clinical symptoms.

In conclusion, these cases detected by newborn mass screening gave us the opportunity to better understand the natural history of prolidase deficiency but also to ask ourselves the question: Is this deficiency related to an adaptive or non-adaptive phenotypic expression? Furthermore, the report of these two cases again emphasizes the scientific value of a well integrated programme.

References

Auray-Blais, C., Giguère, R. and Lemieux, B. Thin layer chromatographic technique in a newborn urinary screening program. In Naruse, H. and Irie, M. (eds.) *Neonatal Screening. Excerpta Medica International Congress Series* 606 (1983) 418–419

Isemura, M., Hanyo, T., Gejyo, F., Nakazawa, R., Igarashi, R., Matsuo, S., Ikeda, K. and Sato, Y. Prolidase deficiency with imidodipeptiduria. A familial case with and without clinical symptoms. *Clin. Chim. Acta* 93 (1979) 401–407

Naughten, E. R., Proctor, S. P., Coulombe, J. T., Levy, H. L. and Ampola, M. G. Congenital prolidase deficiency in affected siblings. Abstract no. 693, Congress A.S.P.-S.P.R. Washington (1982)

J. Inher. Metab. Dis. 7 Suppl. 2 (1984) 147–148

Short Communication

Type Ib Glycogen Storage Disease: An *In Vivo* and *In Vitro* Study of Two Cases

C. Baussan, N. Moatti, M. Brivet and A. Lemonnier
Laboratoire Central de Biochimie, Centre Hospitalier de Bicetre, 78, rue du Général Leclerc, 94270 Le Kremlin-Bicetre, France

Type Ib glycogen storage disease (type Ib GSD) is characterized by clinical and biochemical features of glucose-6-phosphatase deficiency (type Ia GSD). However, the activity of the glucose-6-phosphatase (G-6-Pase, EC 3.1.3.9) is normal in frozen liver specimens and markedly low in fresh tissue. It was postulated by Narisawa *et al.* (1978) that type Ib GSD is caused by a defect in microsomal glucose-6-phosphate (G-6-P) transport leading to a non-functional G-6-Pase *in vivo*. In connection with this, Van Hoof *et al.* (1972) proposed a double isotopic glucose test for the evaluation of the enzyme *in vivo*. In this paper, we report *in vitro* and *in vivo* assays of G-6-Pase in two patients with severe clinical symptoms.

CASE REPORTS

Case 1: This male patient (A.G.) was the fourth child of healthy and non-consanguineous parents. Initial laboratory studies showed fasting hypoglycaemia (0.55 mmol/l) and lactic acidosis (15.7 mmol/l). At 2 months of age, neutropenia appeared and granulocyte counts were from 145 to $450/mm^3$. Recurrent infections ensued. At 5 months of age, he was admitted to hospital for generalized convulsions. Hepatomegaly was noted. During episodes of hypoglycaemia, the serum levels of insulin were normal ($< 8 \mu U/ml$). Blood amino acids were normal. Nocturnal gastric feeding with four diurnal meals was started. Good statural development was noted. Hyperlipaemia recurred and normalized 2 months later. The patient died suddenly at 11 months of age.

Case 2: This female patient (P.L.), born in December 1975, suffered from recurrent attacks of hypoglycaemia since the 2nd day of life. She had hepatomegaly, doll-like facies and moderate growth retardation. Laboratory studies showed hypoglycaemia, with normal insulin level, lactic acidosis and severe hyperlipaemia. A portocaval shunt (PCS) was performed. A striking improvement of the hyperlipaemia was noted but hypoglycaemia and growth retardation persisted. At 5 years of age, lithiasis appeared and hepatic adenomas were revealed by echography. The *in vivo* test was carried out 9 months after PCS.

METHODS

All studies were undertaken after parental consent had been obtained. Liver specimens were obtained by needle biopsy. Glycogen content and G-6-Pase activity were determined in liver tissue according to Hers and Van Hoof (1966). Fresh liver specimens, obtained immediately after biopsy, were homogenized in 0.25 mol/l sucrose as described by Corbeel *et al.* (1981). The *in vivo* assay of G-6-Pase was carried out by the determination of blood $^3H/^{14}C$ ratio after intravenous injection of [2-^3H; U-^{14}C]glucose.

RESULTS AND DISCUSSION

The activities of G-6-Pase in fresh liver specimens of the two patients were 19% and 41% respectively of that measured in the same biopsy after freezing (Table 1). We confirm similar observations (Igarashi *et al.*, 1979; Lange *et al.*, 1980; Corbeel *et al.*, 1981) that in type Ib GSD the G-6-Pase is normal *in vitro* when the assay is performed after disruption of microsomal membranes by thawing.

The *in vivo* test of G-6-Pase gave no decrease in the $^3H/^{14}C$ ratio indicating a non-functional enzyme (Table 1). Data of Sann *et al.* (1980) are in agreement with the previous result, though data of other investigators are not (Kamoun, 1980; Corbeel *et al.*, 1981). But, Sann *et al.* (1980) and Kamoun (1980) did not determine the G-6-Pase activity in fresh liver of their patients. Corbeel *et al.* (1981) found a reduced activity in fresh liver tissue associated with a functional enzyme, *in vivo*, 3 months after PCS. However, the effects of PCS on the biochemical disturbances were different in their patient: an improvement of fasting tolerance and an increase in G-6-Pase activity were observed.

The heterogeneous response to the *in vivo* glucose test corresponds certainly to variant forms of type Ib GSD in relation to the multicomponent nature of G-6-Pase system (Arion *et al.*, 1980). Our two patients are the first reported cases with abnormal functional test of G-6-Pase activity in agreement with low G-6-Pase activity in fresh liver tissue.

Table 1 **Results of *in vitro* and *in vivo* investigations on two patients with type Ib GSD**

	Glycogen content (% of liver mass)	G-6-Pase activity (units/g tissue)		Blood $^3H/^{14}C$ ratio after intravenous injection of [2-^3H; U-^{14}C]glucose (% of initial ratio)[1]	
		Frozen liver	Fresh liver	30 min	60 min
Patient 1 (A.G.)	10.6	6.7	1.3	113	115
Patient 2 (P.L.)	9.3	4.1	1.7	95.3	103.1
Controls[2] (n = 8)				77.8 ± 4.3	59.6 ± 7.2
Adult rats (n = 6)		9.8 ± 1.3	10.2 ± 2.0		

Reference values are mean ± SD
[1] Measured by Dr L. Hue, Université Catholique de Louvain—Laboratoire de Chimie Physiologique
[2] From Van Hoof *et al.* (1972)

References

Arion, W. J., Lange, A. J., Walls, H. E. and Ballas, L. M. Evidence for the participation of independent translocases for phosphate and glucose-6-phosphate in the microsomal glucose-6-phosphatase system. *J. Biol. Chem.* 255 (1980) 10396–10406

Corbeel, L., Hue, L., Lederer, B., De Barsy, T., Van den Berghe, G., Devlieger, H., Jaeken, J., Bracke, P. and Eeckels, R. Clinical and biochemical findings before and after portocaval shunt in a girl with type Ib glycogen storage disease. *Pediatr. Res.* 15 (1981) 58–61

Hers, H. G. and Van Hoof, F. Enzymes of glycogen degradation in biopsy material. *Methods Enzymol.* 8 (1966) 525–532

Igarashi, Y., Otomo, H., Narisawa, K. and Tada, K. A new variant of glycogen storage disease type I: probably due to a defect in the glucose-6-phosphate transport system. *J. Inher. Metab. Dis.* 2 (1979) 45–49

Kamoun, P. P. Is type Ib glycogenosis related to an anomeric preference for glucose-6-phosphate uptake by hepatic microsomes? *Med. Hypotheses* 6 (1980) 1135–1139

Lange, A. J., Arion, W. J. and Beaudet, A. L. Type Ib glycogen storage disease is caused by a defect in the glucose-6-phosphate translocase of the microsomal glucose-6-phosphatase system. *J. Biol. Chem.* 255 (1980) 8381–8384

Narisawa, K., Igarashi, Y., Otomo, H. and Tada, K. A new variant of glycogen storage disease type I probably due to a defect in the glucose-6-phosphate transport system. *Biochem. Biophys. Res. Commun.* 83 (1978) 1360–1364

Sann, L., Mathieu, M., Bourgeois, J., Bienvenu, J. and Bethenod, M. *In vivo* evidence for defective activity of glucose-6-phosphatase in type Ib glycogenosis. *J. Pediatr.* 96 (1980) 691–694

Van Hoof, F., Hue, L., de Barsy, T., Jacquemin, P., Devos, P. and Hers, H. G. Glycogen storage diseases. *Biochimie* 54 (1972) 745–751

J. Inher. Metab. Dis. 7 Suppl. 2 (1984) 149–150

Short Communication

The Lactate Concentration of the Urine, a Parameter for the Adequacy of Dietary Treatment of Patients with Glucose-6-phosphatase Deficiency

J. Fernandes, G. P. A. Smit and R. Berger
Department of Pediatrics, University Hospital, 59 Oostersingel, 9713 EZ Groningen, The Netherlands

Gastric drip feeding (GDF) during the night improves the clinical and metabolic abnormalities of patients with glycogen storage disease due to glucose-6-phosphatase (EC 3.1.3.9) deficiency (Greene *et al.*, 1980; Fernandes *et al.*, 1979; Stanley *et al.*, 1981). The normalization of blood glucose by GDF diminishes lactate overproduction by the liver and, therefore, suppresses the tendency for hyperlactacidaemia. Conversely, a (nearly) normal level of blood lactate is considered to be a parameter for adequate glucose supply by GDF (Stanley *et al.*, 1981). In our experience, however, the blood lactate concentration often fluctuates strongly. The lactate concentration of the urine averages these fluctuations and thus reflects lactate overproduction better than incidental blood lactate values do (Fernandes and Blom, 1976).

PATIENTS AND METHODS

Seventeen patients with glucose-6-phosphatase deficiency (type IA) and one with glucose-6-phosphate translocase deficiency (type IB) were treated with frequent meals at daytime and GDF during 10–12 hours each night, the eldest patient excepted. The meals were starch-enriched and sucrose- and lactose-restricted. The GDF consisted of a liquid lactose-restricted infant formula with maltose added.

Twelve hours' urine was collected from 8 a.m. till 8 p.m. and from 8 p.m. till 8 a.m. next day, synchronously with the frequent-meals regime in daytime and the GDF during the night. Each urine sample was immediately transferred to the collecting bottle and stored at −20 °C. The quantitative collection of urine, easy to carry out in hospital routine, is less suitable for conditions at home and when the child attends school. Then we asked the child to void before breakfast and before starting GDF. We assumed these two urine samples to reflect approximately the lactate concentration during the night and the day, respectively, after having observed the lactate concentrations of 12 hours' urine and the last sample of the same period to be in the same range under steady state conditions. The urinary lactate concentration was used without calculating lactate excretion per day or per kg bodyweight (Fernandes and Blom, 1976). Urinary lactate and creatinine were determined with routine chemical methods.

RESULTS AND DISCUSSION

A low exogenous glucose supply resulted in high lactate concentrations in the urine. This is shown in a longitudinal study of a patient (Figure 1). At high

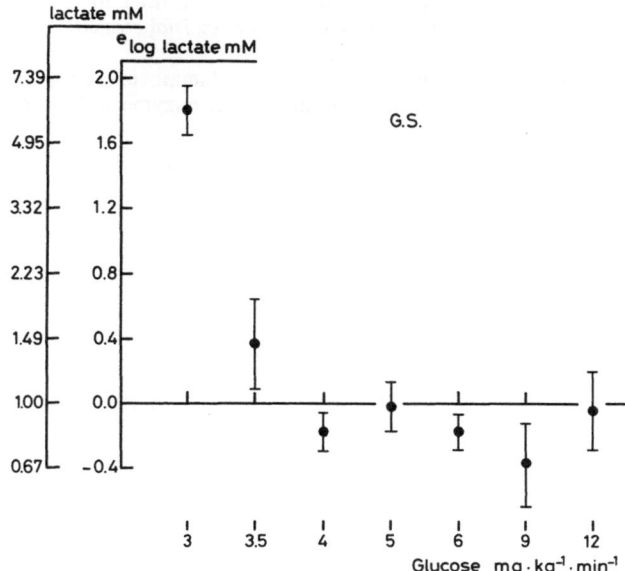

Figure 1 Urinary lactate concentration (mean ± SEM) for various dose levels of glucose in nocturnal gastric drip feeding administered to a patient with glucose-6-phosphatase deficiency. The glucose content of GDF was changed in a random order

glucose infusion rates the lactate concentration decreased to a basal level between 0.3 and 1.0 mmol/l (normal upper limit at 0.3 mmol/l). This was first reached at an infusion rate of 4 mg glucose $kg^{-1} min^{-1}$, which is lower than the theoretical production rate of 6.7 mg $kg^{-1} min^{-1}$, calculated according to Bier *et al.* (1977). In most other patients the urinary lactate concentrations were in the same range, but markedly higher basal concentrations were found in five severely growth-retarded children (height less than 3rd percentile) (results not shown).

The lactate/creatinine ratios were usually below 0.1 (normal range 0.010–0.058). Higher values were measured in five children with height percentiles below 25.

In conclusion we found the urinary lactate concentration to be a useful parameter to estimate the basal glucose requirement of glucose-6-phosphatase-deficient patients. Higher intakes have no additional benefit, as normalization of the lactate concentration in blood and urine can usually not be obtained, nor would this be desirable as it would reduce the availability of lactate as an alternate fuel for the brain in case of inadvertent

Journal of Inherited Metabolic Disease. ISSN 0141–8955. Copyright © SSIEM and MTP Press Limited, Queen Square, Lancaster, UK.

hypoglycaemia (Fernandes *et al.*, 1982). A hyperlactaciduria that persists despite adequate glucose supply is observed in some patients with severe growth retardation. The reason for this apparent correlation is unknown.

References

Bier, D. M., Leake, R. D., Haymond, M. W., Arnold, K. J., Gruenke, L. D., Sperling, M. A. and Kipnis, D. M. Measurement of 'true' glucose production rates in infancy and childhood with 6,6-dideuteroglucose. *Diabetes* 26 (1977) 1016–1023

Fernandes, J. and Blom, W. Urinary lactate excretion in normal children and in children with enzyme defects of carbohydrate metabolism. *Clin. Chim. Acta* 66 (1976) 345–352

Fernandes, J., Berger, R. and Smit, G. P. A. Lactate as energy source for brain in glucose-6-phosphatase deficient child. *Lancet* 1 (1982) 113

Fernandes, J., Jansen, H. and Jansen, T. C. Nocturnal gastric drip feeding in glucose-6-phosphatase deficient children. *Pediatr. Res.* 13 (1979) 225–229

Greene, H. L., Slonim, A. E., Burr, I. M. and Moran, J. R. Type I glycogen storage disease: five years of management with nocturnal intragastric feeding. *J. Pediatr.* 96 (1980) 590–595

Stanley, C. A., Mills, J. L. and Baker, L. Intragastric feeding in type I glycogen storage disease: factors affecting the control of lactic acidemia. *Pediatr. Res.* 15 (1981) 1504–1508

J. Inher. Metab. Dis. 7 Suppl. 2 (1984) 151–152

Short Communication

Sorbitol Dehydrogenase Deficiency in a Family with Congenital Cataracts

Y. S. SHIN, M. RIETH and W. ENDRES
Children's Hospital, University of Munich, FRG

P. HAAS
Department of Ophthalmology, University of Erlangen, FRG

Cataract is one of the important clinical manifestations of galactosaemia due to galactokinase or galactose-1-phosphate uridyltransferase deficiency. It has been known that the accumulation of polyols, sorbitol or galactitol in a lens plays a key role in the formation of diabetic and galactosaemic cataracts (van Heyningen, 1976). It is also well established that the sorbitol pathway involving aldolase reductase (EC 1.1.1.21) and sorbitol dehydrogenase (EC 1.1.1.14) is important in cataract formation (Varma *et al.*, 1977). Recently Vaca *et al.* (1982) reported the first case of red cell sorbitol dehydrogenase deficiency in a family with cataracts. Therefore we have decided to determine the sorbitol dehydrogenase activity in erythrocytes in addition to galactokinase, galactose-1-phosphate uridyltransferase and UDP-galactose epimerase activities in a selected population with congenital cataracts.

METHODS

Sorbitol dehydrogenase was assayed by a two-step radioactive method using [^{14}C]sorbitol. The mixture of the first reaction contained 100 nmol sorbitol (0.1 µCi), 25 µmol Tris–Cl buffer, pH 8.0, 2.5 µmol MgCl$_2$, 1.25 µmol NAD and haemolysates (0.5–1.0 µg Hb) in a total volume of 100 µl. After incubation at 32°C for 20 min the reaction was terminated by heating at 95°C for 4 min. [^{14}C]Fructose in the supernates was quantitatively converted to [^{14}C]fructose-6-phosphate by hexokinase and ATP and separated from [^{14}C]sorbitol on a DEAE-cellulose mini column as used in the galactokinase assay. Galactokinase was assayed by the method described previously (Shin-Buhring *et al.*, 1977). The epimerase activity was determined by a two-step radioactive method of Shin *et al.* (1982).

RESULTS AND DISCUSSION

Through the routine screening of sorbitol dehydrogenase deficiency a family was discovered in which the members with cataracts had a distinctly low activity of sorbitol dehydrogenase in erythrocytes (Table 1). The cataract patients in this family showed a residual activity of sorbitol dehydrogenase 15–20% of the values of healthy subjects or of the patients with congenital cataracts of uncertain origins. Interestingly, the cataract

Table 1 Activities of various enzymes in erythrocytes and the K_m values for sorbitol of sorbitol dehydrogenase

Subject	Cataract	Enzyme activity (nmol min^{-1} (g Hb)$^{-1}$)		
		SD[1]	GK[1]	GE[1]
SD deficiency				
Father	+	21.7 (10.0)[2]	22.1	32.5
Mother	−	133.4 (2.2)	25.0	14.8
Son	+	29.6 (10.0)	27.0	14.9
Daughter	−	117.0	42.0	45.0
GK deficiency				
Father (het.)	−	98.0	13.3	28.7
Mother (het.)	−	80.0	11.4	20.1
Daughter (hom.)	+	78.0	0	28.5
Control				
$n = 18$	−	116.3 ± 29.9[3]	20.0–75.0[4]	30.0 ± 3.2
$n = 14$	+	102.6 ± 28.0	20.0–80.2	26.2 ± 7.5

[1] SD = sorbitol dehydrogenase; GK = galactokinase; GE = epimerase K_m for sorbitol. The control values are approx. 2.0 mmol/l)
[3] Mean ± SD
[4] Range; the activity is age-dependent

Journal of Inherited Metabolic Disease. ISSN 0141–8955. Copyright © SSIEM and MTP Press Limited, Queen Square, Lancaster, UK.

patients with a low sorbitol dehydrogenase activity were all males as shown here and in the family of Vaca *et al.* (1982). We have further determined the K_m values for sorbitol in the patients (Table 1); they were much higher than those in the controls, suggesting a structural alteration in the enzyme in these patients.

It has been observed by Varma and Kinoshita (1974) that in diabetic rats aldose reductase activity was increased and sorbitol dehydrogenase was decreased. This possibly explains the elevated level of sorbitol in the diabetic rat lens (van Heyningen, 1976). Tanimoto *et al.* (1983) recently described an accumulation of sorbitol in the diabetic rabbit lens. It would be important to know whether dietary treatment with a low glucose diet is beneficial to patients with sorbitol dehydrogenase deficiency. Although further studies are necessary with regard to its treatment as well as the nature of the defect, whether it is primary or secondary, it is advisable to screen for sorbitol dehydrogenase deficiency in the population with congenital cataracts.

References

Shin, Y. S., von Rucker, A., Rieth, M. and Endres W. Assay of UDP-galactose 4-epimerase. *Clin. Chem.* 28 (1982) 2332–2333

Shin-Buhring, Y., Osang, M., Ziegler, R. and Schaub, J. A simple assay for galactokinase using DEAE-cellulose column chromatography. *Clin. Chim. Acta* 74 (1977) 1–5

Tanimoto, T., Fukada, H., Sato, H. and Kawamura, J. Sorbitol pathway in lenses of normal and diabetic rabbits. *Chem. Pharmacol. Bull.* 31 (1983) 204–208

Vaca, G., Ibara, B., Bracamontes, M., Garcia-Cruz, D., Sánchez-Corona, J., Medina, C., Wunsch, C., Gonzáles-uiroga, G. and Cantú, J. M. Red cell sorbitol dehydrogenase deficiency in a family with cataracts. *Hum. Genet.* 61 (1982) 338–341

van Heyningen, R. Sugar alcohols in the pathogenesis of galactose and diabetic cataracts. In *The Eye and Inborn Errors of Metabolism. Birth Defects XII* (1976) 295–303

Varma, S. D., Mizuno, A. and Kinoshita, J. H. Diabetic cataracts and flavonoids. *Science* 195 (1977) 205–206

Varma, S. D. and Kinoshita, J. H. Sorbitol pathway in diabetic and galactosemic rat lens. *Biochem. Biophys. Acta* 338 (1974) 632–640

Free Communications *(continued)*

A semi-automatized method for the screening of reductants in urine samples impregnated on paper. *J. R. Alonso-Fernandez, J. Pena and J. M. Fraga*

Incorporation of [^{14}C]glucose into α-1,4 bonds by leukocytes and fibroblasts of patients with type III glycogen storage disease. *A. Gutman and V. Barash*

Prenatal diagnosis of type III glycogenosis. *I. Maire and M. Mathieu*

The use of slowly absorbed carbohydrates in the treatment of GSD (glycogen storage disease). *G. P. A. Smit, R. Berger, S. W. Moses and J. Fernandes*

Ketone body metabolism and hyperlipidaemia and glycogen storage disease (GSD I). *F. Inoue, N. Kodo, S. Hibi, N. Furukawa, A. Kinugasa and T. Kusunoki*

The effects of β-guanidopropionate and of carnitine on glycaemia. *M. G. Piccardo, L. Russo and M. Rosa*

In vitro studies toward replacement therapy in lysosomal diseases: incorporation of lysosomal enzyme added in the medium or provided by coculture with normal cells. *P. Veyron, M. T. Zabot, I. Maire and C. Collombel*

Evidence of polyglandular involvement in Niemann-Pick disease type B. *P. Strisciuglio, S. Di Maio, G. Parenti, A. Franzese, M. L. Sandomenico and G. Andria*

Clinical diagnosis of a new case of ceramidase deficiency (Farber's disease). *B. Cartigny, J. Libert, A. H. Fensom, J. J. Martin, J. L. Dhondt, G. Fontaine and J. P. Farriaux*

Amniotic fluid peptidases in the prenatal detection of cystic fibrosis. *L. G. Dann, S. Baker and K. Blau*

Cystic fibrosis – a disturbed metabolism of energy? *H. Kollberg, A. Bardon and O. Ceder*

Pyruvate dehydrogenase complex activity in normal and in six congenital lactic acidosis fibroblasts with the arylamine acetyl-transferase coupled assay. *C. Marsac, C. Augereau, F. Demaugre, J. M. Saudubray and J. P. Leroux*

Proposals for a co-ordinated scheme for the post-natal diagnosis of inherited metabolic disease. The acutely sick infant. *M. Hjelm and J. W. Seakins*

Maple syrup urine disease: normal, mental and somatic development after prenatal diagnosis (4 years follow up). *C. Romano, R. Cerone, U. Caruso, S. Scaliso and W. Kleijer*

Cystathionine-β-synthase deficiency: annotations after a study of 12 patients. *R. Cerone, S. Scalisi, M. Di Rocco, U. Caruso, G. F. Gargani and C. Romano*

Clinical and biochemical abnormalities in six patients with a presumed C_6-acyl-CoA-dehydrogenase deficiency. *W. Blom, H. R. Scholte and C. J. de Groot*

Some aspects of GC/MS analysis of organic acids in urine. *W. Blom and J. G. M. Huijmans*

The interpretation of complementary examinations of familial deficiency in muscular carnitine: a familial case history. *Ch. Piussan, B. Risbourg, Y. Maingourd, J. Cl. Pautard, C. Lenaerts and M. Mathieu*

Abnormal aromatic acids in the urine of a child with Reye's like syndrome. *F. Rocchiccioli*

Methylglyoxal aciduria in a vitamin B1 deficient breast-fed infant of strict vegetarian. *F. Rocchiccioli and G. Lenoir*

"Urocanase deficiency" in a 7-year-old boy with psychomotor retardation. *A. H. Van Gennip, J. Rajnherc, P. K. de Bree and S. K. Wadman*

Isovaleryl-β-(D)-glucuronide, a new urinary metabolite in isovaleric acidaemia. *L. Dorland, M. Duran, S. K. Wadman, L. Bruinvis, D. Ketting and A. Niederwieser*

Fumaric aciduria: a new organic acid disorder associated with mental retardation and speech impairment. *R. E. Hill, D. T. Wheland and S. McClorry*

J. Inher. Metab. Dis. 7 Suppl. 2 (1984) 153–154

Short Communication

Thiamin-responsive Megaloblastic Anaemia: A Disorder of Thiamin Transport?

V. POGGI, G. LONGO, B. DEVIZIA and G. ANDRIA
Department of Pediatrics, 2nd Medical School, University of Naples, Italy

G. RINDI and C. PATRINI
Institute of Human Physiology, University of Pavia, Italy

E. CASSANDRO
Department of Audiology, 2nd Medical School, University of Naples, Italy

Thiamin-responsive megaloblastic anaemia (TRMA), associated with diabetes mellitus and sensorineural deafness (McKusick 24927) is a very rare disease, so far described in only five patients from four families. (Rogers *et al.*, 1969; Viana and Carvalho, 1978; La Grutta *et al.*, 1980; Haworth *et al.*, 1982). We report the results of some studies carried out in an additional case, suggesting a possible disorder of thiamin transport in TRMA.

CASE REPORT

The patient (P.M.R.), a 5-year-old Italian girl, was the full term product of a G2 P1 Ab0 31-year-old mother whose pregnancy and delivery were uncomplicated. Birth weight was 3.9 kg. At 7.5 months of age a blood cell count revealed a macrocytic anaemia (Hb = 7 g/dl; MCV = 96 fl) treated discontinuously with multiple vitamin preparations providing 20 mg/day of thiamin. This therapy had some success. At 2 years of age glycosuria was detected by chance; a month later juvenile diabetes mellitus was diagnosed and treated with 6 u insulin. At $2\frac{1}{4}$ years of age the patient, hospitalized because of an acute infectious gastroenteritis, was found to have again severe macrocytic anaemia, associated with thrombocytopenia. Treatment with a blood transfusion and multivitamin preparations corrected all haematological abnormalities. At $2\frac{1}{2}$ years of age we first saw the patient, suspected the diagnosis of TRMA and detected a bilateral sensorineural deafness. We demonstrated twice that oral thiamin alone (either thiamin-HCl or benzoyl-oxy-methyl (BOM) thiamin, 50 mg/day) caused a considerable rise of reticulocyte count, haemoglobin concentration and platelet count, and improved megaloblastic changes in the bone marrow. After beginning a regular thiamin supplementation (25 mg/day), the girl did not require insulin therapy any more and her deafness did not progress further.

The family history revealed that parents were not consanguineous and no relatives suffered from unexplained anaemia. The father showed a reduced glucose tolerance at 41 years of age. The mother underwent splenectomy at 19 years of age because of a thrombocytopenia of unknown origin. A maternal uncle had a diagnosis of insulin-dependent diabetes mellitus at age 28 and was shown to have a bilateral sensorineural deafness for the high frequencies.

The following laboratory tests of special interest in this case gave normal results: serum concentrations of vitamin B_{12} and folate, serum iron, total iron binding capacity, HbF, Hb electrophoresis, methylmalonic aciduria, orotic aciduria, organic aciduria, pyruvate dehydrogenase complex activity in cultured skin fibroblasts (Dr S. DiDonato, Milan, Italy).

MATERIALS AND METHODS

Reagents used were as described previously (Patrini and Rindi, 1980).

Fluorometric determination of thiamin and its phosphoesters was performed in plasma, after deproteinization with 70% trichloroacetic acid (TCA), and in acid extract (70% TCA) of red blood cell (r.b.c.) fraction, according to the method described by Patrini and Rindi (1980).

Uptake of [^{14}C]thiamin (specific activity 14 mCi/mmol; Radiochemical Centre, Amersham, England) by r.b.c. was studied by incubating a mixture of 4 ml of washed r.b.c. fraction and 6 ml of isotonic Krebs–Henseleit buffer, pH 7.4, containing 0.2 μmol/l [^{14}C]thiamin, at 37° for 1 h. Radiometric determination of thiaminic compounds in TCA extract of r.b.c. was carried out according to Patrini and Rindi (1980).

Assay of thiamin pyrophosphokinase (TPPKase) activity (EC 2.7.6.2) in r.b.c. haemolysates was performed according to Sanioto *et al.* (1977).

Protein concentration was determined by the method of Lowry.

RESULTS AND DISCUSSION

The main results of special studies on thiamin metabolism and transport are summarized in Table 1. Plasma concentration of total thiamin was profoundly reduced in the patient, while off-therapy, and appeared to be at the lower limit of the control range in her parents. Content of total thiamin in r.b.c. was abnormally low in our proband, at or just below the lower limit of the control range in both parents and in the

Journal of Inherited Metabolic Disease. ISSN 0141-8955. Copyright © SSIEM and MTP Press Limited, Queen Square, Lancaster, UK.

Table 1 Biochemical studies in the patient with thiamin-responsive megaloblastic anaemia and her relatives

	Basal plasma concentration of total thiamin (ng/ml)	Basal r.b.c. content of total thiamin (pg $(10^6$ r.b.c.$)^{-1}$)	Uptake of $[^{14}C]$thiamin by r.b.c. (pmol $(10^9$ r.b.c.$)^{-1}$ h^{-1})	TPPKase activity in r.b.c. haemolysate (nmol (mg protein)$^{-1}$ h^{-1})
Patient	5.11 (1)	4.76 (2)	0.81 ± 0.18 (4)	0.035 (2)
Mother	15.54 (1)	11.76 ± 0.95 (5)	1.03 ± 0.19 (4)	0.034 (2)
Father	17.15 (1)	12.95 ± 1.33 (4)	1.76 ± 0.13 (3)	0.047 (1)
Brother	—	18.20 (1)	1.93 (1)	—
Maternal uncle	—	10.93 (2)	1.46 (2)	0.046 (1)
Controls	21.56 ± 5.45 (20)	17.02 ± 3.20 (21)	2.03 ± 0.40 (20)	0.046 ± 0.004 (4)
range	17.04–33.56	13.08–25.46	1.49–2.73	
	(T = 8.44 ± 2.50;	(T = 0.79 ± 0.23;	(T = 1.09 ± 0.23;	
	TMP = 13.12 ± 3.40)	TMP = 1.85 ± 0.64;	TMP = 0.10 ± 0.08;	
		TPP = 14.37 ± 2.74)	TPP = 0.83 ± 0.20)	

In parentheses, number of observations. Results are expressed as mean or mean ±SD, as appropriate
Abbreviations: T: free thiamin; TMP: thiamin monophosphate; TPP: thiamin pyrophosphate; TPPKase: thiamin pyrophosphokinase

symptomatic maternal uncle, and within the normal range in the brother. For all plasma and r.b.c. specimens obtained from the patient and her relatives we determined also the levels of free thiamin and its phosphoesters. We found them to have a normal distribution, when expressed as a percentage of total thiamin. Three to four days after discontinuing thiamin treatment in the patient, plasma concentration and r.b.c. content of total thiamin were still within the normal range.

Uptake of $[^{14}C]$thiamin by r.b.c. during 1 h incubation was abnormally reduced in the proband and below the control range also in patient's mother and maternal uncle, whereas it appeared to be within normal limits in both the father and the brother. The distribution of labelled thiamin and its phosphoesters in r.b.c. of the proband and her relatives at the end of the incubation was similar to that seen in the controls. We assayed in r.b.c. TPPKase activity, involved in the intracellular thiamin phosphorylation process. This enzyme may also play a role in thiamin transport across biological membranes by keeping low the intracellular concentration of free thiamin and maintaining an inward-oriented gradient. In both the proband and her mother TPPKase activity levels were below −2 SD, though about 75 % of the mean of four controls. Normal enzyme activities were found in both the father and the maternal uncle.

Our results can suggest the following conclusions and speculations.

(1) The possible basic defect of TRMA might be a disorder of thiamin transport across biological membranes of some organs and tissues (i.e. enterocytes, r.b.c., etc.) as suggested by either the low plasma concentration or the reduced r.b.c. content of total thiamin. More direct evidence might be provided by the abnormally low uptake of labelled thiamin by r.b.c. The peculiar clinical symptoms of TRMA might depend on the derangement of specific physiological processes taking place in the tissues where the defect of thiamin transport is localized.

(2) A deficiency of TPPKase activity, apparently partial in r.b.c. under our assay conditions, might contribute to the transport disorder.

(3) Pharmacological doses of thiamin could effectively correct the abnormal levels of the vitamin in plasma and r.b.c. even for a few days after the treatment had been discontinued.

(4) The autosomal recessive inheritance of TRMA is suggested by borderline normal, or clearly abnormal, biochemical tests in some obligate or possible heterozygotes. Some of those subjects also presented with peculiar clinical manifestations of the disease, such as diabetes, reduced glucose tolerance, or deafness, thus suggesting an incompletely recessive inheritance.

References

Haworth, C., Evans, D. I. K., Mitra, J. and Wickramasinghe, S. N. Thiamine responsive anaemia: a study of two further cases. *Br. J. Haematol.* 50 (1982) 549–561

La Grutta, A., Lo Curto, M. and Iachininoto, R. Anemia megaloblastica tiamino sensibile, associata a diabete mellito e sordità. *Riv. Ital. Pediatr.* 6 (1980) 65–70

Patrini, C. and Rindi, G. An improved method for the electrophoretic separation and fluorometric determination of thiamine and its phosphates in animal tissues. *Int. J. Vitam. Nutri. Res.* 50 (1980) 10–18

Rogers, L. E., Porter, F. S. and Sidbury, J. B. Thiamine-responsive megaloblastic anemia. *J. Pediatr.* 74 (1969) 494–504

Sanioto, S. M. L., Reinauer, H. and Hollmann, S. Thiamine pyrophosphokinase activity in liver, heart and brain crude extracts of control and thiamine deficient rats. *Int. J. Vitam. Nutri. Res.* 47 (1977) 315–324

Viana, M. B. and Carvalho, R. I. Thiamine-responsive megaloblastic anemia, sensorineural deafness, and diabetes mellitus: A new syndrome? *J. Pediatr.* 93 (1978) 235–238

J. Inher. Metab. Dis. 7 Suppl. 2 (1984) 155–156

Short Communication

Acid Esterase Deficiency: Comparison of Biochemical Findings in Infantile and Adult Forms

G. T. N. BESLEY and D. M. BROADHEAD
Department of Pathology, Royal Hospital for Sick Children, Edinburgh, UK

E. LAWLOR
Department of Haematology, St. James Hospital, Dublin, Eire

A deficiency of lysosomal acid esterase activity in humans usually results in one of two phenotypically distinct storage disorders (Assmann and Fredrickson, 1983). In Wolman's disease (McKusick 27800) the course is rapid, resulting in death in infancy whereas cholesterol ester storage disease (CESD; McKusick 21500) is relatively benign and patients usually survive well into adulthood. These disorders are relatively rare and few comparative biochemical studies have been reported. In this report, three patients, two with Wolman's disease and one with CESD, have been studied in an attempt to identify a biochemical basis for their phenotypic expression.

MATERIALS AND METHODS

Samples of liver were obtained at necropsy from two patients (3 and 4 months of age) with Wolman's disease. Two needle biopsies were taken from an adult (37 y) with CESD, before and after 6 months treatment with phenobarbitone which resulted in some clinical improvement. Liver samples were stored at $-40°C$ prior to study. Cultured skin fibroblasts were grown in Ham's F10 medium containing 15% fetal calf serum and antibiotics.

Lipids were extracted from liver and fibroblasts basically by Folch extraction. Neutral lipids were separated by t.l.c. and identified with known standards by spraying with anisaldehyde. Quantitative analyses were carried out enzymatically (Gamble *et al.*, 1978; Peridochrom method of Boehringer Corp. Ltd.) on lipids dissolved in isopropanol.

Acid esterase activities were measured on total extracts with glycerol $[1\text{-}^{14}C]$trioleate (Amersham) (Kaplan, 1970) or 4-methylumbelliferyl (4MU) palmitate in the presence of cardiolipin (Guy and Butterworth, 1978) as substrates. Specific radioactivity of $[^{14}C]$triolein was adjusted to 1 mCi/mmol and the lipid purified prior to use. For assay, $[^{14}C]$triolein was dispersed in Triton X-100 by sonication and warming.

RESULTS

The deficiency of acid esterase activity was similar for both Wolman and CESD fibroblasts using either $[^{14}C]$triolein or 4MU-palmitate as substrate. Compared with controls, values for Wolman and CESD fibroblasts respectively were 4% and 3% for triolein and 5% and 4% for 4MU-palmitate. For liver, 4MU-palmitate esterase activities were reduced to 5% and 7% of controls for Wolman's samples (Table 1) and to 9% and 7% for the CESD biopsies. Activities were compared with controls of similar ages as esterase activities in adult livers were approximately three times those of infants. However, using $[^{14}C]$triolein, residual activity in CESD liver was 5% and 4% of controls whereas no activity could be measured in the two Wolman livers.

Cultured fibroblasts from Wolman and CESD patients contained many translucent droplets visible under light microscopy and staining positively with Oil-red O. Analysis of cell extracts by t.l.c. revealed marked storage of cholesterol esters which amounted to 144 and 141 nmol/mg cell protein compared with 0–4 nmol/mg protein in control fibroblasts. Free cholesterol levels were normal in mutant fibroblasts.

Lipid analyses of liver extracts demonstrated (Table 1) marked storage of cholesterol esters in affected tissues. Similar levels, approximately 120 μmol/g wet wt., were recorded in Wolman and CESD livers, amounting to some 90% of total cholesterol. In control livers approximately 20% of cholesterol was esterified. Triglyceride levels were however considerably higher in Wolman's livers, being 10 and 16 times control values, compared with two-fold increase in CESD.

DISCUSSION

Marked storage of cholesterol esters was demonstrated in fibroblast and liver samples from two patients with Wolman's disease and one adult with CESD. Levels were similar in all cases but triglyceride storage was more striking in the Wolman livers. Lipid levels reported here are difficult to compare with those published by others, due to the wide range of values reported on small numbers of samples and the use of a variety of techniques (see Assmann and Fredrickson, 1983). However, our values agree with more recent observations.

Using 4MU-palmitate, residual esterase activities were similar in Wolman and CESD livers, compared with age-matched controls. However, the total lack of activity in Wolman livers, measured with the triglyceride substrate, triolein, may account for the marked storage of triglycerides in these tissues. Conversely it might be argued that high levels of endogenous triglycerides may dilute the radioactive substrate, in theory by about 25%,

Journal of Inherited Metabolic Disease. ISSN 0141–8955. Copyright © SSIEM and MTP Press Limited, Queen Square, Lancaster, UK.

Table 1   Enzyme and lipid levels in Wolman and CESD livers

Sample	Age	Lipid levels (μmol/g wet wt.)			Acid esterase activities (nmol h^{-1} (mg protein)$^{-1}$)	
		Cholesterol		Triglycerides	[^{14}C]Triolein	4MU-Palmitate
		Free	Ester			
Wolman (C.T.)	4 m	25.4	134	324	0	37
Wolman (E.C.)	3 m	12.5	105	204	0	29
Control	12 m	4.5	0.8	12	16.6	436
Control	3 m	4.2	1.5	29	20.3	372
CESD (1)	37 y	18.7	138	42	3.6	90
CESD (2)	37 y	18.3	126	46	3.1	72
Control biopsy	55 y	8.3	1.1	18	—	—
Control P.M.	67 y	5.4	1.7	31	71	1320
Control P.M.	56 y	5.9	1.3	11	78	1440
Control P.M. (fatty cirrhosis)	61 y	5.8	3.0	86	—	—

and thereby appear to lower measured activity. It is suggested, however, that, although Wolman and CESD appear to be allelic, the disorders may arise from different mutations affecting the specificity as well as activity of acid esterase. As a consequence high levels of triglycerides and other substrates may accumulate in Wolman's disease to produce a more debilitating disorder.

We thank Eleanor Cochrane for cell culture and Drs Crowe (Dublin), Galloway (Inverness) and Garcia Novo (Madrid) for referring samples to us.

References

Assmann, G. and Fredrickson, D. S. Acid lipase deficiency: Wolman's disease and cholesterol ester storage disease. In Stanbury, J. B., Wyngaarden, J. B., Fredrickson, D. S., Goldstein, J. L. and Brown, M. S. (eds.) *The Metabolic Basis of Inherited Disease*, 5th Edn., McGraw-Hill, New York, 1983, pp. 803–819

Gamble, W., Vaughan, M., Kruth, H. S. and Avigan, J. Procedure for determination of free and total cholesterol in micro- or nanogram amounts suitable for studies with cultured cells. *J. Lipid Res.* 19 (1978) 1068–1070

Guy, G. J. and Butterworth, J. Acid esterase activity in cultured skin fibroblasts and amniotic fluid cells using 4-methylumbelliferyl palmitate. *Clin. Chim. Acta* 84 (1978) 361–371

Kaplan, A. A simple radioactive assay for triglyceride lipase. *Anal. Biochem.* 33 (1970) 218–225

J. Inher. Metab. Dis. 7 Suppl. 2 (1984) 157–158

Short Communication

Steroid Sulphatase Deficiency. Steroid Sulphatase and Arylsulphatase C Determination in Normal and Affected Fibroblasts

M. PIRAUD, M. T. ZABOT and I. MAIRE

Laboratoire d'Enzymologie et de Cultures Cellulaires (Professeur J. Cotte et M. Mathieu), Hôpital Debrousse, 29 rue Soeur Bouvier, 69322 Lyon Cedex 1, France

Steroid sulphatase deficiency (SSD, McKusick 31205), originally identified as a sex-linked enzyme disorder expressed in the placenta (France and Liggins, 1969), is characterized by low maternal oestrogen excretion and failure of induction of spontaneous labour. The defect persists throughout the life of affected males, who develop in early infancy a severe ichthyosis as the only symptom. The relationship between this ichthyosis and the enzyme deficiency was suggested in 1976 (Jobsis *et al.*) and confirmed in 1978 (Shapiro *et al.*).

It is now known that the deficiency is generalized and expressed in various tissues (skin fibroblasts, leukocytes, lymphocytes, amniotic cells, brain, hair bulb, etc.) as a deficiency of steroid sulphatase (STS, EC 3.1.6.2) and arylsulphatase C (ARS C, EC 3.1.6.1) activities. We do not really know if a single enzyme is responsible for these two activities, or if these two activities share a commom compound involved in two different enzymes.

The methods described in the literature for measuring these activities differ widely, particularly on pH and nature of the buffer and on substrate concentrations. With the aim of optimizing assays for these activities and of determining the most discriminating conditions for detection of SSD in fibroblasts, we studied the influence of pH and phosphate ions on both activities in normal and deficient fibroblasts.

METHODS

Cultured skin fibroblasts between the 4th and 10th passage were used for enzymatic determinations. Cells were harvested by trypsinization, washed and stored at $+4\,^{\circ}C$ (maximum 3 days). Then cells were suspended in distilled water and sonicated (3 seconds maximum at 8 kc/s). Proteins were determined (Lowry *et al.*, 1951) and solutions were adjusted to obtain about 1–2 mg proteins per ml of lysate.

STS activity was measured by a radiochemical method using dehydroepian drosterone sulphate (DHEA-sulphate) as substrate. Tritiated (7-^{3}H) and unlabelled DHEA sulphate were diluted in buffer in order to obtain a 50 µmol/l substrate concentration with a specific activity of 20 mCi/mmol. 100 µl of this reagent were mixed with 100 µl of fibroblast homogenate and incubated for 2 h at 37 °C. Released DHEA was extracted twice by 2 ml of toluene. Extracts were mixed and washed by 3 ml of distilled water. The toluene layer was separated from the aqueous layer by freezing.

Radioactivity of 3 ml supernatant toluene was counted with 5 ml of Picofluor 15. A blank without incubation was performed on each fibroblast homogenate.

ARS C activity was measured by a fluorimetric method, using 4-methylumbelliferyl sulphate (4-MUS) as substrate. The reaction mixture consisted of 50 µl of fibroblast lysate and 100 µl of substrate solution (concentration in the reaction mixture 0.5 mmol/l) in buffer. The reaction was allowed to proceed for 1 h at 37 °C and stopped by the addition of 2 ml 0.5 mol/l bicarbonate–carbonate buffer pH 10.7. The amount of fluorescence released was measured at 448 nm, after excitation at 362 nm, and compared to 4-methylumbelliferone standards. Blanks were performed in the same conditions, but without incubation.

Buffers: pH influence was studied using either buffer with phosphate ions (pH 5–6.5, citrate 0.1 mol/l–phosphate 0.2 mol/l; pH 7–8.5, phosphate 0.2 mol/l) or buffer without phosphate ions (pH 5–6.5, citrate 0.2 mol/l; pH 7–8.5, TRIS 0.2 mol/l).

RESULTS

Figure 1a shows pH influence on ARS C activity using normal and SSD fibroblasts. When phosphate ions were absent in buffer, no deficiency was noticed with SSD fibroblasts; when phosphate ions were present, ARS C activity was maximal at pH 8 in normal fibroblasts, and no activity was found with SSD fibroblasts, whatever the pH. K_m of ARS C for 4-MUS in phosphate buffer pH 8 was 0.5 mmol/l.

Figure 1b shows that STS activity presented an optimal pH of 8.0 with or without phosphate ions and that the deficient cells gave clearcut results whatever the conditions used.

Two DHEA sulphate concentrations (25 and 50 µmol/l) and two incubation times (1 and 2 h) were tested. The more sensitive results were obtained with 25 µmol/l DHEA sulphate and 2 h of incubation.

DISCUSSION AND CONCLUSION

Phosphate ions are necessarily required for ARS C determination, as demonstrated in Figure 1a. In absence of phosphate ions, arylsulphatases A and B are not inhibited and a deficiency of ARS C in SSD fibroblasts could not be demonstrated. Using ARS C (in presence of phosphate ions) or STS assays, the detection of the

Journal of Inherited Metabolic Disease. ISSN 0141-8955. Copyright © SSIEM and MTP Press Limited, Queen Square, Lancaster, UK.

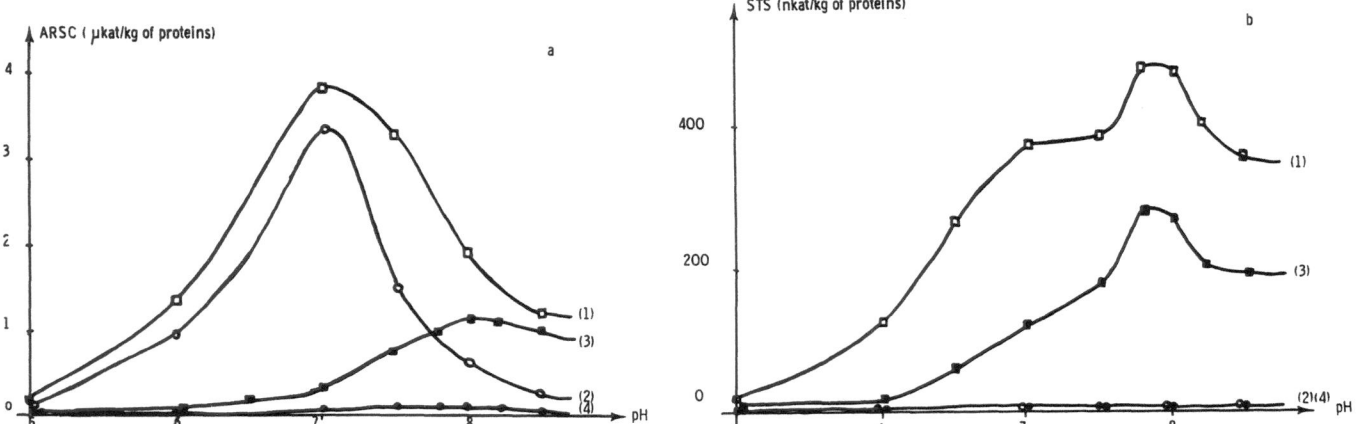

Figure 1 Arylsulphatase C (a) and steroid sulphatase (b) activities in normal and SSD fibroblasts:pH influence (1) normal fibroblasts – buffer without phosphate ions (—□—), (2) SSD fibroblasts – buffer without phosphate ions (—○—), (3) normal fibroblasts – buffer with phosphate ions (—■—), (4) SSD fibroblasts – buffer with phosphate ions (—●—)

defect is possible with a wide range of pH values (Figure 1a, b) but pH 8 is optimal. For the choice of the substrate concentration, we suggest the use of 4-MUS at the concentration of K_m i.e. 2.5 mmol/l in the test.

Sensitive conditions are realized for STS assay when 5–25 % of the radioactive substrate are transformed. In our conditions, the best compromise was obtained with a substrate concentration of 25 µmol/l, and an incubation time of 2 h.

Generally, conditions used by other authors for these enzymatic determinations in fibroblasts are different, if not far, from ours. Though non-optimal, these conditions allow SSD diagnosis, except when ARS C determination is performed without phosphate ions.

References

France, J. T. and Liggins, G. C. Placental sulfatase deficiency. *J. Clin. Endocrinol. Metab.* 29 (1969) 138–143

Jobsis, A. C., Van Duuren, C. Y., De Vries, G. P., Koppe, J. G., Rijken, Y., Van Kempen, G. M. J. and De Groot, W. P. Trophoblast sulphatase deficiency associated with X chromosomal ichthyosis. *Ned. Tijdschr. Geneeskd.* 120 (1976) 1980

Lowry, O. H., Rosebrough, N. J., Farr, A. L. and Randall, R. J. Protein measurement with the Folin phenol reagent. *J. Biol. Chem.* 193 (1951) 265–275

Shapiro, L. J., Weiss, R., Buxman, M. M., Vidgoff, J. and Dimond, R. L. Enzymatic basis of typical X-linked ichthyosis. *Lancet* 2 (1978) 756–757

J. Inher. Metab. Dis. 7 Suppl. 2 (1984) 159–160

Short Communication

Steroid Sulphatase Deficiency is Present in Patients with the Syndrome 'Ichthyosis and Male Hypogonadism' and with 'Rud Syndrome'

G. ANDRIA, A. BALLABIO, G. PARENTI, S. DI MAIO and A. PICCIRILLO*
*Departments of Pediatrics and *Department of Dermatology, 2nd Medical School, University of Naples, Via S. Pansini 5, 80131 Napoli, Italy*

Ichthyosis is a prominent feature of many genetic syndromes, generally classified only on the basis of clinical, histological and genetic criteria (McKusick, 1983). A definite biochemical defect has been actually demonstrated only in very few of them including the classical X-linked ichthyosis (McKusick 30810), which is associated with a generalized deficiency of steroid sulphatase and arylsulphatase C activities, probably due to the same molecule (see Shapiro, 1983 for review). In late pregnancy steroid sulphatase deficiency can cause diminished oestriol production by the placenta, thus leading to difficulties of labour and delivery such as cervical dystocia.

A different entity, classified as 'ichthyosis and male hypogonadism' (McKusick 30820) has been so far described in four families (see McKusick, 1983 for references). Apart from ichthyosis and hypogonadism, anosmia and mental retardation were also reported in a large pedigree (Perrin *et al.*, 1976). Ichthyosis, oligophrenia and epilepsy are also typical features of the so-called 'Rud syndrome', frequently associated with hypogonadism. Rud syndrome, however, is an ill-defined category and is not reported in McKusick's catalogue (1983), although it was included in another catalogue of congenital syndromes (Bergsma, 1979). We recently observed two siblings, previously classified as affected by 'ichthyosis and male hypogonadism' (Di Maio *et al.*, 1982) and a young adult male with 'Rud syndrome', who turned out to have a steroid sulphatase deficiency in cultured skin fibroblasts.

CASE REPORTS

Case 1, C.C., a 9 5/12 year-old boy, was the eldest of three sibs; his brother (R.C.) was affected by the same syndrome. The patient was born by forceps delivery at 41 weeks of gestation. He presented with ichthyosis at the age of 3 months. Milestones of development were delayed. Clinical examination showed ichthyosis, with dry, scaly and brown skin mainly on the neck, trunk, extensor surface of the limbs and flexures, bilateral cryptorchidism, micropenis and very mild mental retardation. Anosmia was demonstrated by using qualitative and quantitative tests (Henkin and Bartter, 1966). Histological examination of the affected skin showed hyperkeratosis and a normal appearing granular layer.

Endocrinological studies were carried out. LHRH test showed a normal increase of FSH and LH levels. HCG stimulation test showed an abnormal response of testosterone, but a therapeutic trial with HCG (2000 u/w for 6 weeks) revealed a normal increase in testosterone levels. Treatment with HCG also resulted in a partial descent of testes. These results were consistent with a diagnosis of hypogonadotropic hypogonadism of possible hypothalamic origin.

Case 2, R. C., a 6 10/12 year-old boy, is the younger brother of C.C. He was born by Caesarean section, because of breech presentation. Clinical presentation and endocrinological tests were exactly the same as in his brother.

Case 3, L. V., a 18 6/12 year-old young adult male, was referred to us by a dermatologist with a diagnosis of 'Rud syndrome'. He presented with a history of epilepsy, mild oligophrenia and ichthyosis since infancy. An older brother was reportedly affected by congenital ichthyosis. A sister suffered from 'petit mal' seizures. Physical examination revealed short stature (<5th centile), micropenis (stretched length 8.5 cm: < 2 SD for age) with normal sized testes, and ichthyosis involving arms, legs and trunk. Histological examination of the skin showed hyperkeratosis and a normal appearing granular layer.

It was possible to perform only few endocrinological tests that revealed normal testosterone levels and a low basal concentration of FSH, consistent with a possible hypogonadotropic hypogonadism.

RESULTS AND DISCUSSION

We assayed steroid sulphatase and arylsulphatase C activities in cultured skin fibroblasts obtained from our three patients (see Table 1). We found both enzymatic activities to be profoundly deficient, at levels comparable to those of three cases with classical X-linked ichthyosis.

These results suggest the following main conclusions:

(1) Some male patients, diagnosed as having either the syndrome 'ichthyosis and male hypogonadism' or 'Rud syndrome', may have a marked steroid sulphatase deficiency, as observed in X-linked ichthyosis. Therefore this enzymatic activity should be assayed in all male subjects previously classified only on clinical grounds as examples of the first two syndromes.

(2) Hypogenitalism, under various clinical expressions (cryptorchidism, micropenis, infertility)

159

Journal of Inherited Metabolic Disease. ISSN 0141-8955. Copyright © SSIEM and MTP Press Limited, Queen Square, Lancaster, UK.

Table 1   Steroid sulphatase and arylsulphatase C activities in cultured skin fibroblasts

	Enzymatic activities	
	Steroid sulphatase[1]	Arylsulphatase C[2]
Ichthyosis and hypogonadism		
C.C.	13.6	0.10
R.C.	Undetectable	0.12
Rud syndrome		
L.V.	11.0	0.47
X-Linked ichthyosis		
Case 1	Undetectable	0.31
Case 2	1.6	0.14
Case 3	42.8	0.01
Male controls $(n = 6; \bar{x} \pm \text{SD})$	485.0 ± 99.6	2.04 ± 0.30

[1] pmol dehydroepiandrosterone (g protein)$^{-1}$ h^{-1} (Epstein *et al.* (1981) modified)
[2] nmol 4-methylumbelliferone (mg protein)$^{-1}$ h^{-1} (Meyer *et al.* (1979) modified)

is probably a frequent feature of steroid sulphatase deficiency; therefore all patients with proven steroid sulphatase deficiency deserve a thorough investigation of their gonadic function.

It is surprising that even recent reviews on X-linked ichthyosis (Shapiro, 1983; Harkness *et al.*, 1982) do not mention this symptom. Traupe and Happle (1983), starting from a different approach, published a study drawing the same conclusions as ours. They re-examined 25 patients with steroid sulphatase deficiency and found cryptorchidism in seven patients.

Some clinical features, observed in our patients, also suggest the following speculations:

(1) Rud syndrome, whose authenticity is still questioned, is probably a heterogeneous category. It might also include some patients with steroid sulphatase deficiency, a well-known cause of birth complications, possibly leading to oligophrenia and epilepsy.

(2) Anosmia, present in two of our patients, might be an expression of a hypothalamic damage, possibly also responsible for the hypogonadism. It is noteworthy that anosmia was also a quite constant feature in many male members of a large pedigree (Perrin *et al.*, 1976) with ichthyosis, hypogonadism and mental retardation. Steroid sulphatase, however, was not assayed in those patients. We propose that anosmia should be carefully inquired about in all subjects with steroid sulphatase deficiency, since it may be overlooked.

(3) Kallmann syndrome, in most cases inherited as an X-linked trait, is also characterized by the presence of anosmia and hypogonadism. It would be worth looking for ichthyosis and checking steroid sulphatase levels in patients with Kallmann syndrome, too.

References

Bergsma, D. (ed.) *Birth Defects Compendium*, 2nd edn. The National Foundation March of Dimes, Alan R. Liss, New York, 1979, p. 741

Di Maio, S., Sandomenico, M. L., Zaccaria, S., Franzese, A., Nunziata, L., Lubrano, P., Mariani, A. and Tenore, A. Ittiosi e ipogonadismo in due fratelli. *Ital. J. Pedriatr.* 8 (1982) 555

Epstein, E. H. Jr and Leventhal, M. E. Steroid sulfatase of human leukocytes and epidermis and the diagnosis of recessive X-linked ichthyosis. *J. Clin. Invest.* 67 (1981) 1257–1262

Harkness, R. A. Current clinical problems in placental steroid sulphatase or arylsulphatase C deficiency and the related 'cervical dystocia' and X-linked ichthyosis. *J. Inher. Metab. Dis.* 5 (1982) 142–144

Henkin, R. I. and Bartter, F. C. Studies on olfactory thresholds in normal man and in patients with adrenal cortical insufficiency: the role of adrenal cortical steroids and serum sodium concentration. *J. Clin. Invest.* 45 (1966) 1631–1639

Lowry, O. H., Rosebrough, N. J., Farr, A. L. and Randall, R. J. Protein measurement with Folin phenol reagent. *J. Biol. Chem.* 193 (1951) 265–275

McKusick, V. A. *Mendelian Inheritance in Man*, 5th edn, Johns Hopkins Univ. Press, Baltimore, 1983, p. 1060

Meyer, J. Ch., Grundmann, H. P. and Schnyder, U. W. Determination of arylsulfatase C in hair follicles. *Arch. Dermatol. Res.* 266 (1979) 95–97

Perrin, J. C. S., Idemoto, J. Y., Sotos, J. F., Maurer, W. F. and Steinberg, A. G. X-Linked syndrome of congenital ichthyosis, hypogonadism, mental retardation and anosmia. *Birth Defects* 5 (1976) 267–274

Shapiro, L. J. Steroid sulfatase deficiency and X-linked ichthyosis. In Stanbury, J. B., Wyngaarden, J. B., Fredrickson, D. S., Goldstein, J. L. and Brown, M. S. (eds.) *The Metabolic Basis of Inherited Disease*, 5th Edn. McGraw-Hill, New York, 1983, pp. 1027–1039

Traupe, H. and Happle, R. Clinical spectrum of steroid sulfatase deficiency: X-linked recessive ichthyosis, birth complication, and cryptorchidism. *Eur. J. Pediatr.* 140 (1983) 19–21